Optical Diagnostics: Biomedical Applications

Optical Diagnostics: Biomedical Applications

Editor: Macie Holloway

FOSTER
ACADEMICS
www.fosteracademics.com

www.fosteracademics.com

FOSTER ACADEMICS

Cataloging-in-Publication Data

Optical diagnostics : biomedical applications / edited by Macie Holloway.
p. cm.
Includes bibliographical references and index.
ISBN 978-1-64646-591-0
1. Optical fiber detectors--Diagnostic use. 2. Lasers--Diagnostic use. 3. Lasers--Therapeutic use.
4. Diagnostic imaging. 5. Optical fibers in medicine. 6. Lasers in medicine. 7. Imaging systems in medicine.
I. Holloway, Macie.
R857.O6 O68 2023
616.075 4--dc23

Foster Academics,
118-35 Queens Blvd., Suite 400,
Forest Hills, NY 11375, USA

ISBN 978-1-64646-591-0 (Hardback)

Contents

Preface

Optical diagnostics is a specialized field of diagnostics that makes use of optical imaging. It is a technique that enables medical practitioners to look inside the body in a non-invasive manner. Optical imaging makes use of visible light and the special properties of photons to obtain detailed images of organs, tissues, cells and molecules. Optical diagnostics help in diagnosing various pathological disorders of biological tissues. There are several biomedical applications of optical diagnostics. The major advantage of optical imaging is that it offers minimally invasive or non-invasive methods for looking inside the body. Optical diagnostics also reduces a patient's exposure to harmful radiation. It can be used to measure metabolic changes that can act as early indicators of abnormal functioning of organs and tissues. A combination of optical imaging with other imaging techniques like MRI or X-rays can provide enhanced information to monitor complex diseases. The objective of this book is to give a general view of optical diagnostics and its biomedical applications. Researchers and students in this field will be assisted by this book.

The information shared in this book is based on empirical researches made by veterans in this field of study. The elaborative information provided in this book will help the readers further their scope of knowledge leading to advancements in this field.

Finally, I would like to thank my fellow researchers who gave constructive feedback and my family members who supported me at every step of my research.

Editor

1

Ovarian Cancer Targeting Phage for In Vivo Near-Infrared Optical Imaging

Mallika Asar [1], Jessica Newton-Northup [2], Susan Deutscher [2,3] and Mette Soendergaard [1,*]

[1] Department of Chemistry, Western Illinois University, 214 Currens Hall, Macomb, IL 61455, USA; m-asar@wiu.edu

[2] Department of Biochemistry, University of Missouri, 117 Schweitzer Hall, Columbia, MO 65211, USA; newtonj@missouri.edu (J.N.-N.); deutschers@missouri.edu (S.D.)

[3] Harry S. Truman Memorial Veterans Hospital, 1 Hospital Drive, Columbia, MO 65201, USA

* Correspondence: m-soendergaard@wiu.edu

Abstract: Ovarian cancer is often diagnosed at late stages due to current inadequate detection. Therefore, the development of new detection methods of ovarian cancer is needed. This may be achieved by phage nanoparticles that display targeting peptides for optical imaging. Here, two such phage clones are reported. Ovarian cancer binding and specificity of phage clones (pJ18, pJ24) and peptides (J18, J24) were investigated using fluorescent microscopy and modified ELISA. Further, AF680-labeled phage particles were subjected to biodistribution and optical imaging studies in SKOV-3 xenografted mice. Fluorescent microscopy and ELISA of phage and peptides showed significantly increased binding to SKOV-3 cells compared to controls. Additionally, these studies revealed that J18 exhibits specificity for ovarian cancer SKOV-3 and OVCAR-3 cell lines. Further, peptides displayed increased SKOV-3 binding compared to N35 (non-relevant peptide) with EC_{50} values of 22.2 ± 10.6 μM and 29.0 ± 6.9 (mean ± SE), respectively. Biodistribution studies of AF680-labeled phage particles showed tumor uptake after 4 h and excretion through the reticuloendothelial system. Importantly, SKOV-3 tumors were easily localized by optical imaging after 2 h and 4 h and displayed good tumor-to-background contrast. The fluorescent tumor signal intensity was significantly higher for pJ18 compared to wild type (WT) after 2 h.

Keywords: phage; imaging; ovarian cancer; molecular targeting; nanoparticles; peptides

1. Introduction

Ovarian cancer is the most fatal gynecological malignancy, accounting for more than 14,000 deaths annually in the U.S. The majority of patients are diagnosed at stages III and IV, at which point five-year survival rates are 72% and 27%, respectively [1]. However, a more optimistic prognosis is presented to patients diagnosed with local disease, for which five-year survival rates are over 90%. These statistics emphasize the importance of early detection and diagnosis. At present, the standard ovarian cancer detection method is the measurement of glycoprotein CA-125 serum levels [2,3]. However, only 80% of advanced ovarian cancers and 50% of stage I tumors secrete detectable levels of CA-125. Additionally, CA-125 is associated with other conditions such as benign ovarian cysts, endometriosis, and inflammatory disease, and is found in several normal tissues [3–5]. Thus, new methods of ovarian cancer detection and diagnosis are needed.

Bacteriophage (phage) is employed in phage display, a high throughput technology utilized to identify peptide and antibody-based ligands [6–8]. Phage display has been used to discover novel peptides that target and image cancer biomarkers and cells, including the ErbB-2 receptor, galectin-3, PC-3 prostate carcinoma, and SKOV-3 ovarian adenocarcinoma cells [9–14]. While free peptide ligands may be used in targeted cancer imaging, phage as nanoparticles offer advantages in regard to their large size, which allows labeling with numerous fluorophores or radiotracers. Such labeling leads to signal amplification and provides increased sensitivity [15]. Further, phage particles exhibit increased stability and biodistribution compared to single ligands [16]. Finally, phage nanoparticles may be easily genetically modified and produced in large quantities using standard biotechnological approaches, including recombinant DNA technology and propagation in liquid *E. coli* culture. Phage nanoparticles have been utilized as tumor imaging agents of various targets such as Lewis lung carcinoma and prostate cancer in mouse models using optical imaging [13,17]. In fact, phage mediated cancer-targeting coupled with optical imaging, provide additional advantages, such as low toxicity compared to radionuclides. Although the use of fluorophores with emission wavelengths in the visible spectrum is problematic due to tissue depth limitations [18], near-infrared fluorophores (700–900 nm) emit light that penetrates human tissue at a depth of circa 1–3 cm [19,20]. While this depth of tissue penetration prevents imaging of certain tumors, ovarian cancer metastases are most often located along the peritoneal lining, and may, therefore, be imaged using this technique [19].

Here, we report the development of two phage nanoparticles (pJ18 and pJ24) that display 15-mer ovarian cancer-targeting peptides. The phage were previously identified using a two-tier phage display selection against xenografted ovarian tumors in mice. Micropanning experiments revealed that pJ18 and pJ24 exhibited the highest cancer-to-normal cell-binding ratio and these phage were thus selected for further studies [10]. In this study, phage and single peptides were evaluated separately using in vitro cell-based assays and fluorescent microscopy, which revealed affinity in the μmolar range and specificity for ovarian cancer cells. The phage clones were labeled with near-infrared fluorophore Alexa Fluor 680 (AF680) and investigated in regard to tumor targeting and imaging of human ovarian tumors in xenografted nude mice. Phage pJ18 successfully imaged tumors with sufficient tumor-to-background uptake, suggesting that this clone may be used for subsequent utilization in detection and diagnosis of ovarian cancer.

2. Materials and Methods

2.1. Chemicals and Reagents

Chemicals were purchased from ThermoFisher Scientific (Waltham, MA, USA) unless otherwise stated.

2.2. Cell Lines and Cell Culture

The human ovarian adenocarcinoma (SKOV-3), human ovarian adenocarcinoma (OVCAR-3), human melanoma (MDA-MB-435), and human embryonic kidney (HEK293) cell lines were obtained from American Type Tissue Culture (Manassas, VA, USA). SKOV-3 cells were maintained in McCoy's 5A supplemented with 10% fetal bovine serum (FBS) and 50 μg/mL gentamicin at 37 °C in 5% CO_2. All other cell lines were maintained in RPMI 1640 (custom) supplemented with 10% fetal bovine serum (FBS), 2 mM L-glutamine, and 1.7 μM insulin at 37 °C in 5% CO_2.

2.3. Animals and Handling

Female 4–6-week-old nude nu/nu mice (n = 2; Harlan, Indianapolis, IN, USA) were injected subcutaneously (shoulder) with 1×10^7 SKOV-3 cells under anesthesia (3.5% isoflurane, Baxter Healthcare Corp., Deerfield, IL, USA), and tumors (1 cm) were established over 8 weeks. After optical imaging studies, the animals were sacrificed by cervical dislocation. The NIH Guidelines for the Care and Use of Laboratory Animals and the Policy and Procedures for Animal Research of the Harry S. Truman Veterans Memorial Hospital were followed, and all animal studies were approved by the Institutional Animal Care and Use Committee (IACUC; 6823) at Harry S. Truman Veterans Memorial Hospital.

2.4. Phage

A linear 15-amino acid fUSE5 phage display library (a gift from Dr. George P. Smith [21]) was previously employed in a two-tier selection protocol against SKOV-3 cells, as previously reported to select and identify phage pJ18 and pJ24 [10]. Phage were amplified in *E. coli* K91 Blue Kan (K91BK) and isolated as previously described [22]. In brief, *E. coli* K91BK colonies infected with phage were propagated overnight in NZY medium with 100 μg/mL kanamycin and 20 μg/mL tetracycline at 37 °C and 225 rpm. The culture was then centrifuged at 5000× *g* for 15 min, and the phage were precipitated from the supernatant using 0.15 volume polyethylene glycol (PEG)/NaCl overnight at 4 °C. Next, phage were collected by centrifugation (8000× *g*, 15 min), resuspended in tris buffered saline (TBS), and precipitated once more using 0.15 volume PEG/NaCl. The virions were then immediately collected by centrifugation (8000× *g*, 15 min), and then resuspended in 1 mL TBS. The concentration of virions was determined by measuring the absorbance at 269 nm and 320 nm as described previously [22].

2.5. Peptides

Peptides (J18: RSLWSDFYASASRGP, J24: RRLPHLMPFEGSVFL, and N35: APGPTFLD) were synthesized with a biotin group linked to a GSG-amino acid spacer at the NH_2-terminus (biotin-GSG-peptide) by solid-phase Fmoc chemistry (396 multiple peptide synthesizer, Advanced Chem Tech, Louisville, KY, USA). Peptides were purified on a C18 column (Novapack Reverse Phase, Waters, Milford, MA, USA) by reverse-phase high-pressure liquid chromatography (RP-HPLC; Beckmann Coulter System Gold HPLC, Beckmann Coulter, Fullerton, CA, USA), and identified by electrospray ionization mass spectrometry (Mass Consortium Corp, San Diego, CA, USA). Peptides were lyophilized and stored at −20 °C.

2.6. Fluorescent Microscopy

Binding of phage pJ18, pJ24, wild type (WT), and dimethyl sulfoxide (DMSO; vehicle) to SKOV-3 cells were evaluated using fluorescent microscopy. SKOV-3 cells were maintained on microscope chamber slides (Nest Scientific, Rahway, NJ, USA) to 80% confluency. Cell medium was aspirated and washed thrice with TBS. Cells were fixed using 0.2% Triton X-100 and 10% formalin in TBS and washed extensively. Phage pJ18, pJ24, and WT (10^{11} V/mL) in 1% bovine serum albumin (BSA) TBS were incubated with biotinylated anti-Fd filamentous phage antibody (Fitzgerald, Acton, MA, USA) and streptavidin-fluorescein isothiocyanate (FITC) conjugate for 1 h. The phage complex was then added to SKOV-3 cells for 1 h. Cells were washed repeatedly with TBS and mounted using ProLong™ Diamond Antifade Mountant with 4′,6-diamidino-2-phenylindole (DAPI). Bound phage were detected using a Keyence BZ-X800 fluorescent microscope (Keyence, Itasca, IL, USA).

Cells (SKOV-3, OVCAR-3, MDA-MB-435, and HEK293) were grown to 80% confluency on chamber slides (Lab-Tek, Rochester, NY, USA). Growth medium was aspirated and 10 μM biotinylated J18 or J24 in phosphate buffered saline (PBS) were added for 1 h at 37 °C. Next, the slides were washed (PBS), fixed with 10% formalin, and then washed (PBS) repeatedly. The cells were blocked (10% FBS, 0.3 M glycine, 0.01% Tween-20, PBS) for 1 h, and bound peptides were probed with a mouse monoclonal anti-biotin antibody labeled with Cy3 (Sigma Aldrich, St. Louis, MO, USA) for 1 h. The slides were washed (PBS, 0.05% Tween-20), and bound peptides were detected using an epifluorescent Nikon T1-SM inverted microscope (Nikon, Melville, NY, USA).

The fluorescent intensity per cell was quantified by determining the corrected total cell fluorescence (CTCF) using ImageJ software (v1.52a, National Institute of Health, Bethesda, MD, USA) [23]. The mean fluorescent intensity per cell (region of interest; ROI) was adjusted for the mean background (non-cell) fluorescent intensity.

2.7. Modified ELISA

The binding ability of phage pJ18, pJ24, and WT, and biotinylated peptides J18, J24, and a non-relevant peptide N35 (negative control) to SKOV-3 cells were analyzed using an in vitro assay. Cells were grown in 96-well tissue culture plates (TPP, Trasadingen, Switzerland) to 80% confluency.

For phage, the cell medium was aspirated, and the cells were fixed using 0.2% Triton X-100 and 10% formalin. Cells were then washed with TBS, and 10^9 or 10^{10} V/mL pJ18, pJ24, or WT phage (1% BSA; TBS) was pre-incubated with biotinylated anti-Fd filamentous phage antibody (Fitzgerald, Acton, MA, USA) and streptavidin-horse radish peroxidase (HRP)-conjugate, and added to the cells for 1 h. The cells were washed (TBS) and incubated with HRP substrate 2, 2′-azino-bis(3-ethylbenzothiazoline-6-sulphonic acid) (ABTS) for 30 min. Phage binding was detected by measuring the absorbance at 405 nm on a SpectraMax 250 microplate reader (Molecular Devices, San Jose, CA, USA).

To determine peptide binding, 10 nM to 300 μM of biotinylated J18, J24, or N35 (non-relevant peptide) in PBS were incubated with the cells for 1 h at 37 °C, after which the plates were washed repeatedly (1% BSA, PBS) and fixed with 10% formalin. After extensive washing, the cells were blocked (10% FBS, 0.3 M glycine, 0.05% Tween-20 in PBS), and the bound peptides were probed by incubation with streptavidin-conjugated HRP for 1 h. Next, the plate was washed (PBS, 0.05% Tween-20), and ABTS was added and allowed to develop for 20 min. Bound peptides were detected by measuring the absorbance at 405 nm using a μ Quant Universal Microplate Spectrophotometer (Bio-Tek Instruments, Winooski, VT, USA), and the half-maximal effective concentration (EC_{50}) was calculated using GraphPad Prism software (vs. 8.0, San Diego, CA, USA).

2.8. Fluorescent Labeling of Phage

The near-infrared fluorophore Alexa Fluor 680 (AF680; carboxylic acid, succinimidyl ester 5-isomer; Invitrogen, Carlsbad, CA, USA) was dissolved in 2% dimethyl sulfoxide (DMSO) and incubated with phage (0.29 mM coat protein VIII) in 0.5 M Na_3 citrate, 0.1 M $NaHCO_3$ pH 8.5 for 4 h at room temperature in the dark. The reaction was terminated overnight at 4 °C by addition of 270 mM ethanolamine, pH 9. Excess hydrolyzed AF680 was removed by dialyzing labeled phage against TBS, pH 7.5 (Slide-A-Lyzer cassette, 10 kDa molecular weight cutoff, ThermoFisher Scientific, Rockford, IL, USA).

2.9. Biodistribution and Near-Infrared Optical Imaging of AF680-Labeled Phage

AF680-labeled pJ18, pJ24 or WT (10^{12} transducing units; TU) were injected into the tail-vein of SKOV-3 xenografted mice and allowed to circulate. For biodistribution experiments, the mice were sacrificed after 4 h, perfused with PBS, and tumors, organs, and tissues were excised. For optical imaging experiments, the mice were under gas anesthesia (3.5% isoflurane, Baxter Healthcare Corp. Deerfield, IL, USA), and fluorescence reflectance images were obtained before injection (0 h), and 2 h and 4 h after injection. Images were attained, and the fluorescent intensity was measured using a Xenogen IVIS 200 System and analyzed by Living Image software (vs. 4.3.1, Perkin Elmer, Waltham, MA, USA) [23].

2.10. Statistical Analysis

Two-way analysis of variance (ANOVA) and Student's *t*-test were performed to analyze the statistical significance of the fluorescent quantification, modified phage ELISA, and fluorescent intensity for the optical imaging experiment using Prism GraphPad Software (vs. 8.0, San Diego, CA, USA). A p-value of ≤ 0.05 was considered significant.

3. Results

3.1. Fluorescent Microscopy

Phage and peptide binding to various cell lines was assessed using fluorescent microscopy. Phage pJ18, pJ24, and WT (10^{11} V/mL) were incubated with SKOV-3 cells, and the binding was gauged by biotinylated anti-Fd filamentous phage antibody and FITC. Results showed that pJ18 and pJ24 exhibited significantly increased binding to SKOV-3 cells compared to WT and DMSO (Figure 1).

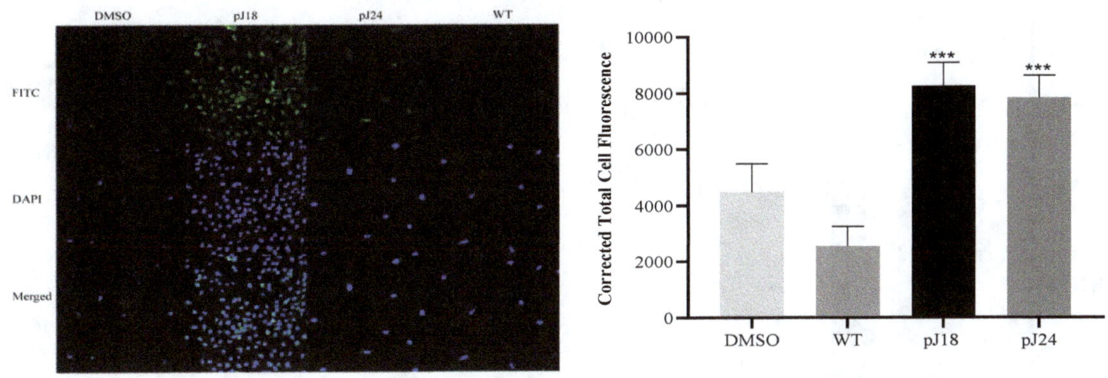

(a) (b)

Figure 1. Fluorescent microscopy of phage binding to SKOV 3 cells. (**a**) Cells were incubated with 10^{11} V/mL pJ18, pJ24, wild type (WT), or dimethyl sulfoxide (DMSO) (vehicle) and probed by a biotinylated anti-Fd filamentous phage antibody and streptavidin-fluorescein isothiocyanate (FITC). Cells were further stained with ProLong™ Diamond Antifade Mountant with 4′,6-diamidino-2-phenylindole (DAPI) and detected using a Keyence BZ X800 fluorescent microscope (Keyence, Itasca, IL, USA). (**b**) The corrected total cell fluorescence was determined using ImageJ software, and showed that pJ18 and pJ24 exhibited higher fluorescence compared to WT and DMSO. Phage pJ18 and pJ24 also showed significantly higher fluorescence compared to DMSO (not shown). A *p*-value of <0.05 was considered significant. *** $p < 0.001$. Green (FITC-phage); blue (DAPI).

Individual peptides, J18 and J24, were synthesized with an N-terminal GSG-spacer and a biotin group and employed in fluorescent microscopy studies to further evaluate the binding characteristics and to verify that the interaction was mediated by the displayed peptides and not by inherent phage proteins. The binding of J18 and J24 were assessed against both cancerous (SKOV-3, OVCAR-3, MDA-MB-435) and non-cancerous (HEK293) cell lines. In brief, peptides were incubated with each cell line and probed with a mouse monoclonal anti-biotin antibody labeled with Cy3. These studies revealed that peptide J18 displayed significantly increased binding for ovarian cancer SKOV-3 and OVCAR-3 cell lines while exhibiting minimal affinity for breast cancer MDA-MB-435 and embryonic kidney HEK293 cells. Peptide J24 showed significantly higher binding to SKOV-3 cells and little to no binding to other cell lines (Figure 2).

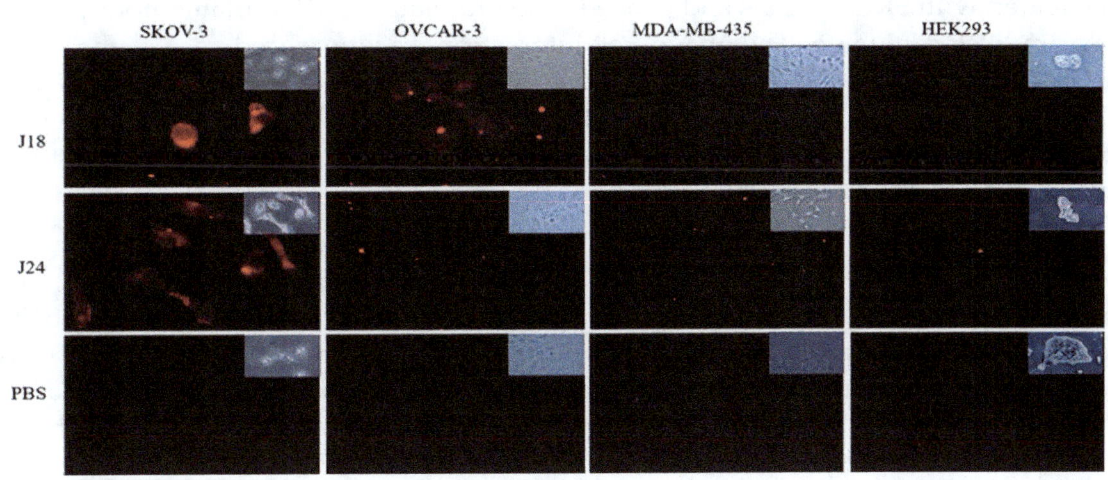

(a)

Figure 2. *Cont.*

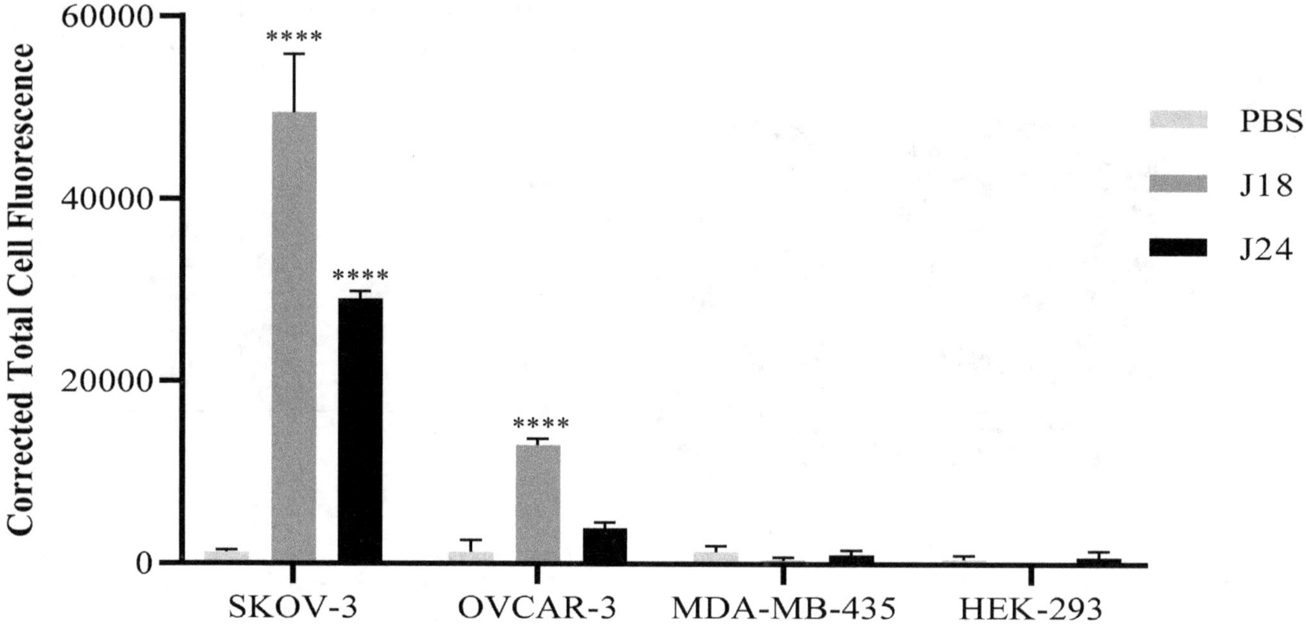

(**b**)

Figure 2. (**a**) Fluorescent microscopy of peptide binding to SKOV-3, OVCAR-3, MDA-MB-435, and HEK293 cells. Cells were incubated with 10 μM biotinylated J18, J24, or PBS for 1 h at 37 °C. Bound peptides were probed by a mouse monoclonal anti-biotin antibody and detected using an epifluorescent Nikon T1-SM inverted microscope (Nikon, Melville, NY, USA). (**b**) The corrected total cell fluorescence was determined using ImageJ software. Results showed that peptide J18 displayed higher fluorescence compared to PBS (vehicle) for SKOV-3 and OVCAR-3 cells. Peptide J24 demonstrated higher fluorescence to SKOV-3 cells. A p-value of < 0.05 was considered significant. **** $p < 0.0001$. Red (cy3-peptides).

3.2. Modified ELISA

In order to further evaluate the SKOV-3 binding properties of both phage and peptides, these were subjected to in vitro cell binding assays. For analysis of phage binding, 10^9 or 10^{10} V/mL pJ18, pJ24, or WT were incubated with SKOV-3 cells and probed by biotinylated anti-Fd filamentous phage antibody and streptavidin-HRP conjugate. The phage–cell interaction was measured spectrophotometrically at 405 nm after the addition of ABTS. Phage pJ18 and pJ24 (10^9 V/mL) failed to show increased binding to SKOV-3 cells compared to WT. However, at 10^{10} V/mL pJ18 and pJ24 both exhibited significantly increased SKOV-3 binding compared to WT, indicating that the interaction is mediated by the displayed peptides, rather than by inherent non-specific binding of the virion (Figure 3).

To further validate that the displayed peptides mediate the binding interaction, and not the intrinsic phage proteins, a cell-based dose-response assay was carried out. For this, SKOV-3 cells were incubated with different concentrations of biotinylated peptides (10 nM to 300 μM), after which binding was probed by streptavidin-HRP and detected spectrophotometrically at 405 nm after addition of ABTS (Figure 4). Peptides J18 and J24 displayed increased binding to SKOV-3 cells in comparison to a non-relevant peptide (negative control; N35) and exhibited EC_{50} values of 22.2 ± 10.6 μM and 29.0 ± 6.9 (mean ± SE), respectively.

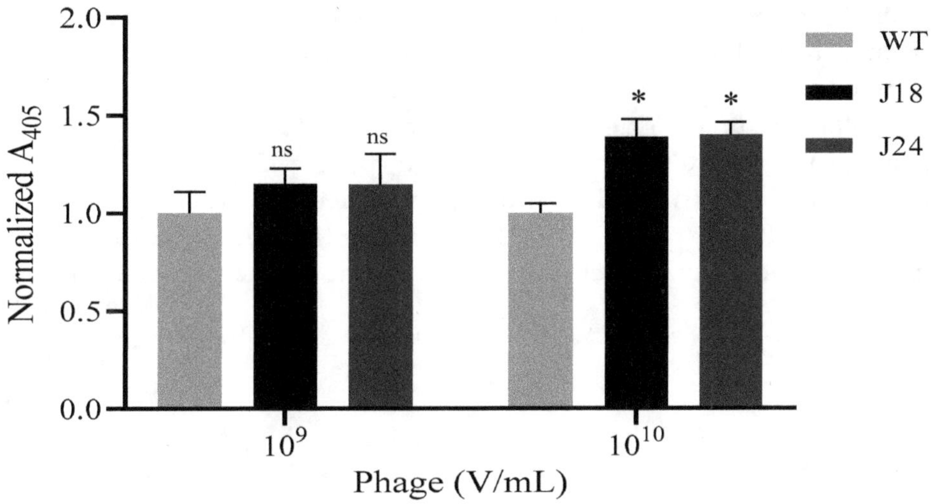

Figure 3. Binding of phage to ovarian carcinoma (SKOV-3) cells. Cells were grown to 80% confluency on 96-well plates, fixed using 0.2% Triton X-100 and 10% formalin, and then incubated with 10^9 or 10^{10} V/mL pJ18, pJ24, or WT phage. Phage binding was probed by biotinylated anti-Fd filamentous phage antibody and streptavidin-HRP, and detected spectrophotometrically at 405 nM after addition of 2, 2′-azino-bis(3-ethylbenzothiazoline-6-sulphonic acid) (ABTS). Binding of phage pJ18 and pJ24 to SKOV-3 cells was significantly higher at 10^{10} V/mL compared to WT. Measurements were performed on a SpectraMax 250 microplate reader (Molecular Devices, San Jose, CA, USA). A p-value of <0.05 was considered significant. * $p < 0.05$.

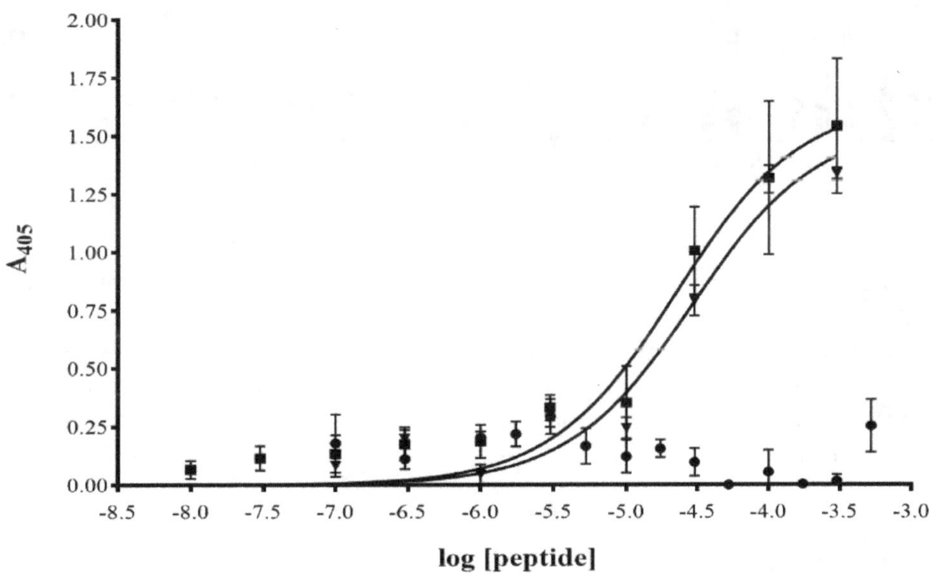

Figure 4. Binding properties of biotinylated peptides J18, J24, and N35 to ovarian carcinoma (SKOV-3) cells. Cells were grown to 80% confluency on 96-well plates and then incubated with varying concentrations (10 nM to 300 μM) of J18 (■), J24 (▼), and N35 (•) for 1 h at 37 °C. Plates were washed with PBS and fixed with 10% formalin. Biotinylated peptides were detected by HRP-conjugated streptavidin and measurement of absorbance at 405 nM after the addition of HRP-substrate ABTS. EC50 values for J18 and J24 were calculated to be 22.2 ± 10.6 μM, and 29.0 ± 6.9 μM (mean ± SE), respectively. Measurements were performed on a μ Quant Universal Microplate Spectrophotometer (Winooski, VT, USA).

3.3. Phage Biodistribution Studies

The biodistribution of AF680-labeled phage clones pJ18, pJ24, and WT was investigated in female nude mice bearing xenografted SKOV-3 tumors. Phage were injected into the tail-vein of the animals;

after 4 h the mice were sacrificed by cervical dislocation, and the fluorescent intensity in the tumors and normal tissues was measured (Figure 5). Both phage clones pJ18 and pJ24 exhibited fluorescent tumor uptake after 4 h; however, the levels were not significantly higher compared to WT. pJ24 exhibited significantly higher uptake in lung, kidneys, and liver compared to WT phage. The reticuloendothelial system was the major route of excretion for all phage (pJ18, pJ24, and WT), which was apparent from increased uptake primarily in the liver, lungs, and spleen. However, the kidneys also showed increased fluorescent intensity for pJ18 and pJ24, indicating that renal clearance is a minor excretion route. Uptake of phage in the heart, muscle, and brain did not differ between the clones.

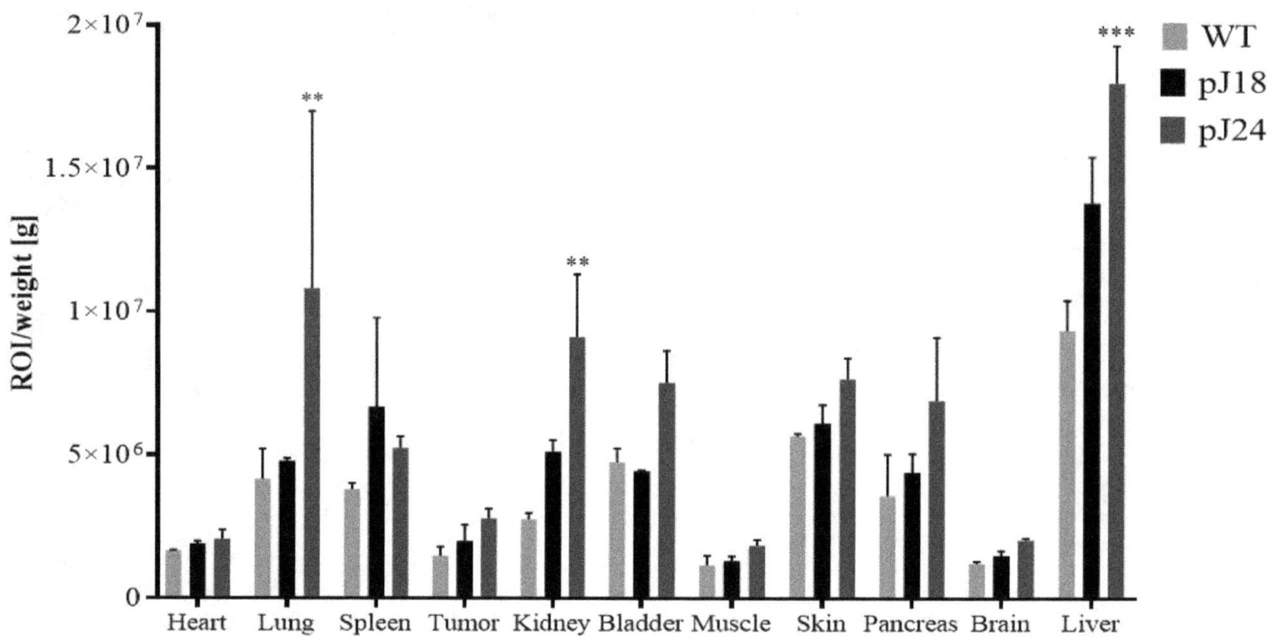

Figure 5. Biodistribution of AF680-labeled pJ18, pJ24, and WT phage in SKOV-3 xenografted nude female mice. Mice ($n = 2$) were injected with 10^{12} virions of phage. After 4 h the animals were sacrificed, and the organs, tissues, and tumors were excised and weighed. The fluorescent intensity was measured using a Xenogen IVIS 200 System. Fluorescent uptake was normalized to the weight of each organ and reported as fluorescent intensity per gram. Fluorescent intensity/g was significantly higher for pJ24 in the lungs, kidneys, and liver as compared to WT. A p-value of <0.05 was considered significant. ** $p < 0.01$, *** $p < 0.001$.

3.4. Near-Infrared Optical Imaging

Near-infrared optical imaging of nude mice carrying xenografted SKOV-3 tumors was performed to investigate the imaging properties of phage clones pJ18 and pJ24 (Figure 6a). AF680-labeled phage (pJ18, pJ24, or WT) were tail-vein injected into the animals and circulated for up to 4 h. The mice were imaged before the injection (0 h) to determine autofluorescence, as well as 2 h and 4 h post-injection. The obtained images revealed that the SKOV-3 tumors were easily localized and exhibited sufficient tumor-to-background contrast (Figure 6a). The fluorescent tumor signal intensity of each ROI was significantly higher in comparison to WT for pJ18 at 2 h post-injection. The tumor uptake decreased after 4 h for all phage clones. Although the signal intensity remained higher for pJ18 compared to WT, the difference was no longer significant (Figure 6b).

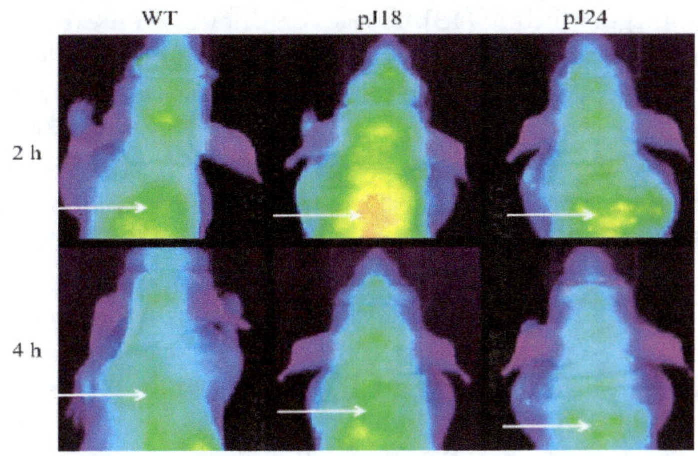

(a)

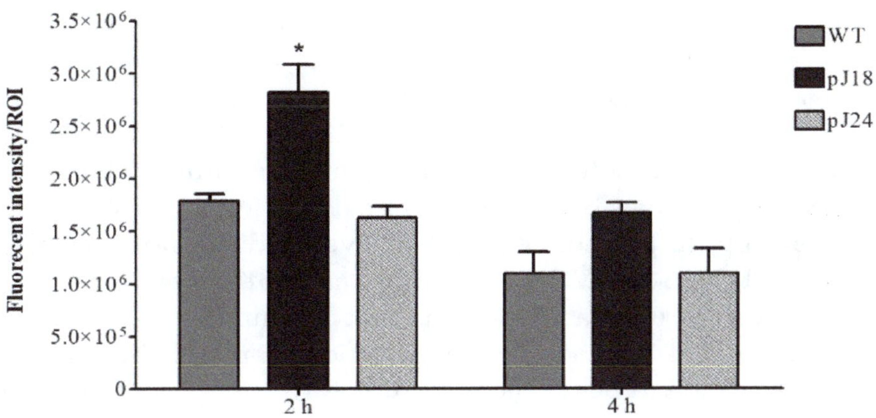

(b)

Figure 6. In vivo optical imaging of SKOV-3 xenografted tumors in female nude mice ($n = 2$) using AF680-labeled pJ18, pJ24, and WT phage. The mice were injected with 10^{12} virions of phage and imaged under anesthesia at 2 h and 4 h post-injection. (**a**) Fluorescence reflectance images of SKOV-3 xenografted mice. A white arrow indicates tumor location. (**b**) Quantification of fluorescent signal intensity of the region of interest (ROI). Fluorescence reflectance images were obtained using a Xenogen IVIS 200 System, and the fluorescent signal intensity was quantified using ImageJ software. Fluorescent intensity/ROI was significantly higher for pJ18 after 2 h compared to WT. A p-value of <0.05 was considered significant. * $p < 0.05$.

4. Discussion

Bacteriophage offer advantages as molecular imaging agents, in that they may be easily produced in *E. coli* and genetically modified to display various ligands. Additionally, phage may be utilized in both the development and delivery of such modalities. First, these nanoparticles may be employed in phage display technology to select and identify peptide-based ligands. Second, once such ligands have been validated, peptide-displaying phage may be used as biological nanoparticles that mediate binding to a molecular target, and that may at the same time carry various imaging agents. Phage particles have previously been successfully labeled with fluorophores, radiotracers, and iron, and used in optical [9,13] and radio imaging [24], as well as magnetic resonance imaging of molecular targets [25]. The large size of Fd filamentous phage also allows labeling with up to hundreds of imaging molecules per virion, typically on coat protein VIII (cpVIII), thereby providing signal amplification [15]. The spatial separation of the fluorophore on cpVIII and display of the foreign peptides on genetically modified coat protein III (cpIII) diminish any steric hindrance between the groups, thereby minimally affecting peptide-mediated target binding [13]. However, phage often exhibit non-specific hydrophobic binding [26–28]. For this reason, it is vital to validate that the displayed peptide mediates phage binding, and not inherent coat proteins. To do so, the modified ELISA and fluorescent microscopy experiments were carried out using peptide-displaying and WT phage, as well as single peptides.

Fluorescent microscopy was used to investigate phage binding to ovarian adenocarcinoma (SKOV-3) cells, and revealed that both clones, pJ18 and pJ24, displayed increased binding compared to WT. These results indicate that SKOV-3 binding of pJ18 and pJ24 is mediated by the respectively displayed peptides, as only minimal binding was observed for a WT phage, which is void of a foreign peptide. In order to further validate this observation, fluorescent microscopy studies were carried out using individual biotinylated peptides (J18 and J24) against both cancerous (SKOV-3, OVCAR-3, MDA-MB-435) and non-cancerous (HEK293) cell lines. The results showed that peptide J18 exhibited affinity for ovarian cancer cell lines (SKOV-3 and OVCAR-3), but only minimal binding to breast cancer (MDA-MB-435) and embryonic kidney (HEK293) cells. To the contrary, peptide J24 only exhibited binding to SKOV-3 cells, with negligible binding to other cell lines. Taken together, these results suggest that the selected peptides J18 and J24 bind ovarian cancer-specific antigens, and may, as a result, be utilized as ovarian carcinoma imaging agents. Further, the different binding characteristics of J18 and J24 for SKOV-3 and OVCAR-3 cells indicate that the peptides may target different antigens. SKOV-3 cells are known to exhibit more invasive potential compared to OVCAR-3, and to express higher levels of epidermal growth factor receptor (EGFR) [29–31]. The higher affinity of J18 for SKOV-3 may, therefore, suggest that the peptides bind an antigen with high and low expression profiles in the two cell lines, respectively, such as EGFR. The minimal binding to MDA-MB-435 cells, which lack EGFR expression, further supports this notion [32]. However, additional studies are needed to validate this observation. The high SKOV-3-to-OVCAR-3 binding ratio of J24 may also indicate that the peptide targets an antigen that is involved in invasiveness and that is comparatively overexpressed in the more aggressive SKOV-3 cell line [30,31]. For these reasons, peptide J18 may be binding to an antigen present in a wider array of ovarian cancer types and could, therefore, be useful in more broad applications, while J24 may be utilized to provide a more specialized targeting strategy.

As pJ18 and pJ24 was selected against SKOV-3 cells in a two-tier *in vivo* phage display selection [10], binding of the phage to this cell line was further investigated using a modified ELISA. The results revealed that at a concentration of 10^9 V/mL pJ18, pJ24, and WT showed similar binding to SKOV-3 cells. Nevertheless, at 10^{10} V/mL pJ18 and pJ24, both exhibited significantly increased binding compared to WT. The latter results (10^{10} V/mL) suggest, as previously noted, that the phage–SKOV-3 cell interaction is mediated by the displayed peptides, and not by non-specific binding of the virion. However, these results also indicate that 10^9 V/mL of pJ18 and pJ24 is insufficient to mediate detectable cell binding.

Phage from the fUSE5 phage display library express one to five peptides on genetically modified cpIII [33], and thus a phage concentration of 10^9 V/mL correlates to a peptide concentration of 1.7–8.3 pM. Therefore, to further evaluate the binding interaction, a cell-based dose-response assay using peptide concentrations (10 nM to 300 μM) above those used in the phage-based assay (1.7–8.3 pM) was performed. Both peptides J18 and J24 displayed saturation binding kinetics to SKOV-3 cells with EC_{50} values of 22.2 ± 10.6 μM and 29.0 ± 6.9 (mean ± SE), respectively. In comparison, a non-relevant peptide (N35; negative control) showed only minimal binding, from which it was not possible to calculate an EC_{50} value. The EC_{50} values of J18 and J24 are consistent with previously reported peptides that were identified by phage display technology [9,34]. In fact, phage that display peptides with EC_{50} values in the micromolar range have previously been used in optical imaging of xenografted tumors in mice [9]. Finally, the saturation binding kinetics further indicate that the peptide–cell interactions are specific [35], which confirms the previous notion that phage pJ18 and pJ24 binding is mediated by the displayed peptides, and not by non-specific phage proteins.

In order to evaluate the pharmacokinetics of phage pJ18 and pJ24, these were labeled with the near-infrared fluorophore AF680 and employed in biodistribution studies. After 4 h, fluorescent tumor uptake was detected for all phage clones (pJ18, pJ24, and WT). However, for pJ18 and pJ24 the tumor uptake was not significantly higher compared to WT. The low tumor levels may be a result of rapid pharmacokinetics and could suggest that optimal uptake occurs at earlier time points. Most other organs (lung, spleen, kidney, bladder, skin, and liver) showed increased fluorescent levels. In fact, pJ24 showed significantly higher uptake in the lungs, liver, and kidneys indicating elevated background binding compared to WT. Comparing the hydrophobicity of pJ18 and pJ24 according to the Wimley–White hydrophobicity scale [36], it is evident that pJ24 is comparatively more hydrophobic. Hydrophobicity is associated with the binding of nanoparticles to plasma proteins [37,38], and even slight increases in hydrophobicity have been shown to influence and extend biodistribution times [39,40]. For all phage, the liver exhibited increased fluorescent uptake compared to other organs, indicating that the phage were excreted through the reticuloendothelial system (RES). This observation was expected, as nanoparticles are cleared primarily through the RES [41,42], which was further confirmed by elevated uptake by the spleen and lungs. However, the kidneys also displayed increased fluorescent intensity, especially for pJ24. These results suggest that the kidneys may be a minor excretion route for both pJ18 and pJ24, but not for WT phage, which showed only minimal uptake in these organs. Previous biodistribution studies of phage have shown similar results regarding reticuloendothelial excretion [9,13,43–45]. While the large size and biochemical properties of nanoparticles, including phage, are known to greatly affect biodistribution and excretion [46], the display of peptides have shown to partly re-direct the clearance [13]. Taking these observations into account, the pharmacokinetic results in this study may indicate that peptides J18 and J24 are steering the excretion system towards the kidneys. Phage uptake in other organs (heart, muscle, and brain) was comparatively lower and did not differ between the clones. The low uptakes were possibly caused by the tight junctions that connect heart and muscle cells and challenge extravasation of large particles into these tissues. Additionally, the blood–brain barrier excludes the vast majority of particles above 400 kDa, which significantly limits the ability of phage to enter the brain [47].

Near-infrared optical imaging of SKOV-3 xenografted nude mice was carried out to evaluate the tumor imaging capabilities of AF680-labeled pJ18, pJ24, and WT. The images revealed that the tumors were easily localized and showed satisfactory tumor-to-background contrast. Peak tumor fluorescent intensity was obtained after 2 h for all phage clones, and at this time point, the signal intensity was significantly higher for pJ18 compared to WT. In correlation to the biodistribution study, the tumor uptake of pJ18 and pJ24 after 4 h was similar to that of WT. These observations may be due to high uptake and clearance rates, which for pJ18 is further supported by the similarly low levels in other tissues at this time point. However, the imaging study showed that pJ24 failed to demonstrate increased tumor uptake at any time point. This observation may indicate that pJ24 exhibits optimal tumor uptake at a time point before 2 h or after 4 h of circulation. The surface charge and displayed functional groups of nanoparticles are known to influence both cellular uptake and excretion; consequently, the small difference in positive charge at physiological pH of peptide J18 (charge +1 at pH 7) and J24 (charge +1.1 at pH 7) may be the reason behind the observed differences [41].

Overall, this optical imaging study shows that the peptides, J18, and J24, influence the binding characteristics of the phage particles. Phage clone pJ18 enables specific targeting and imaging of SKOV-3 tumors in xenografted mice. Thus, this phage nanoparticle may be utilized in future studies to improve current detection strategies of ovarian cancer.

Peptide displaying phage, pJ18 and pJ24, were previously selected using phage display technology for binding to human ovarian adenocarcinoma SKOV-3 cells [10]. Here, fluorescent microscopy and modified ELISA showed increased and specific binding of phage, pJ18 and pJ24, and peptides, J18 and J24, to ovarian cancer cells compared to controls. In vivo studies revealed successful tumor targeting of AF680-labeled pJ18, enabling easy tumor visualization. In conclusion, this study demonstrates the ability of pJ18 to target and image xenografted ovarian tumors *in vivo*. Therefore, this phage clone may be utilized in further studies as an ovarian cancer-targeting nanoparticle to improve the detection and diagnosis of the disease.

Author Contributions: Conceptualization, M.S. and S.D.; methodology, M.A., M.S., and J.N.-N.; software, M.S. and J.N.-N.; Formal analysis, M.S., M.A., and J.N.-N.; writing—original draft preparation, M.S.; writing—review and editing, M.S. and S.D.; supervision, M.S. and S.D.; project administration, M.S. and S.D.; funding acquisition, S.D.

Acknowledgments: The authors would like to acknowledge the contributions of Lisa D. Watkinson, Terry L. Carmack, and the VA Biomolecular Imaging Core.

References

1. Siegel, R.L.; Miller, K.D.; Jemal, A. Cancer statistics, 2018. *CA A Cancer J. Clin.* **2018**, *68*, 7–30. [CrossRef] [PubMed]
2. Zurawski, V.R., Jr.; Orjaseter, H.; Andersen, A.; Jellum, E. Elevated serum CA 125 levels prior to diagnosis of ovarian neoplasia: Relevance for early detection of ovarian cancer. *Int. J. Cancer* **1988**, *42*, 677–680. [CrossRef] [PubMed]
3. Miralles, C.; Orea, M.; Espana, P.; Provencio, M.; Sanchez, A.; Cantos, B.; Cubedo, R.; Carcereny, E.; Bonilla, F.; Gea, T. Cancer antigen 125 associated with multiple benign and malignant pathologies. *Ann. Surg. Oncol.* **2003**, *10*, 150–154. [CrossRef] [PubMed]
4. Kim, B.; Park, Y.; Kim, B.; Ahn, H.J.; Lee, K.-A.; Chung, J.E.; Han, S.W. Diagnostic performance of CA 125, HE4, and risk of Ovarian Malignancy Algorithm for ovarian cancer. *J. Clin. Lab. Anal.* **2019**, *33*, e22624. [CrossRef] [PubMed]
5. Jacobs, I.J.; Skates, S.J.; MacDonald, N.; Menon, U.; Rosenthal, A.N.; Davies, A.P.; Woolas, R.; Jeyarajah, A.R.; Sibley, K.; Lowe, D.G.; et al. Screening for ovarian cancer: A pilot randomised controlled trial. *Lancet* **1999**, *353*, 1207–1210. [CrossRef]
6. Smith, G.P. Filamentous fusion phage: Novel expression vectors that display cloned antigens on the virion surface. *Science* **1985**, *228*, 1315–1317. [CrossRef]
7. McCafferty, J.; Griffiths, A.D.; Winter, G.; Chiswell, D.J. Phage antibodies: Filamentous phage displaying antibody variable domains. *Nature* **1990**, *348*, 552–554. [CrossRef]
8. Huston, J.S.; Levinson, D.; Mudgett-Hunter, M.; Tai, M.S.; Novotny, J.; Margolies, M.N.; Ridge, R.J.; Bruccoleri, R.E.; Haber, E.; Crea, R.; et al. Protein engineering of antibody binding sites: Recovery of specific activity in an anti-digoxin single-chain Fv analogue produced in *Escherichia coli*. *Proc. Natl. Acad. Sci. USA* **1988**, *85*, 5879–5883. [CrossRef]
9. Soendergaard, M.; Newton-Northup, J.R.; Deutscher, S.L. In vitro high throughput phage display selection of ovarian cancer avid phage clones for near-infrared optical imaging. *Comb. Chem. High Throughput Screen.* **2014**, *17*, 859–867. [CrossRef]
10. Soendergaard, M.; Newton-Northup, J.R.; Deutscher, S.L. In vivo phage display selection of an ovarian cancer targeting peptide for SPECT/CT imaging. *Am. J. Nucl. Med. Mol. Imaging* **2014**, *4*, 561–570.
11. Zou, J.; Glinsky, V.V.; Landon, L.A.; Matthews, L.; Deutscher, S.L. Peptides specific to the galectin-3 carbohydrate recognition domain inhibit metastasis-associated cancer cell adhesion. *Carcinogenesis* **2005**, *26*, 309–318. [CrossRef] [PubMed]
12. Kumar, S.R.; Deutscher, S.L. Galectin-3-Targeting Peptides as Novel In Vivo tumor-Imaging and Targeting Agents. In Proceedings of the Tumor Microvasculature Environment AACR Meeting, Florence, Italy, 2006.
13. Newton, J.R.; Kelly, K.A.; Mahmood, U.; Weissleder, R.; Deutscher, S.L. In vivo selection of phage for the optical imaging of PC-3 human prostate carcinoma in mice. *Neoplasia* **2006**, *8*, 772–780. [CrossRef] [PubMed]
14. Kumar, S.R.; Quinn, T.P.; Deutscher, S.L. Evaluation of an 111In-radiolabeled peptide as a targeting and imaging agent for ErbB-2 receptor expressing breast carcinomas. *Clin. Cancer Res.* **2007**, *13*, 6070–6079. [CrossRef] [PubMed]
15. Rakonjac, J.; Bennett, N.J.; Spagnuolo, J.; Gagic, D.; Russel, M. Filamentous Bacteriophage: Biology, Phage Display and Nanotechnology Applications. *Curr. Issues Mol. Biol.* **2011**, *13*, 51–75. [PubMed]
16. Abbineni, G.; Modali, S.; Safiejko-Mroczka, B.; Petrenko, V.A.; Mao, C. Evolutionary Selection of New Breast Cancer Cell-Targeting Peptides and Phage with the Cell-Targeting Peptides Fully Displayed on the Major Coat and Their Effects on Actin Dynamics during Cell Internalization. *Mol. Pharmacol.* **2010**, *7*, 1629–1642. [CrossRef] [PubMed]

17. Kelly, K.A.; Waterman, P.; Weissleder, R. In vivo imaging of molecularly targeted phage. *Neoplasia* **2006**, *8*, 1011–1018. [CrossRef] [PubMed]
18. Hilderbrand, S.A.; Weissleder, R. Near-infrared fluorescence: Application to in vivo molecular imaging. *Curr. Opin. Chem. Biol.* **2010**, *14*, 71–79. [CrossRef]
19. Aina, O.H.; Marik, J.; Gandour-Edwards, R.; Lam, K.S. Near-infrared optical imaging of ovarian cancer xenografts with novel alpha 3-integrin binding peptide "OA02". *Mol. Imaging* **2005**, *4*, 439–447. [CrossRef]
20. Pysz, M.A.; Gambhir, S.S.; Willmann, J.K. Molecular imaging: Current status and emerging strategies. *Clin. Radiol.* **2010**, *65*, 500–516. [CrossRef]
21. Scott, J.K.; Smith, G.P. Searching for peptide ligands with an epitope library. *Science* **1990**, *249*, 386–390. [CrossRef]
22. Smith, G.P. Smith Lab Homepage. Available online: http://www.biosci.missouri.edu/smithGP/PhageDisplayWebsite/PhageDisplayWebsiteIndex.html (accessed on 26 February 2014).
23. Abramoff, M.D.; Magalhaes, P.J.; Ram, S.J. Image Processing with Image. *J. Biophotonics Int.* **2004**, *11*, 36–42.
24. Li, Z.B.; Jin, Q.L.; Huang, C.W.; Dasa, S.; Chen, L.H.; Yap, L.P.; Liu, S.L.; Cai, H.C.; Park, R.; Conti, P.S. Trackable and Targeted Phage as Positron Emission Tomography (PET) Agent for Cancer Imaging. *Theranostics* **2011**, *1*, 371–380. [CrossRef] [PubMed]
25. Ghosh, D.; Lee, Y.; Thomas, S.; Kohli, A.G.; Yun, D.S.; Belcher, A.M.; Kelly, K.A.; M13-templated magnetic nanoparticles for targeted in vivo imaging of prostate cancer. M13-templated magnetic nanoparticles for targeted in vivo imaging of prostate cancer. *Nat. Nanotechnol.* **2012**, *7*, 677–682. [CrossRef]
26. Giordano, R.J.; Cardo-Vila, M.; Lahdenranta, J.; Pasqualini, R.; Arap, W. Biopanning and rapid analysis of selective interactive ligands. *Nat. Med.* **2001**, *7*, 1249–1253. [CrossRef] [PubMed]
27. Spear, M.A.; Breakefield, X.O.; Beltzer, J.; Schuback, D.; Weissleder, R.; Pardo, F.S.; Ladner, R. Isolation, characterization, and recovery of small peptide phage display epitopes selected against viable malignant glioma cells. *Cancer Gene Ther.* **2001**, *8*, 506–511. [CrossRef]
28. Adey, N.B.; Mataragnon, A.H.; Rider, J.E.; Carter, J.M.; Kay, B.K. Characterization of phage that bind plastic from phage-displayed random peptide libraries. *Gene* **1995**, *156*, 27–31. [CrossRef]
29. Choi, J.H.; Choi, K.C.; Auersperg, N.; Leung, P.C. Gonadotropins upregulate the epidermal growth factor receptor through activation of mitogen-activated protein kinases and phosphatidyl-inositol-3-kinase in human ovarian surface epithelial cells. *Endocr.-Relat. Cancer* **2005**, *12*, 407–421. [CrossRef]
30. Choi, J.-H.; Choi, K.-C.; Auersperg, N.; Leung, P.C.K. Gonadotropins Activate Proteolysis and Increase Invasion through Protein Kinase A and Phosphatidylinositol 3-Kinase Pathways in Human Epithelial Ovarian Cancer Cells. *Cancer Res.* **2006**, *66*, 3912–3920. [CrossRef]
31. Ellerbroek, S.M.; Halbleib, J.M.; Benavidez, M.; Warmka, J.K.; Wattenberg, E.V.; Stack, M.S.; Hudson, L.G. Phosphatidylinositol 3-Kinase Activity in Epidermal Growth Factor-stimulated Matrix Metalloproteinase-9 Production and Cell Surface Association. *Cancer Res.* **2001**, *61*, 1855–1861.
32. Anido, J.; Matar, P.; Albanell, J.; Guzman, M.; Rojo, F.; Arribas, J.; Averbuch, S.; Baselga, J. ZD1839, a specific epidermal growth factor receptor (EGFR) tyrosine kinase inhibitor, induces the formation of inactive EGFR/HER2 and EGFR/HER3 heterodimers and prevents heregulin signaling in HER2-overexpressing breast cancer cells. *Clin. Cancer Res. Off. J. Am. Assoc. Cancer Res.* **2003**, *9*, 1274–1283.
33. Smith, G.P.; Scott, J.K. Libraries of peptides and proteins displayed on filamentous phage. *Methods Enzym.* **1993**, *217*, 228–257.
34. Ma, C.; Yin, G.; Yan, D.; He, X.; Zhang, L.; Wei, Y.; Huang, Z. A novel peptide specifically targeting ovarian cancer identified by in vivo phage display. *J. Pept. Sci.* **2013**, *19*, 730–736. [CrossRef] [PubMed]
35. Hulme, E.C.; Trevethick, M.A. Ligand binding assays at equilibrium: Validation and interpretation. *Br. J. Pharmacol.* **2010**, *161*, 1219–1237. [CrossRef] [PubMed]
36. Wimley, W.C.; White, S.H. Experimentally determined hydrophobicity scale for proteins at membrane interfaces. *Nat. Struct. Biol.* **1996**, *3*, 842–848. [CrossRef] [PubMed]
37. Cedervall, T.; Lynch, I.; Foy, M.; Berggard, T.; Donnelly, S.C.; Cagney, G.; Linse, S.; Dawson, K.A. Detailed identification of plasma proteins adsorbed on copolymer nanoparticles. *Angew. Chem. Int. Ed. Engl.* **2007**, *46*, 5754–5756. [CrossRef] [PubMed]

38. Gessner, A.; Waicz, R.; Lieske, A.; Paulke, B.; Mader, K.; Muller, R.H. Nanoparticles with decreasing surface hydrophobicities: Influence on plasma protein adsorption. *Int. J. Pharm.* **2000**, *196*, 245–249. [CrossRef]
39. Cullis, P.R.; Chonn, A.; Semple, S.C. Interactions of liposomes and lipid-based carrier systems with blood proteins: Relation to clearance behaviour in vivo. *Adv. Drug Deliv. Rev.* **1998**, *32*, 3–17.
40. Chonn, A.; Semple, S.C.; Cullis, P.R. Association of blood proteins with large unilamellar liposomes in vivo. Relation to circulation lifetimes. *J. Biol. Chem.* **1992**, *267*, 18759–18765.
41. Li, S.D.; Huang, L. Pharmacokinetics and biodistribution of nanoparticles. *Mol. Pharm.* **2008**, *5*, 496–504. [CrossRef]
42. Wang, M.; Thanou, M. Targeting nanoparticles to cancer. *Pharm. Res.* **2010**, *62*, 90–99. [CrossRef]
43. Yip, Y.L.; Hawkins, N.J.; Smith, G.; Ward, R.L. Biodistribution of filamentous phage-Fab in nude mice. *J. Immunol. Methods* **1999**, *225*, 171–178. [CrossRef]
44. Smith, M.W.; Al-Jayyoussi, G.; Gumbleton, M. Peptide sequences mediating tropism to intact blood-brain barrier: An in vivo biodistribution study using phage display. *Peptides* **2012**, *38*, 172–180. [CrossRef] [PubMed]
45. Zou, J.; Dickerson, M.T.; Owen, N.K.; Landon, L.A.; Deutscher, S.L. Biodistribution of filamentous phage peptide libraries in mice. *Mol. Biol. Rep.* **2004**, *31*, 121–129. [CrossRef] [PubMed]
46. Alexis, F.; Pridgen, E.; Molnar, L.K.; Farokhzad, O.C. Factors affecting the clearance and biodistribution of polymeric nanoparticles. *Mol. Pharm.* **2008**, *5*, 505–515. [CrossRef] [PubMed]
47. Pardridge, W.M. The blood-brain barrier: Bottleneck in brain drug development. *NeuroRX J. Am. Soc. Exp. Neurother.* **2005**, *2*, 3–14. [CrossRef] [PubMed]

2

Identification and Characterization of Nasal Polyposis and Mycoplasma Superinfection by Scanning Electron Microscopy and Nasal Cytology with Optical Microscopy

Arturo Armone Caruso [1], Veronica Viola [2], Salvatore Del Prete [3], Sabato Leo [4], Daniela Marasco [3], Andrea Fulgione [5], Daniele Naviglio [2,*] and Monica Gallo [6,*]

1 ENT Department, AIAS Structure of Afragola, Contrada Leutrec snc, 80021 Naples, Italy; armocar@libero.it
2 Department of Chemical Sciences, University of Naples Federico II, via Cintia, 21, 80126 Naples, Italy; violaveronica@outlook.it
3 Service Biotech s.r.l., 80132 Napoli, Italy; saldep@gmail.com (S.D.P.); danielamarasco.servicebiotech@gmail.com (D.M.)
4 ENT Outpatient Clinic at Scafati Hospital ASL SA, 84018 Salerno, Italy; sabato.leo@libero.it
5 Department of Agricultural Science, University of Naples Federico II, Via Università 100, 80045 Portici (NA), Italy; andrea.fulgione@unina.it
6 Department of Molecular Medicine and Medical Biotechnology, University of Naples Federico II, via Pansini, 5, 80131 Naples, Italy
* Correspondence: naviglio@unina.it (D.N.); mongallo@unina.it (M.G.)

Abstract: Nasal polyposis is characterized by benign, non-cancerous and painless growths originating in the tissue of the nasal cavities and paranasal sinuses. Polyps arise from chronic inflammation due to asthma, recurrent infections, allergies, drug sensitivity or immune disorders. They can obstruct the nasal cavities and thus cause respiratory problems, a reduction in the sense of smell and susceptibility to infections. Furthermore, nasal polyps can recur. Hence the importance of using valid diagnostic methods. In this work, the diagnostic investigation carried out by scanning electron microscopy (SEM) and nasal cytology led, for the first time, to the identification of a mycoplasma superinfection on nasal polyposis.

Keywords: mycoplasma; nasal cytology; nasal polyposis; optical microscopy; scanning electron microscopy

---

1. Introduction

Nasal polyposis (NP) is a common disease in 4% of the population. The nasal polyps derive from an inflammatory process of the mucosa that covers the nasal cavity wall. The polyps tend to grow and, therefore, to obstruct the nasal passages and the paranasal sinuses. The underlying causes of polyp formation are not yet fully known. However, any condition that triggers chronic inflammation in the nasal cavities or sinuses, such as infections, allergies and cellular rhinitis, can increase the risk of polyp formation [1–3]. Although it is a minor illness, nasal polyposis has a very negative influence on patients' well-being, often influencing their lifestyle [4–6]. Moreover, the disease, although treatable, is burdened with frequent recurrences. In this work, for the first time, a case of a patient with nasal polyposis and mycoplasma [7] superinfection has been reported, in which the clinical investigation was performed using the scanning electron microscope (SEM) and the optical microscope for nasal cytology.

2. Clinical Case

A 55-year-old female was observed due to significant breathing difficulties. After the completion of the rite of privacy and informed consent to the carrying out of investigations, the physical examination was performed by means of a Nasopharyngoscope XION Medical (Berlin, Germany) diameter of 4 mm previously disinfected, according to the regulations in force. The examination documented the presence of nasal polyposis bilaterally, confirmed by axial scan (Figure 1).

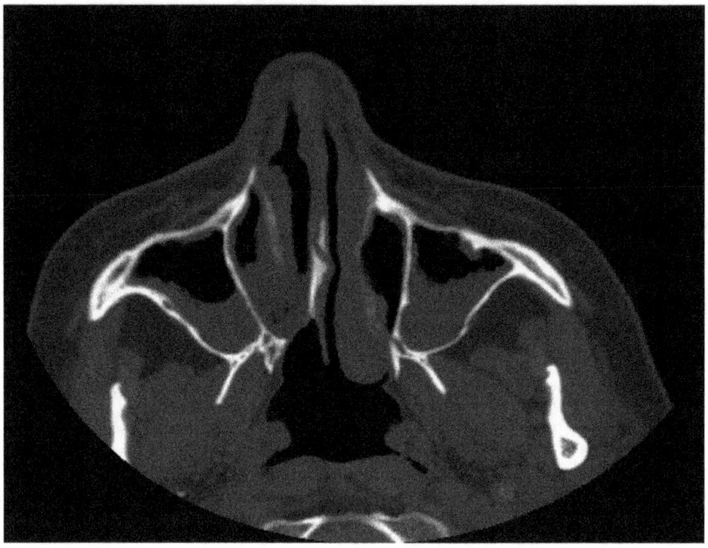

Figure 1. Axial scan of the facial massif where the polypoid formation is seen in both nostrils and maxillary sinuses.

Furthermore, considering some characteristics of the physical examination (presence of exudate), nasal mucosa samples were taken by nasal scraping®. To establish the criterion of recurrence of the polyposis itself, the sampling was applied to a polarized and colored slide according to the Pappernheim (May-Grunwald-Giemsa) panoptic, and then observed under an optical microscope at 100× magnification in oil immersion. In addition, a second sampling was performed for nasal scraping® and placed on a 13 mm round slide for Scanning Electron Microscopy (SEM).

Subsequently, a nasal swab was performed and placed in Brain-Heart totipotent liquid growth culture medium. This swab was placed in 48 h culture and then scanned in electron microscopy, as per practices described in Materials and Methods.

3. Mycoplasma and Superantigens

Mycoplasma is a kind of bacterial pathogen that causes vertebrate diseases. Due to its size, diagnosis by light microscopy is not easy. Currently, X-rays are performed, followed by serology, and amplification of the PCR and/or culture, but all these investigations are particularly difficult at an early stage of the disease. Conversely, thanks to its deep scanning capability, SEM can observe the entire internal structure of the mycoplasma cells. A study by Sato et al. (2012) shows the applicability of the atmospheric scanning electron microscope for the study of mycoplasmas and for the diagnosis of mycoplasma infection at an early stage [8]. As is known, SEM does not exploit photons of light such as optical microscopy but uses an electron beam that strikes the sample. Thanks to the wavelength of electrons much lower than that of photons, the resolving power of a SEM is much higher than that of an optical microscope. Moreover, even the depth of field of an SEM is much higher allowing perfect images even for three-dimensional samples, with a high thickness [9,10]. Mycoplasma is "presented" to T-cells and recognized by a mechanism that is common to superantigens (bacterial, viral and neoplastic), while it is different from that of common soluble antigens. As is known, superantigens, even though they are not mitogenic sensu strictiori, induce the proliferation of T-lymphocytes even at low concentrations (lower than those of soluble antigens). Based on the results of experimental research, the mechanisms by which it is thought that mycoplasma can contribute to the development of human diseases, in genetically predisposed subjects, are essentially the following: (1) "Acute" release of cytokines; (2) Induction of autoimmunity; (3) Immuno-depression; (4) Selection of the T-lymphocyte population. These toxins are, in fact, able to activate T-lymphocytes interacting with the major histocompatibility complex (MHC-II) interaction that results in the release of pro-inflammatory cytokines. Firstly, IL-5, capable of inducing chemotaxis, migration and activation of eosinophils and delaying apoptosis, when they act as superantigens in the lateral wall of the nose in the case of chronic hyperplastic sinusitis with nasal polyposis [11,12]. Variations in the immune response to mycoplasmic antigens may be responsible for various levels of disease severity. Indeed, the superantigen would be responsible for the formation of nasal polyps [13,14].

As reported in the literature, the mycoplasms [7,15] are the smallest known bacterial forms, they are devoid of a cell wall and belong to the class of mollicutes, order of the mycoplasmatales. The mycoplasms that create disturbances to the respiratory tract are usually *Mycoplasma pneumoniae*. Pneumonia occurs only in 10–15% of cases out of 12 million, and in most cases (30–40%) involves tracheobronchitis and atypical pneumonia, or 15% of all pneumonia cases. If a mycoplasma infection is suspected, various samples should be collected per culture [9,16]. A sample is used to inoculate agar media enriched with preformed protein sources, peptones or yeast and cholesterol extracts, in the form of serum. Phenol red is added to the culture medium as a pH indicator, with thallium acetate and penicillin to inhibit the growth of other microorganisms. The sample thus inoculated in agar should be placed at 5% CO_2 and 95% air. The second soil will be passed on a two-phase soil and then passed to agar. The growth of mycoplasma agar colonies takes on a typical fried egg shape. The diagnosis of mycoplasma infection is mainly performed on clinical grounds. Bacteria can be grown from excreted samples or pharyngeal exudate swabs, but this procedure takes several weeks to produce results. There are alternative tests carried out on blood, more precisely on cold agglutinins, but this test is not always true, because many subjects are false-negative. Mycoplasms are an extracellular pathogen. It does not invade the respiratory epithelium but adheres to the host cells by means of specialized ends P1, protein adhesin, which adheres to neuraminic acid residues and is responsible for the virulence. Once adhered to the tissue they form hydrogen peroxide to dig the underlying mucosa. Some mycoplasmic antigens act as superantigens creating an aggravation of the pathology. Thanks to biomolecular methods (pCR number of options are available for conclusive detection of the presence of mycoplasmas in escretous fluid) that are usually preferred to isolation methods on soil as we described before; it is also highlighted by more complex microscopic techniques such as confocal vision, where they appear grouped in colonies with a typical fried egg appearance, or with SEM microscopy where individual colonial constituents can also be seen and often appear to interact parasitic with other bacterial forms. Under the SEM microscope, they are clearly visible as spheroidal elements with a diameter between 0.1 and 0.2 μm, often grouped in circular or dome-shaped aggregates or even in cluster formations. Finally, mycoplasma have a slower replication capacity [9] than the classic tuberculosis, while increasing the culture time up to 15 days more or less, they mainly attack immunocompromised individuals being opportunistic and non-parasitic pathogens. Therefore, these mycoplasmas are more difficult to identify and constitute a new class of pathogens [17–19] SEM can be an innovative and fast means for the easy identification of these pathogens.

4. Bacterial Biofilms

As is known, bacteria can exist in two distinct forms, planktonic or biofilm. Biofilm existence improves bacterial survival through several mechanisms. Therefore, it is the state in which 99% of bacteria prefer to exist, forming tightly organized microcolonies enclosed in the extracellular matrix [20]. Biofilms have been implicated in multiple significant infectious processes for the practice of otolaryngology, and scanning electron microscopy (SEM) is among the most recent and most reliable modalities for biofilm detection [21]. Evidence suggests that genetic modifications of the host in innate and adaptive immunity drive biofilm susceptibility leading to a subset of patients with chronic rhinosinusitis (CRS) with recurrent and recalcitrant disease [22]. In fact, while the role of biofilms in CRS has been studied for several years, the interest of the research has now been directed towards the clarification of new methods of biofilm detection, microbial diversity and new therapeutic approaches. Recent studies on biofilm superantigens aim to clarify the immunological mechanisms of inflammation of the upper airways, in particular the type 2 response observed in nasal polyposis [23].

5. Materials and Methods

Cytological Method: a written informed consent was obtained from the patient. The cytologic sampling was carried out, after fulfilling the privacy requirements and informed consent, by means of a scraping technique, i.e., by crawling a rhino (Nasal-scraping®) 2–3 times on the mucous surface of the central area of the inferior turbinate. The nasal mucosal cells were placed on an electrostatically charged cytology slide (Superfrost Plus Menzel-Gläser, Thermo Scientific, Milan, Italy). The cells were then stained according to the panoptic method (3 min in pure May-Grunwald dye (Carlo Erba, Milan, Italy), 6 min in 50% May-Grunwald dye, 1 min in bidistilled water (Carlo Erba, Milan, Italy); and 30 min in Giemsa solution (Carlo Erba, Milan, Italy) diluted 1:10 *v/v*). The slide was then covered with a glass cover with dimensions of 24 × 50 mm and observed under an optical microscope (Nikon Eclipse 50i) at 100× oil-immersion enlargement. The images were recorded using a Nikon DS1 camera and digitized using a NIS-D elements computer support. Observation by optical microscope allowed to observe the presence of bacterial colonies and eosinophilic cells, using May-Grunwald-Giemsa differential staining which makes it possible to distinguish red blood cells and leukocytes, thus allowing to identify some pathologies of the blood cells (Figures 2 and 3).

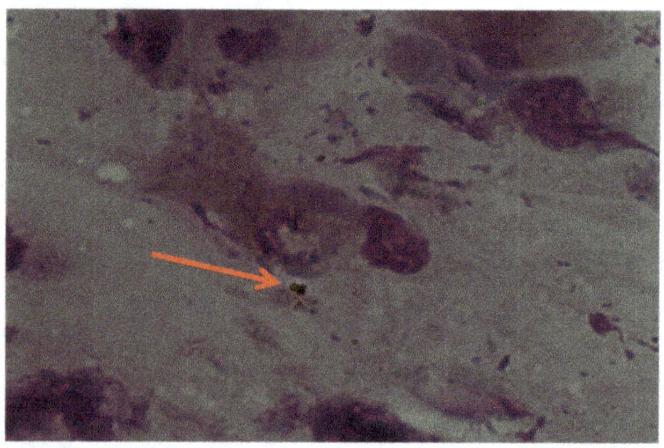

Figure 2. Optical microscope image. The red arrow shows the presence of masses indicating a suspected infection (100× image enlargement, oil immersion).

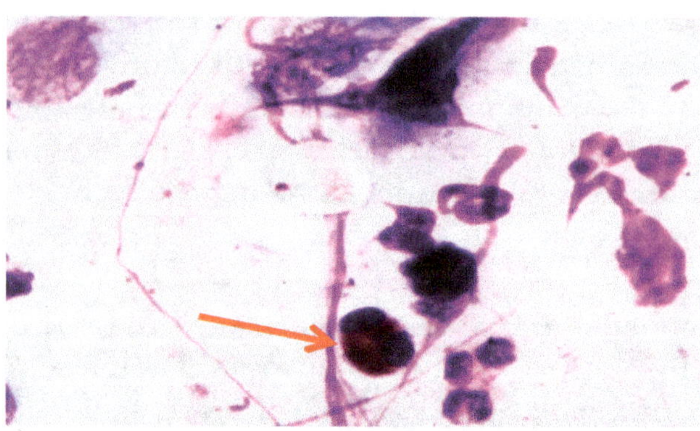

Figure 3. Optical microscope image. The red arrow shows the presence of eosinophils (100× image enlargement, oil immersion). In cases of allergic rhinitis, eosinophils are pathognomonic elements.

SEM method applied to the practice of nasal scraping® cytology and buffer was grown in Brain-Heart liquid culture medium 48 h. The samples were prepared in this sense, both the nasal cytological sampling using nasal scraping® and the culture, were applied on a 13 mm DIA round glass, were fixed in 2% glutaraldehyde, washed in PBS (Phosphate Buffered Saline) at pH 7.4 for 15 min for 3 times, and treated in osmio 4% for 2 h. Subsequently, the samples were subjected to 2 washings in PBS at pH 7.4 each at 30 min. Finally, the sample thus treated was dehydrated in alcohol at increasing concentrations; 30% at 25 min, 50% at 25 min, 70% at 20 min and 96% at 20 min for 2 times. Once dehydrated, the sample was placed in a critical point in CO_2 (critical point at 31 °C and 73 atmosphere).

The treatment of the samples allowed to visualize at various magnifications the bacterial species colonizing the nasal mucosa and the typical inflammatory cells; moreover, the culture has placed attention on the pathogens involved in the phlogosis [24,25] of the nasal mucosa of the patient under examination (Figures 4 and 5). These pathogens were compatible with the bacterial genus of Mycoplasmas.

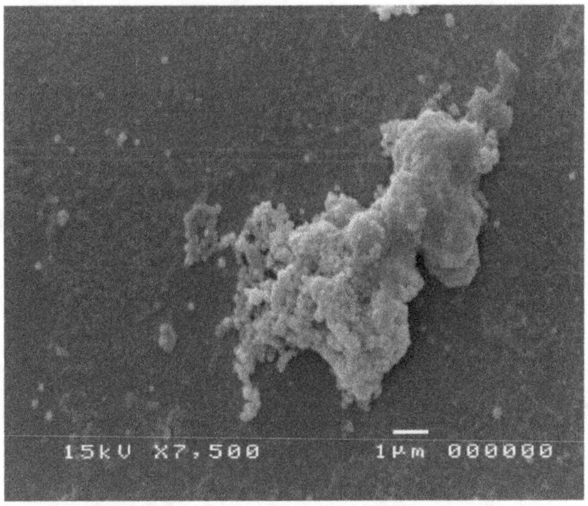

Figure 4. SEM image showing a mycoplasma colony (image enlargement 10,000×).

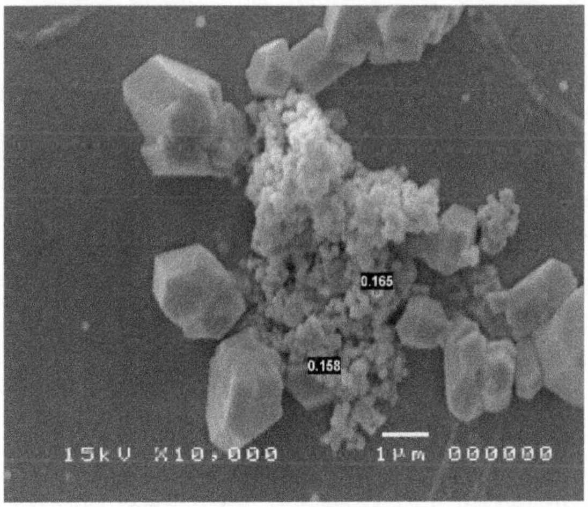

Figure 5. SEM image showing a colony of mycoplasma in colony caught in crystals (image enlargement 10,000×).

6. Discussion

The use of a suction device to remove large volumes of mucus helps to increase the chances of obtaining representative sinus microflora. Spurious recovery of mycoplasmas, due to endoscope contamination, is possible, as well as the possibility that glutaraldehyde may not adequately kill mycoplasma. Indeed, it is known that activated alkaline glutaraldehyde is one of the most widely used high-level disinfectants worldwide. However, several reports have highlighted the potential for nontuberculous mycobacteria to develop high-level resistance to this product [26]. In our case, on the other hand, a sample was taken with a sterile swab, which demonstrated the presence of numerous small masses compatible with an infection by optical microscopy. The SEM observation has documented the presence of a spheroidal shape with dimensions between 0.176 and 0.182 microns. The forms were compatible with those of Mycoplasma. Therefore, cytochemical investigations based on the use of SEM have confirmed that the isolated bacterium belongs to this pathogen.

In conclusion, it has been observed that the patient affected by mycoplasma showed nasal polyposis [24,25,27], and presence of eosinophilic cells was justified by the role played by the ability of mycoplasma to act as superantigen [16,27]. Eosinophilic cells exist everywhere in nasal mucosa when the patient has allergic rhinitis. Therefore, in cases of allergic rhinitis, eosinophils are pathognomonic elements. Consequently, the investigations conducted showed that a comparative study of nasal cytology using optical microscopy and SEM is a precision diagnostic path that can direct the specialist towards an adequate therapy. Therefore, the use of SEM microscopy and nasal cytology represent a valid and innovative support to research and can be proposed as methods of choice in clinical diagnosis.

Author Contributions: Conceptualization, A.A.C., S.D.P. and S.L.; methodology, A.A.C., S.D.P. and S.L.; validation, A.A.C., D.N. and M.G.; formal analysis, V.V. D.M. A.F.; writing—original draft preparation, A.A.C., S.L. and M.G.; writing—review and editing, A.A.C. and M.G.; supervision, A.A.C., D.N. and M.G. All authors reviewed and approved the final version of the manuscript.

References

1. Newton, J.R.; Ah-See, K.W. A review of nasal polyposis. *Ther. Clin. Risk Manag.* **2008**, *4*, 507. [CrossRef] [PubMed]
2. Pietruszewska, W.; Olejniczak, I.; Józefowicz-Korczyaska, M.; Gryczyński, M. Etiology of nasal polyps: An update. *Otolaryngol. Polska* **2006**, *60*, 551–557.
3. Stevens, W.W.; Schleimer, R.P.; Kern, R.C. Chronic Rhinosinusitis with Nasal Polyps. *J. Allergy Clin. Immunol. Pract.* **2016**, *4*, 565–572. [CrossRef] [PubMed]
4. Gelardi, M.; Iannuzzi, L.; Tafuri, S.; Passalacqua, G.; Quaranta, N. Allergic and non-allergic rhinitis: Relationship with nasal polyposis, asthma and family history. *Acta Otorhinolaryngol. Ital.* **2014**, *34*, 36–41. [PubMed]
5. Brescia, G.; Zanotti, C.; Parrino, D.; Barion, U.; Marioni, G. Nasal polyposis pathophysiology: Endotype and phenotype open issues. *Am. J. Otolaryngol.* **2018**, *39*, 441–444. [CrossRef]
6. Tan, B.K.; Chandra, R.K.; Pollak, J.; Kato, A.; Conley, D.B.; Peters, A.T.; Grammer, L.C.; Avila, P.C.; Kern, R.C.; Stewart, W.F.; et al. Incidence and associated premorbid diagnoses of patients with chronic rhinosinusitis. *J. Allergy Clin. Immunol.* **2013**, *131*, 1350–1360. [CrossRef]
7. Waites, K.B.; Xiao, L.; Liu, Y.; Balish, M.F.; Atkinson, T.P. Mycoplasma pneumoniae from the Respiratory Tract and Beyond. *Clin. Microbiol. Rev.* **2017**, *30*, 747–809. [CrossRef]
8. Sato, C.; Manaka, S.; Nakane, D.; Nishiyama, H.; Suga, M.; Nishizaka, T.; Miyata, M.; Maruyama, Y. Rapid imaging of mycoplasma in solution using Atmospheric Scanning Electron Microscopy (ASEM). *Biochem. Biophys. Res. Commun.* **2012**, *417*, 1213–1218. [CrossRef]
9. Jurkovic, D.A.; Newman, J.T.; Balish, M.F. Conserved Terminal Organelle Morphology and Function in Mycoplasma penetrans and Mycoplasma iowae. *J. Bacteriol.* **2012**, *194*, 2877–2883. [CrossRef]
10. Park, H.J.; Kang, K.M.; Dybvig, K.; Lee, B.L.; Jung, Y.W.; Lee, I.H. Interaction of cationic antimicrobial peptides withMycoplasma pulmonis. *FEBS Lett.* **2013**, *587*, 3321–3326. [CrossRef]
11. Cole, B.C.; Atkin, C.L. The Mycoplasma arthritidis T-cell mitogen MAM: A model superantigen. *Immunol. Today* **1991**, *12*, 271–276. [CrossRef]
12. Fleischer, B. Superantigens. *Apmis* **1994**, *102*, 3–12. [CrossRef] [PubMed]
13. Bernstein, J.M.; Ballow, M.; Schlievert, P.M.; Rich, G.; Allen, C.; Dryja, D. A superantigen hypothesis for the pathogenesis of chronic hyperplastic sinusitis with massive nasal polyposis. *Am. J. Rhinol.* **2003**, *17*, 321–326. [CrossRef] [PubMed]

14. Logunov, D.I.; Shchebliakov, D.V.; Zubkova, O.V.; Shmarov, M.M.; Rakovskaia, I.V.; Gintsburg, L.A.; Gudkov, A.V.; Naroditskiĭ, B.S. Lipid-associated membrane lipopeptides of M. arginini activate NF-kB by interacting with TLR2/1, TLR2/6, and TLR2/CD14. *Mol. Genet. Microbiol. Virol.* **2009**, *2*, 25–28.
15. Choi, Y.-J.; Jeon, J.-H.; Oh, J.-W. Critical combination of initial markers for predicting refractory Mycoplasma pneumoniae pneumonia in children: A case control study. *Respir. Res.* **2019**, *20*, 193–199. [CrossRef] [PubMed]
16. Cowan, M.K. *Microbiology: A Systems Approach*; McGraw-Hill: New York, NY, USA, 2018.
17. Fang, K.-N.; Wang, J.; Ni, J.-W. Correlation between Mycoplasma pneumoniae DNA replication level and disease severity in children with severe Mycoplasma pneumoniae pneumonia. *Chin. J. Contemp. Pediatr.* **2019**, *21*, 876–880.
18. Zimmer, F.M.L.; Moura, H.; Barr, J.R.; Ferreira, H.B. Intracellular changes of a swine tracheal cell line infected with a Mycoplasma hyopneumoniae pathogenic strain. *Microb. Pathog.* **2019**, *137*, 103717. [CrossRef]
19. Rogozinski, L.E.; Alverson, B.K.; Biondi, E.A. Diagnosis and treatment of Mycoplasma pneumoniae in children. *Minerva Pediatr.* **2017**, *69*, 156–160.
20. Ramakrishnan, Y.; Shields, R.C.; ElBadawey, M.R.; A Wilson, J. Biofilms in chronic rhinosinusitis: What is new and where next? *J. Laryngol. Otol.* **2015**, *129*, 744–751. [CrossRef]
21. Boase, S.; Foreman, A.; Cleland, E.; Tan, L.; Melton-Kreft, R.; Pant, H.; Hu, F.Z.; Ehrlich, G.D.; Wormald, P.-J. The microbiome of chronic rhinosinusitis: Culture, molecular diagnostics and biofilm detection. *BMC Infect. Dis.* **2013**, *13*, 210. [CrossRef]
22. Cryer, J.; Schipor, I.; Perloff, J.R.; Palmer, J.N. Evidence of Bacterial Biofilms in Human Chronic Sinusitis. *ORL* **2004**, *66*, 155–158. [CrossRef] [PubMed]
23. Maina, I.W.; Patel, N.N.; Cohen, N.A. Understanding the Role of Biofilms and Superantigens in Chronic Rhinosinusitis. *Curr. Otorhinolaryngol. Rep.* **2018**, *6*, 253–262. [CrossRef] [PubMed]
24. Li, P.; Zhang, Y.; Li, X.; Zhou, W.; Li, X.; Jiang, F.; Wu, W. Mycoplasma hyopneumoniae Mhp597 is a cytotoxicity, inflammation and immunosuppression associated nuclease. *Vet. Microbiol.* **2019**, *235*, 53–62. [CrossRef] [PubMed]
25. Kornspan, J.D.; Tsur, M.; Tarshis, M.; Rottem, S.; Brenner, T. Mycoplasma hyorhinis induces proinflammatory responses in mice lymphocytes. *J. Basic Microbiol.* **2015**, *55*, 679–684. [CrossRef]
26. Burgess, W.; Margolis, A.; Gibbs, S.; Duarte, R.S.; Jackson, M. Disinfectant Susceptibility Profiling of Glutaraldehyde-Resistant Nontuberculous Mycobacteria. *Infect. Control. Hosp. Epidemiol.* **2017**, *38*, 784–791. [CrossRef]
27. Schaunaman, N.; Sanchez, A.; Dimasuay, K.G.; Pavelka, N.; Numata, M.; Alam, R.; Martin, R.J.; Chu, H.W. Interleukin 1 Receptor-Like 1 (IL1RL1) Promotes Airway Bacterial and Viral Infection and Inflammation. *Infect. Immun.* **2019**, *87*. [CrossRef]

3

Measurement of Oral Epithelial Thickness by Optical Coherence Tomography

Dario Di Stasio [1,†], Dorina Lauritano [2,*,†], Hasan Iquebal [3], Antonio Romano [1], Enrica Gentile [1] and Alberta Lucchese [1]

1 Multidisciplinary Department of Medical-Surgical and Dental Specialties, University of Campania—Luigi Vanvitelli, 80138 Naples, Italy
2 Department of Medicine and Surgery, Centre of Neuroscience of Milan, University of Milano-Bicocca, 20126 Milan, Italy
3 ECU School of Dental Medicine, 1851 MacGregor Downs Road, Greenville, NC 27834, USA
* Correspondence: dorina.lauritano@unimib.it
† These authors contributed equally to this work.

Abstract: Optical coherence tomography (OCT) is a real-time, in-situ, non-invasive imaging device that is able to perform a cross-sectional evaluation of tissue microstructure based on the specific intensity of back-scattered and reflected light. The aim of the present study was to define normal values of epithelial thickness within the oral cavity. OCT measurements of epithelial thickness were performed in 28 healthy patients at six different locations within the oral cavity. Image analysis was performed using Image J 1.52 software. The healthy epithelium has a mean thickness of 335.59 ± 150.73 μm. According to its location within the oral cavity, the epithelium showed highest values in the region of the buccal mucosa (659.79 μm) and the thinnest one was observed in the mouth's floor (100.07 μm). OCT has been shown to be useful for the evaluation of oral mucosa in vivo and in real time. Our study provides reference values for the epithelial thickness of multiple sites within the oral cavity. Knowledge of the thickness values of healthy mucosa is, therefore, of fundamental importance.

Keywords: in vivo; oral mucosa; optical coherence tomography

---

1. Introduction

Optical coherence tomography (OCT) is an imaging diagnostic device which measures the intensity of backscattered and reflected light so that it can produce high-resolution microscopic images of biological tissues [1], with an axial and lateral resolution estimated, respectively, at 13–17 and 17–22 μm [2].

OCT usually has an interferometer-based operating mechanism, with a low-coherence-length broadband light source. A low-coherence diode produces a light beam of variable wavelength in the infrared spectrum and it is conveyed by an optical probe. The initial light beam is divided into two: an optic fiber splitter between the biological tissue and reference arms of a Michelson or Mach–Zehnder interferometer. The two light beams converge again in the optical fiber after being diffused backwards from the tissue and reflected by the reference mirror, thus causing interference. A photodetector or spectrometer (depending on the type of OCT) registers this interference, transforms the signal from a luminous to a digital one and scans its information: finally, a computer receives the signal for graphical processing. According to the structure of the reference arm optics, OCT can be classified into time domain (TD) and frequency domain (FD)-OCT [3,4].

The TD-OCT or time-domain OCT (as it measures the time the light takes to be reflected) is an early and simple device but it allows the creation of approximately 400 axial scans per second [1]. According to the different components they employ, OCT devices can provide several types of analysis.

In particular, three types of microscopic exploration can be produced by OCT technology:

1. the A-scan type, which uses a single light beam and defines the depth of the findings observed thanks to their reflectivity;
2. the B-scan type, which, on the contrary, employs multiple A-scans on the x- and z-axes that provide a cross-sectional 2D view of the observed structure and the obtained image is also called longitudinal;
3. the C-scan type, which is also a 2D cross-sectional view on the x- and y-axes, but the image obtained is called "en face";
4. Matching a series of B-scan and C-scan images, it is possible to create a 3D reconstruction of the observed structures [1].

The FD-OCT is divided into swept-source (SS) and spectral domain (SD)-OCT according to the output characteristics and the structure of the light source receiving components [5]. The hardware characteristics from the light source, the spectrometer, and the optical components of FD-OCT inevitably create nonlinearity in the k-domain [6]. This nonlinearity to the k-domain diminishes the depth resolution in the FD-OCT system using the inverse Fourier transform relationship of the interference pattern. Several compensation methods have been created to overcome this nonlinearity [7]. One of these consists of inserting the interferometer into the SS-OCT system, receiving the linearized interference pattern to the k-domain and using the pattern as a trigger signal [8]. SS-OCT, compared to other OCT technologies, is faster and consequently widely used because of its speed [9,10]. Moreover, SS-OCT devices have shown an improved sensitivity roll-off and attenuation of OCT signal, and can detect more structural signals from deeper tissues compared to SD-OCT [11].

Previous investigations demonstrated a progressive thickening from normal epithelium through the different grades of dysplasia to early invasive carcinoma in vocal fold lesions [12] and in the oral cavity [13]. OCT images provided microanatomic information about the epithelium, basement membrane, and lamina propria, and have proved to be a valid and practicable method for the determination of epithelial thickness in vivo [14–16]. There are also other devices for in the vivo imaging of the oral mucosa such as high-frequency ultrasonography (US) [17]. A direct comparison between OCT and high-frequency ultrasound (US) [18,19] highlighted that the spatial resolution of OCT is significantly better.

On this basis, the aim of the present study was to measure normal values of epithelial thickness within the oral cavity by SS-OCT.

2. Materials and Methods

A total of 28 patients, referred to the Oral Pathology Unit at the University of Campania, "Luigi Vanvitelli", in Naples (Italy), were selected to evaluate the epithelial thickness of the oral mucosa. All subjects gave their informed consent for inclusion before they participated in the study. The Ethical Committee of the same university approved the study (n.0000689/2014, approved on 4 September 2014). Inclusion criteria were healthy volunteers with clinically normal mucous membranes, who did not report any other systemic diseases, non-smokers and aged over 18. Pregnant women were excluded from this study.

OCT measurements of epithelial thickness were performed at the exact same site in all patients, bilaterally at 6 different locations within the oral cavity, namely, the gingiva (Figure 1a), the labial mucosa (Figure 1b), the buccal mucosa (Figure 1c), the ventral surface of the tongue (Figure 1d), the floor of the mouth (Figure 1e), and the tongue dorsum (Figure 1f). Three repeated scans were performed in the same location.

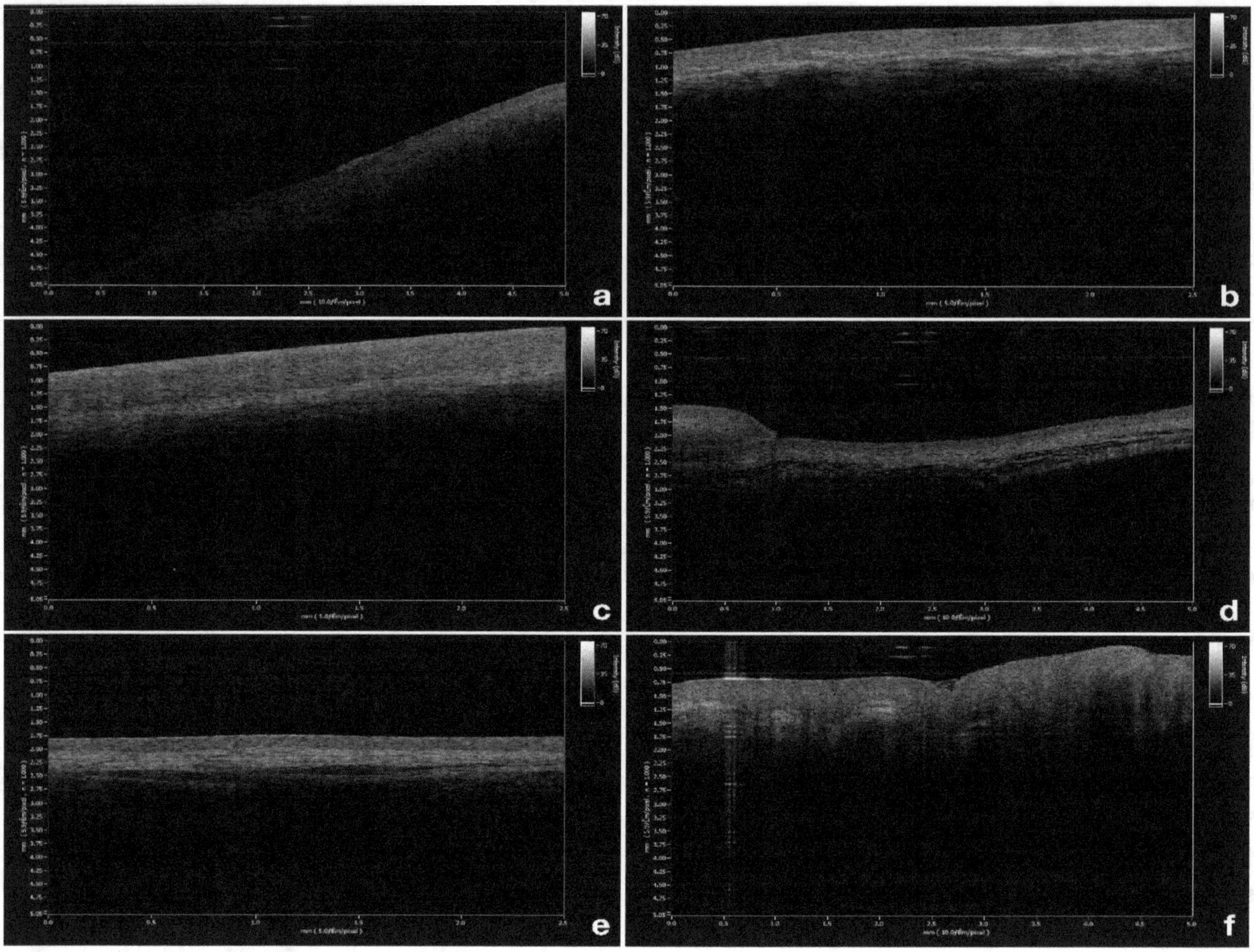

Figure 1. (**a**) Optical coherence tomography (OCT) image of healthy gingiva; (**b**) OCT image of healthy labial mucosa; (**c**) OCT image of healthy buccal mucosa; (**d**) OCT image of healthy ventral surface of the tongue; (**e**) OCT image of healthy floor of the mouth; (**f**) OCT image of healthy tongue dorsum.

2.1. Epithelial Thickness Mesurement

Image analysis was performed using Image J 1.52 software [20]. Images were processed in order to obtain the measurements of epithelial thickness.

The measurements were carried out as follows: 1. Open ImageJ software. 2. Drag and drop the picture into the software interface. 3. A segment was drawn along the ruler at the left side margin of the image using the "straight line" tool provided by the software. The examiners drew a distance of 0.5 mm along the ruler. The software calculates the distance in pixels of the selected segment. 4. Analyze menu > set scale > known distance (500) > unit of length (μm). The software automatically recalculates the number of pixels/mm (0.088 pixels/μm). 5. Epithelial thickness outline was created using the "straight line" tool and tracing a line starting from the most recognizable superficial point of epithelium up to the recognizable signal change in terms of gray scale with the computer mouse in cases of desktop computers or trackpad in cases of laptops; this is made possible by the fact that the epithelium reveals a less intense signal than the lamina propria in the B-mode OCT scan. 6. Analyze menu > measure. The length in μm was then calculated.

Two different operators performed the computerized measurements; repeated measurements to minimize errors have been made. The two authors were blinded to the readings of the other authors. Just the lead author had access to the results of the measurements. One-way ANOVA has been used to highlight differences between repeated measurements between the left and right side of the oral cavity.

2.2. OCT System

Optical coherence tomography (OCT) is a non-invasive imaging device that can be employed for both real-time and in-situ investigations, able to perform a cross-sectional evaluation of tissue microstructure based on the specific intensity of back-scattered and reflected light [21]. This study used a swept-source OCT instrument (IVS-300) by Santec™, with a grip type probe of the same manufacturer directly applied to the oral mucosa after application of ultrasound gel with a working distance of 10 mm. Centre wavelength was 1310 (± 30) nm, axial resolution of the system was ≤ 12 μm (in tissue); lateral resolution was 22 μm. Both 2D and 3D imaging modes were used by the default native software Inner Vision™ (Windows 7 OS based) and a native OCT viewer elaborated all images. The scan mode was set for 5 × 5mm on the X and Y axis and a pixel size of 500 and Z offset 24 (the number of the pixels to shift the A-lines of the frame to correct for the path length difference between the OCT sample arm and reference arm in air) [22].

2.3. Statistical Analysis

Demographic parameters and the epithelial thickness of each location were collected and analyzed through descriptive statistics. Kurtosis and skewness were employed to further evaluate the distribution of the measured values of epithelial thickness. Differences between the six different anatomical locations were determined by the non-parametric Mann–Whitney U test. The software R was used for all computations and p values ≤ 0.05 were considered statistically significant.

3. Results

A total of 504 OCT images per side from six different locations within the oral cavity were obtained from 28 white healthy volunteers with a mean age of 35.57 years (range, 20–59 years) and a sex distribution of 35.7% men and 64.3% women.

According to its location within the oral cavity, the epithelium showed a variable thickness. Details regarding measured sites are reported in Table 1. The highest and the thinnest values were observed, respectively, in the region of the buccal mucosa, −659.79 μm, and in the mouth's floor, −100.07 μm. The difference in epithelial thickness between the different anatomical locations was statistically significant—$p \leq 0.05$ (Figure 2). The healthy epithelium has a mean thickness of 335.59 ± 150.73 μm. There were no significant differences between the left and right side of the oral cavity, as the ANOVA analysis of the measurements per image underlined. Therefore, thanks to the repeated measurements, it is possible to exclude an interobserver variability in this study.

Table 1. Values of epithelial thickness within the oral cavity.

Anatomic Location		Thickness (μm)	SD
gingiva	Mean	285.04	± 32.98
	Min	218.30	
	Max	333.33	
labial mucosa	Mean	339.83	± 36.44
	Min	271.19	
	Max	405.56	
buccal mucosa	Mean	545.40	± 62.45
	Min	373.75	
	Max	659.79	
ventral surface of the tongue	Mean	239.79	± 37.30
	Min	159.09	
	Max	318.00	
floor of the mouth	Mean	124.09	± 13.53
	Min	100.07	
	Max	144.44	
tongue dorsum	Mean	479.32	± 83.56
	Min	333.33	
	Max	650.02	

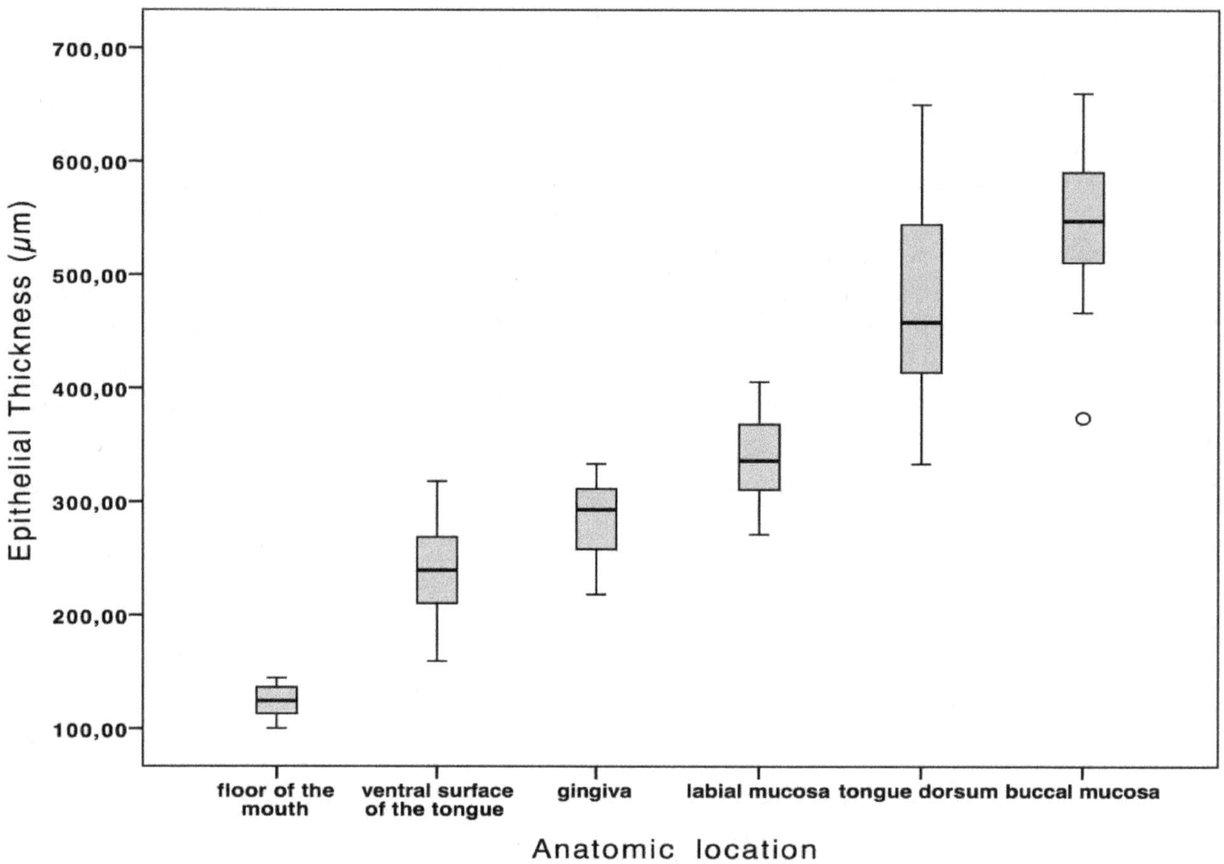

Figure 2. The box plot shows the normal values of epithelial thickness according to anatomic location. The difference in epithelial thickness between the different anatomical locations was statistically significant—$p \leq 0.05$.

Through the OCT examination of a healthy buccal mucosa, it was possible to clearly establish the stratified squamous epithelium (SS) along the mucosal surface, underlying the lamina propria (LP), and the transition between these tissues along the basement membrane (BM) boundary.

The appearance of these tissues is strictly related to their optical density and scattering properties; that is why the lower optical density of buccal mucosa epithelium is darker, as evident in a lower signal intensity. Conversely, the optically denser LP appears brighter than the BM one, caused by a higher signal intensity. The lower contrast is a typical characteristic of a keratinized epithelium. Moreover, there are very few differences between the OCT image of the gingival mucosa and its own lamina (LP) at a depth of 285.04 ± 32.98 μm.

4. Discussion

In vivo, non-invasive imaging techniques such as magnetic resonance imaging [9], confocal laser microscopy [23–25] and ultrasound imaging [17] have found widespread applications in medicine. Each of these techniques measures a different physical property and has a resolution and penetration range that prove advantageous for specific applications. One of the main limitations of this technique is that the quality of the images remains strongly user dependent [1] and the large, rigid probe, which makes examination of the posterior and less-accessible locations of the oral cavity difficult [14].

The literature has shown that OCT is a valid method for determining epithelial thickness in vivo [15,26]. With this technique, indeed, it is possible to perform the non-invasive cross-sectional imaging of biological tissues by measuring their optical reflections [9]. Therefore, it is essential to know the dimensions of the different layers of normal mucosal tissue in different anatomical sites within the oral cavity in order to consider OCT a valuable imaging technique for analyzing the oral mucosa.

Within the oral cavity, healthy epithelium varies from 75 to 550 µm in thickness depending on the anatomic site [27,28]. Prestin et al. [14] were the first to provide reference values for epithelial thickness within the oral cavity. In the present study, we presented data on the epithelial thickness of additional oral cavity sites compared to those presented by Prestin et al.

Furthermore, Tsai et al. [13] studied four groups of oral mucosa samples, namely, healthy mucosa, epithelial hyperplasia, moderate dysplasia and squamous cell carcinoma of the oral cavity (OSCC), combining the results obtained with histology. The authors showed the analysis and statistical results of the SS-OCT scan images using three diagnostic indicators (the standard deviation of a scan signal profile in mode A, the exponential decay constant of a spatial scanning frequency spectrum in mode A and epithelial thickness). The obtained data revealed that in abnormal oral mucosa samples, the standard deviation becomes larger, the spatial frequency spectrum decay constant becomes smaller and the epithelium becomes thicker.

In addition, Kraft et al. [29] were able to demonstrate a progressive thickening from normal epithelium through the different grades of dysplasia to early invasive carcinoma in vocal fold lesions. Hence, with the help of OCT, the grade of dysplasia can be determined approximately by morphometric measurement of epithelial thickness.

On the basis of this, the thickness of the epithelium and the integrity of the basement membrane, identifiable with the aid of OCT, could be a valid aid for the clinician to obtain information on the possible nature and grade of the dysplasia of oral cavity lesions.

5. Conclusions

OCT has been shown to be a simple method for the evaluation of oral mucosa in vivo. Our study provides reference values for the epithelial thickness of multiple sites within the oral cavity. As evidenced by the literature, increased epithelial thickness values may be related to pathological changes. Knowledge of the thickness values of healthy mucosa is, therefore, of fundamental importance for this purpose. Excisional biopsy followed by histological examination is still the gold standard for a reliable assessment of oral cavity lesions. Despite the limitations of this study, due in part to the sample size, the present data allow us to consider OCT as a promising technique to detect and monitor different pathological conditions and have the potential to provide an in-vivo, real-time, non-invasive method for the early diagnosis of cancer and precancer.

Author Contributions: Conceptualization, D.D.S. and A.L.; Methodology, E.G. and D.L.; Software, A.R.; Validation D.D.S., A.L. and D.L.; Investigation, A.R.; Resources, E.G.; Data Curation, A.L. and D.D.S.; Writing—Review and Editing, D.D.S. and D.L.; Visualization, I.H.; Supervision, A.L.

References

1. Gentile, E.; Maio, C.; Romano, A.; Laino, L.; Lucchese, A. The potential role of in vivo optical coherence tomography for evaluating oral soft tissue: A systematic review. *J. Oral Pathol. Med.* **2017**, 1–13. [CrossRef] [PubMed]
2. Feldchtein, F.I.; Gelikonov, V.M.; Iksanov, R.R.; Gelikonov, G.V.; Kuranov, R.V.; Sergeev, A.M.; Gladkova, N.D.; Ourutina, M.N.; Reitze, D.H.; Warren, J.A.; et al. In vivo OCT imaging of hard and soft tissue of the oral cavity. *Opt. Express* **1998**, *3*, 239–250. [CrossRef] [PubMed]
3. Steele, T.O.; Meyers, A. Early Detection of Premalignant Lesions and Oral Cancer. *Otolaryngol. Clin. N. Am.* **2011**, *44*, 221–229. [CrossRef] [PubMed]
4. Hsieh, Y.-S.; Ho, Y.-C.; Lee, S.-Y.; Chuang, C.-C.; Tsai, J.; Lin, K.-F.; Sun, C.-W. Dental optical coherence tomography. *Sensors (Basel).* **2013**, *13*, 8928–8949. [CrossRef] [PubMed]
5. Jung, U.; Cho, N.; Kim, S.-H.; Jeong, H.; Kim, J.; Ahn, Y.-C. Simple Spectral Calibration Method and Its Application Using an Index Array for Swept Source Optical Coherence Tomography. *J. Opt. Soc. Korea* **2011**, *15*, 386–393. [CrossRef]

6. Kim, K.H.; Park, B.H.; Maguluri, G.N.; Lee, T.W.; Rogomentich, F.J.; Bancu, M.G.; Bouma, B.E.; de Boer, J.F.; Bernstein, J.J. Two-axis magnetically-driven MEMS scanning catheter for endoscopic high-speed optical coherence tomography. *Opt. Express* **2007**, *15*, 18130. [CrossRef] [PubMed]
7. Huber, R.; Adler, D.C.; Fujimoto, J.G. Buffered Fourier domain mode locking: Unidirectional swept laser sources for optical coherence tomography imaging at 370,000 lines/s. *Opt. Lett.* **2006**, *31*, 2975. [CrossRef] [PubMed]
8. Choi, W.J.; Wang, R.K. In vivo imaging of functional microvasculature within tissue beds of oral and nasal cavities by swept-source optical coherence tomography with a forward/side-viewing probe. *Biomed. Opt. Express* **2014**, *5*, 2620. [CrossRef]
9. Huang, D.; Swanson, E.A.; Lin, C.P.; Schuman, J.S.; Stinson, W.G.; Chang, W.; Hee, M.R.; Flotte, T.; Gregory, K.; Puliafito, C.A. Optical coherence tomography. *Science* **1991**, *254*, 1178–1181. [CrossRef]
10. Alibhai, A.Y.; Or, C.; Witkin, A.J. Swept Source Optical Coherence Tomography: A Review. *Curr. Ophthalmol. Rep.* **2018**, 7–16. [CrossRef]
11. Wang, F.; Zhang, Q.; Deegan, A.J.; Chang, J.; Wang, R.K. Comparing imaging capabilities of spectral domain and swept source optical coherence tomography angiography in healthy subjects and central serous retinopathy. *Eye Vis.* **2018**, *5*, 19. [CrossRef] [PubMed]
12. Arens, C.; Glanz, H.; Wönckhaus, J.; Hersemeyer, K.; Kraft, M. Histologic assessment of epithelial thickness in early laryngeal cancer or precursor lesions and its impact on endoscopic imaging. *Eur. Arch. Otorhinolaryngol.* **2007**, *264*, 645–649. [CrossRef] [PubMed]
13. Tsai, M.-T.; Lee, H.-C.; Lee, C.-K.; Yu, C.-H.; Chen, H.-M.; Chiang, C.-P.; Chang, C.-C.; Wang, Y.-M.; Yang, C.C. Effective indicators for diagnosis of oral cancer using optical coherence tomography. *Opt. Express* **2008**, *16*, 15847–15862. [PubMed]
14. Prestin, S.; Rothschild, S.I.; Betz, C.S.; Kraft, M. Measurement of epithelial thickness within the oral cavity using optical coherence tomography. *Head Neck* **2012**, *34*, 1777–1781. [CrossRef] [PubMed]
15. Ridgway, J.M.; Armstrong, W.B.; Guo, S.; Mahmood, U.; Su, J.; Jackson, R.P.; Shibuya, T.; Crumley, R.L.; Gu, M.; Chen, Z.; et al. In Vivo Optical Coherence Tomography of the Human Oral Cavity and Oropharynx. *Arch. Otolaryngol. Neck Surg.* **2006**, *132*, 1074. [CrossRef] [PubMed]
16. Wilder-Smith, P.; Lee, K.; Guo, S.; Zhang, J.; Osann, K.; Chen, Z.; Messadi, D. In vivo diagnosis of oral dysplasia and malignancy using optical coherence tomography: Preliminary studies in 50 patients. *Lasers Surg. Med.* **2009**, *41*, 353–357. [CrossRef] [PubMed]
17. Di Stasio, D.; Lauritano, D.; Paparella, R.; Franco, R.; Montella, M.; Serpico, R.; Lucchese, A. Ultrasound imaging of oral fibroma: A case report. *J. Biol. Regul. Homeost. Agents* **2017**, *31*, 23–26. [PubMed]
18. Vogt, M.; Knüttel, A.; Hoffmann, K.; Altmeyer, P.; Ermert, H. Comparison of high frequency ultrasound and optical coherence tomography as modalities for high resolution and non invasive skin imaging. *Biomed. Tech. (Berl).* **2003**, *48*, 116–121. [CrossRef] [PubMed]
19. Warszawik-Hendzel, O.; Olszewska, M.; Maj, M.; Rakowska, A.; Czuwara, J.; Rudnicka, L. Non-invasive diagnostic techniques in the diagnosis of squamous cell carcinoma. *J. Dermatol. Case Rep.* **2015**, *9*, 89–97. [CrossRef]
20. Rueden, C.T.; Schindelin, J.; Hiner, M.C.; DeZonia, B.E.; Walter, A.E.; Arena, E.T.; Eliceiri, K.W. ImageJ2: ImageJ for the next generation of scientific image data. *BMC Bioinformatics* **2017**, *18*, 1–26. [CrossRef]
21. Di Stasio, D.; Lauritano, D.; Romano, A.; Salerno, C.; Minervini, G.; Minervini, G.; Gentile, E.; Serpico, R.; Lucchese, A. In vivo characterization of oral pemphigus vulgaris by optical coherence tomography. *J. Biol. Regul. Homeost. Agents* **2015**, *29*, 39–41. [PubMed]
22. de Boer, J.F.; Leitgeb, R.; Wojtkowski, M. Twenty-five years of optical coherence tomography: The paradigm shift in sensitivity and speed provided by Fourier domain OCT [Invited]. *Biomed. Opt. Express* **2017**, *8*, 3248. [CrossRef] [PubMed]
23. Lucchese, A.; Gentile, E.; Romano, A.; Maio, C.; Laino, L.; Serpico, R. The potential role of in vivo reflectance confocal microscopy for evaluating oral cavity lesions: A systematic review. *J. Oral Pathol. Med.* **2016**, *45*, 723–729. [CrossRef] [PubMed]
24. Grassia, V.; Gentile, E.; Di Stasio, D.; Jamilian, A.; Matarese, G.; D'Apuzzo, F.; Santoro, R.; Perillo, L.; Serpico, R.; Lucchese, A. In vivo confocal microscopy analysis of enamel defects after orthodontic treatment: A preliminary study. *Ultrastruct. Pathol.* **2016**, *40*, 317–323. [CrossRef] [PubMed]

25. De Rosa, A.; Di Stasio, D.; Lauritano, D.; Santoro, R.; Marotta, A.; Itro, A.; Lucchese, A. Non-invasive analysis of bleaching effect of hydrogen peroxide on enamel by reflectance confocal microscopy (RCM): Study of series of cases. *Odontology* **2019**, *107*, 285–290. [CrossRef] [PubMed]
26. Lee, A.M.D.; Cahill, L.; Liu, K.; MacAulay, C.; Poh, C.; Lane, P. Wide-field in vivo oral OCT imaging. *Biomed. Opt. Express* **2015**, *6*, 2664. [CrossRef] [PubMed]
27. Paulsen, F.; Thale, A. Epithelial-connective tissue boundary in the oral part of the human soft palate. *J. Anat.* **1998**, *193*, 457–467. [CrossRef]
28. Klein-Szanto, A.J.; Schroeder, H.E. Architecture and density of the connective tissue papillae of the human oral mucosa. *J. Anat.* **1977**, *123*, 93–109.
29. Kraft, M.; Glanz, H.; von Gerlach, S.; Wisweh, H.; Lubatschowski, H.; Arens, C. Clinical value of optical coherence tomography in laryngology. *Head Neck* **2008**, *30*, 1628–1635. [CrossRef]

4

Low-Coherence Interferometric Fiber-Optic Sensors with Potential Applications as Biosensors

Marzena Hirsch [1,†], Daria Majchrowicz [1,†], Paweł Wierzba [1], Matthieu Weber [2], Mikhael Bechelany [2] and Małgorzata Jędrzejewska-Szczerska [1,*]

1 Department of Metrology and Optoelectronics, Faculty of Electronics, Telecommunications and Informatics, Gdańsk University of Technology, Narutowicza Street 11/12, 80-233 Gdańsk, Poland; hirsch.marzena@gmail.com (M.H.); majchrowiczdaria@gmail.com (D.M.); pwierzba@eti.pg.gda.pl (P.W.)

2 Institut Européen des Membranes, UMR-5635, Université de Montpellier, École Nationale Supérieure de Chimie de Montpellier, Centre national de la recherche scientifique, Place Eugène Bataillon, Montpellier 34095, France; matthieu.weber@umontpellier.fr (M.W.); mikhael.bechelany@univ-montp2.fr (M.B.)

* Correspondance: mjedrzej@eti.pg.gda.pl

† These authors contributed equally to this work.

Academic Editor: Vittorio M. N. Passaro

Abstract: Fiber-optic Fabry-Pérot interferometers (FPI) can be applied as optical sensors, and excellent measurement sensitivity can be obtained by fine-tuning the interferometer design. In this work, we evaluate the ability of selected dielectric thin films to optimize the reflectivity of the Fabry-Pérot cavity. The spectral reflectance and transmittance of dielectric films made of titanium dioxide (TiO_2) and aluminum oxide (Al_2O_3) with thicknesses from 30 to 220 nm have been evaluated numerically and compared. TiO_2 films were found to be the most promising candidates for the tuning of FPI reflectivity. In order to verify and illustrate the results of modelling, TiO_2 films with the thickness of 80 nm have been deposited on the tip of a single-mode optical fiber by atomic layer deposition (ALD). The thickness, the structure, and the chemical properties of the films have been determined. The ability of the selected TiO_2 films to modify the reflectivity of the Fabry-Pérot cavity, to provide protection of the fibers from aggressive environments, and to create multi-cavity interferometric sensors in FPI has then been studied. The presented sensor exhibits an ability to measure refractive index in the range close to that of silica glass fiber, where sensors without reflective films do not work, as was demonstrated by the measurement of the refractive index of benzene. This opens up the prospects of applying the investigated sensor in biosensing, which we confirmed by measuring the refractive index of hemoglobin and glucose.

Keywords: Fabry-Pérot interferometers; atomic layer deposition; titanium dioxide thin film; fiber-optic sensor; interference

---

1. Introduction

Optoelectronic instruments based on spectroscopic techniques (e.g., absorption [1,2], Raman [3,4], optical tomography [5,6]) are currently applied in medicine, especially for diagnosis and imaging. However, these measurement methods are expensive, as they often require high-end measurement equipment, expensive consumables (e.g., reagents, dedicated trays, or substrates) and complex methods of sample preparation. Moreover, highly skilled laboratory staff is needed in order to ensure the quality of the measurements performed, which considerably restricts the use of optoelectronic methods in medical diagnosis.

Therefore, there is a real need to develop relatively inexpensive measuring devices that can be used by hospital staff, preferably at the point-of-care (e.g., bedside).

The use of fiber-optic sensors as low-cost measuring devices in biology and medicine represent an attractive alternative. This type of sensor has been the subject of intense research, as it offers several advantages over conventional sensors, such as very high resolution, high accuracy, and small dimensions [7,8]. In fact, fiber-optic sensors possess several advantages in comparison to electronic sensors. Their design often makes use of dielectric materials, which makes them insensitive to electric and magnetic fields generated by other medical devices. Furthermore, they are resistant to most chemical reagents and ionizing radiations. Fiber-optic sensors can be tailored to measure various species and quantities, and they are inexpensive to produce. Finally, the small dimensions of such sensors (below hundreds of micrometers) reduce their impact on the investigated area, allowing for extremely precise measurements [9,10].

Low-coherence interferometry is an excellent detection technique, as it enables the fiber-optic sensors to be insensitive to changes in the intensity of optical signal in the transmission system (because all the information about the measured values is included in the frequency component of the measuring signal spectrum [11,12]). Fiber-optic Fabry-Pérot interferometers (FPI) can be used as efficient optical sensors, and excellent measurement sensitivity can be obtained by the fine-tuning of the interferometer design [13–15].

In the recent years, the advancement of nanotechnology has opened new routes to manufacture thin-films, nanostructures, and nanocomposites materials. Innovative techniques which exploit these routes allow for the elaboration of precise (nano)structures to be achieved, stimulating interest in the properties of these materials and their potential applications.

Atomic layer deposition (ALD) is a vapor phase deposition technique enabling the synthesis of ultrathin films of inorganic materials, with a subnanometer thickness control [16]. ALD can be used to coat 3D substrates with a conformal and uniform film of a high-quality material, a unique capability amongst thin film deposition techniques. Consequently, ALD-grown materials can be applied in various applications such as microelectronics [17], photovoltaics [18], or optical sensing [19]. ALD is based on self-limiting reactions taking place at the surface of the substrate in a cycle-wise fashion. A typical ALD cycle consists of alternate pulses of a precursor and co-reactant gasses in the reactor chamber, separated by purge steps. The properties of the synthetized nanostructures can be tuned by adjusting the process conditions—e.g. the chemistry of the precursor(s) and the co-reactants, the temperature, the number of cycles, or the nature of the substrate [20–23].

Novel interferometer layouts can be considered (as depicted in Figure 1), where a thin film is grown on the end-face of a standard single-mode (SM) fiber. This film deposition creates two distinctive layouts. In the first layout, the deposited film itself is the sensing cavity of the Fabry-Pérot interferometer (Figure 1a). In the second layout, the deposited film acts as a partially transparent mirror improving the reflection at the boundary between the extrinsic cavity and the optical fiber (Figure 1b). Another view of this second layout is the fact that an extrinsic cavity is delimited by two single-mode fibers with the deposited films (Figure 1c).

In this work, we investigated the possible applications of ALD-grown films on SM fibers in low-coherence fiber-optic Fabry-Pérot sensing interferometers. We evaluate the ability of different thin films—namely titanium dioxide (TiO_2) and aluminum oxide (Al_2O_3)—with different thicknesses to tune the reflectivity of the Fabry-Pérot cavity, and we illustrate this modelling work with an experimental fiber using a TiO_2 film.

We first introduce the theory behind the concepts of FPI. Our theoretical modelling work is focused on the first interferometer layout (as shown in Figure 1a), since its properties bring a valuable insight to the expected performance of the other layout, especially the one depicted in Figure 1b. Next, as the best modelling results were obtained with TiO_2 films, we experimentally investigated the ability of an ALD-grown TiO_2 thin film to tune the reflectivity of the FPI cavity, by measuring the influence of TiO_2 thin films on the intensity of reflected interfering beams. Following that, we performed measurements of the refractive index of water, benzene, hemoglobin, and glucose. The main objective of this part of the study was assessment of suitability of the sensor for applications in biosensing. Short-term stability of the TiO_2 layers was checked and the refractive index values were compared with reference values to ascertain the correct operation of the sensor.

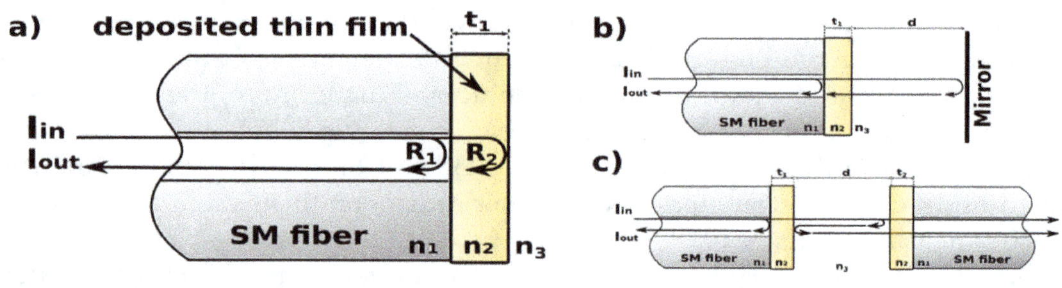

Figure 1. Different designs of fiber-optic Fabry-Pérot interferometers: (**a**) Interferometer with thin film sensing cavity; (**b**) and (**c**) Interferometers with extrinsic sensing cavity operating in reflective and transmission modes, respectively. n_1—refractive index of the fiber; n_2—refractive index of the film; n_3—refractive index of the medium in the cavity; t_1, t_2—thickness of the thin films; d—length of the cavity.

The investigated materials Al_2O_3 and TiO_2 belong to the metal oxides group. These materials are both transparent, and they recently became the subject of growing interest for electronic and optoelectronic sensors. In fact, the sensing properties of oxide thin films are exploited as gas, humidity, and temperature sensors, as well as biosensors [24–26].

2. Theory

The Fabry-Pérot interferometers (FPIs) presented in Figure 1b,c can be considered as multi-cavity interferometers. The propagation of optical radiation in such interferometers is often described using the Gaussian beam formalism. However, FPIs with cavities formed by films manufactured by ALD can be analyzed using a simplified model. As the thickness of the deposited films is limited and as the refractive index difference between the film and the media is relatively small, the Gaussian beam propagating in such films does not expand appreciably. Consequently, in the model, the films manufactured by ALD can be replaced by planar reflective surfaces, whose reflection and transmission coefficients can be calculated using the plane wave approach [27]. This results in a tractable single-cavity model in which the information about the cavities formed by the deposited films is preserved in the values of corresponding reflection and transmission coefficients.

The reflectivity R_1 at the boundary of the optical fiber and the deposited film, and the reflectivity R_2 at the boundary between the film and the surrounding medium, can be calculated using the Fresnel equations:

$$R_1 = \left(\frac{n_2 - n_1}{n_1 + n_2}\right)^2, \tag{1}$$

$$R_2 = \left(\frac{n_3 - n_2}{n_2 + n_3}\right)^2 \tag{2}$$

Using (1) and (2), the reflectivity $\Re$ of the deposited film can be expressed as:

$$\Re = \frac{R_1 + R_2 - 2\sqrt{R_1 R_2}\cos\delta}{1 + R_1 R_2 - 2\sqrt{R_1 R_2}\cos\delta} \tag{3}$$

The phase difference introduced in the interferometer is expressed by Equation (4):

$$\delta = \frac{4\pi}{\lambda} t n_2 \tag{4}$$

where λ—wavelength; t—thickness of the deposited film; $n_{1,2,3}$—refractive indices of the optical fiber core, the deposited film, and the surrounding media (as shown in Figure 1).

Establishing a precise value of the refractive index for the thin films is challenging, as it depends on the thickness and the growth conditions. Furthermore, some materials exhibit birefringence in the bulk form, whereas the thin films behave as isotropic materials [28–30].

Considering Al_2O_3 material, the values of the refractive index reported in the literature exhibit a substantial dependence on the deposition method and growth conditions [18–20]. In our model, the refractive index of Al_2O_3 was based on our group experimental data and calculated from Equation (5) [23,31]:

$$n^2_{Al_2O_3} = 1 + \frac{1.4313493\lambda^2}{\lambda^2 - (0.0726631)^2} + \frac{0.65054713\lambda^2}{\lambda^2 - (0.1193242)^2} + \frac{5.3414021\lambda^2}{\lambda^2 - (18.028251)^2}. \quad (5)$$

Next, the Refractive index of TiO_2 was calculated, using Equation (6) below [32]:

$$n^2_{TiO_2} = 5.193 + \frac{0.2441}{\lambda^2 - 0.0803}. \quad (6)$$

The wavelengths λ are expressed in μm in Equations (5) and (6).

3. Modelling

The spectral characteristics of the TiO_2 and Al_2O_3 thin films have been calculated using the equations presented in Section 2 for various thicknesses (30, 80, 120, 170, and 220 nm). The refractive index of the medium in the cavity n_3 was set to 1.00. The reflectance and transmission have been studied for wavelengths in the range from 500 nm to 1700 nm. The results obtained for TiO_2 and Al_2O_3 films are presented in Figures 2 and 3, respectively.

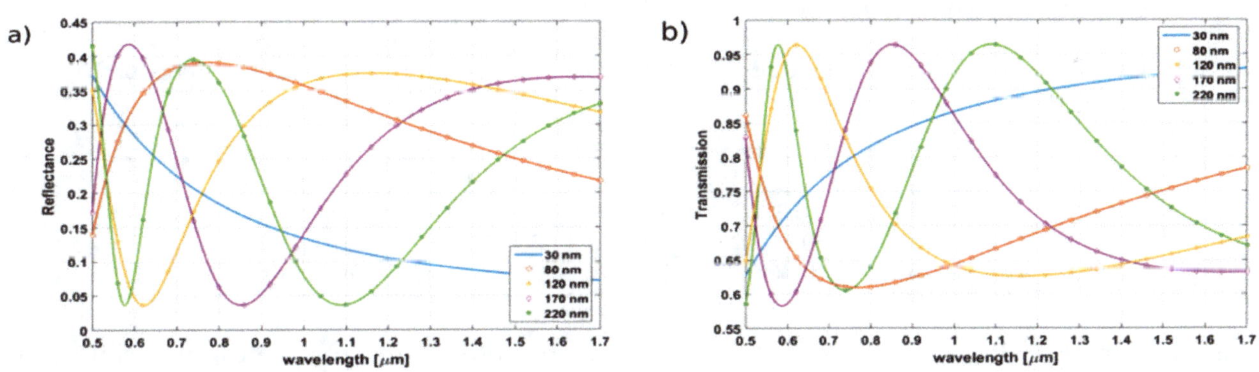

Figure 2. (**a**) Calculated reflectance and (**b**) calculated transmission for TiO_2 films of thicknesses ranging from 30 to 220 nm.

For the thinnest films of both oxides (30 nm), it can be seen that the spectral reflectance slowly decreases when increasing the wavelength. However, for thicker films, the optical behavior is different, as wide but distinct fringes can be noticed (for both oxides). Considering the same film thickness, the fringes of the reflectance appear faster for materials presenting higher refractive indexes (in our calculations, the assumed values of n are 2.46 for TiO_2 and 1.75 for Al_2O_3 (at 1300 nm)). The fringes present in the spectra obtained for thicker films are due to the interferences taking place in the film. This effect can be exploited for the design of an interferometer where the thin film itself acts as the sensing medium. However, the measurement techniques most commonly used to process signals from FPI require that the spectrum of the source should cover at least half of the fringe [27]. This condition is difficult to fulfil for the investigation of thin films, as it would require a broadband source with a spectral width over 150 nm, which is difficult to implement. The wavelength range considered is also not very convenient for standard telecommunication optical fibers. Therefore, extracting the data from a FPI sensor using such a thin film as an active medium would require adapting the standard technologies currently used for spectral analysis. However, when considering the sensitivity of TiO_2 thin films to humidity, temperature, and specific chemical compounds, this material could find applications in such Fabry-Pérot sensors.

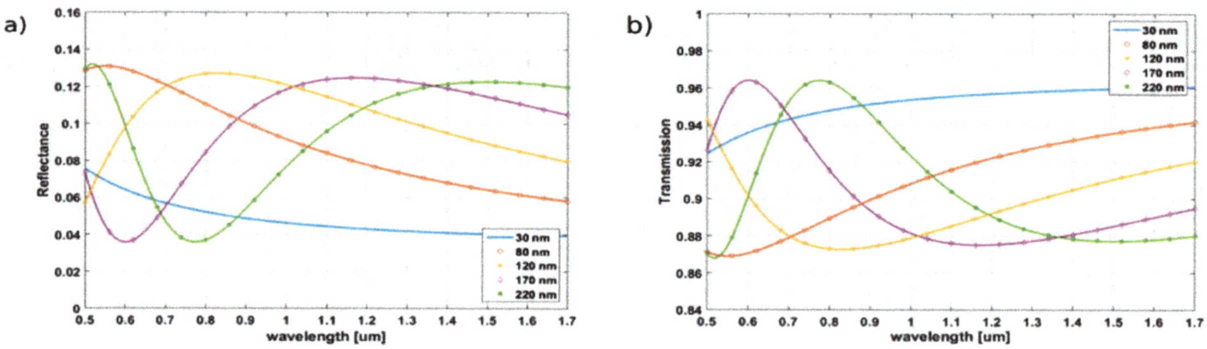

Figure 3. (**a**) Calculated reflectance and (**b**) calculated transmission for Al_2O_3 films of thicknesses ranging from 30 to 220 nm.

The maximum reflectance obtained is higher for TiO_2 (up to 0.417) then for Al_2O_3 (R_{max} = 0.131). However, even if the reflectance value predicted for Al_2O_3 thin films is lower than the one of TiO_2, it still provides significantly higher level of reflection than a simple boundary between an optical fiber and air cavity (R = 0.036), especially for films thicker than 100 nm.

When considering standard single-mode optical fibers such as SMF-28, wavelengths between 1200 and 1600 nm are typically used. In this range, the maximum reflectance is achieved for films presenting thicknesses between 120 and 220 nm (Table 1).

Table 1. Comparison of calculated values of reflectance and optimal film thickness t chosen for the highest reflection at selected wavelengths.

λ (nm)	R_{TiO_2}	$R_{Al_2O_3}$
900	0.3769, t = 80 nm	0.1258, t = 120 nm
1300	0.3679, t = 120 nm	0.1226, t = 170 nm
1550	0.3663, t = 220 nm	0.1225, t = 220 nm

The numerical values presented in the Table 1 were determined for the highest reflectance at selected wavelengths (the ones that are most commonly used when working with optical fibers). However, even if a much thinner film is used, the reflectance of the interferometer's mirror will significantly increase compared to the one of a clean-cut fiber.

Considering the time-consuming nature of the ALD process, where the thickness of the layer depends on the number of performed cycles, using a thinner film allows us to considerably minimize the time required for the fabrication of the sensor. Taking this point into consideration for the experimental evaluation of the performance of ALD layer in optical fiber FPI, a thin TiO_2 film of 80 nm thickness has been prepared on the tip of an optical fiber.

4. Materials

4.1. ALD of TiO_2

All depositions have been carried out in a custom-built ALD reactor described elsewhere [33]. Titanium isopropoxide ((*i*PrO)$_4$Ti) precursor was purchased from Sigma Aldrich and used as received. The co-reactant was millipore water. The substrates used were p-type (100) silicon wafers

(MEMC Korea Company, Cheonan, South Korea) and SMF-28 optical fibers (Thorlabs, Newton, MA, USA). To remove the organic contaminants, the substrates were pre-cleaned in acetone and ethanol, and de-ionized water for 5 min in an ultrasonic bath before the depositions.

ALD of TiO_2 was achieved using sequential exposures of $(iPrO)_4Ti$ and H_2O at 120 °C separated by purge steps of argon with a flow rate of 100 sccm. The process consisted of 5 s pulse ($(iPrO)_4Ti$), 30 s exposure, and 40 s purge with dry argon and a 3 s pulse (H_2O), 30 s exposure and 60 s purge. 4000 ALD cycles were carried out in order to achieve the deposition of TiO_2 of ≈80 nm.

Interestingly, it has been shown in previous studies that the amorphous, anatase, and rutile phases of TiO_2 can be obtained by tuning the ALD process parameters, and that the films with different crystallinity phases presented different optical properties [34]. Furthermore, the refractive index of the film has been determined by spectroscopic ellipsometry and a value of 2.0 has been obtained (at lambda = 633 nm). This value is in agreement with the ones found in the literature for TiO_2 films prepared with similar ALD processes (n increases typically from 2.0 to 2.5 with the increasing deposition temperature).

4.2. Characterization of the Films

Chemical and structural characterizations have been performed using Scanning Electron Microscopy (SEM, Hitachi S-4800, Tokyo, Japan), X-ray diffraction (PANAlytical Xpert-PRO diffractometer equipped with an X'celerator detector using Ni-filtered Cu-radiation, Almelo, The Netherlands), and Raman (Raman OMARS 89 (DILOR), Kyoto, Japan). To determine the TiO_2 film thickness after the ALD deposition, ex-situ spectroscopic ellipsometry (SE) measurements were carried out using a Semilab GES5E visible ellipsometer (1.2–5.0 eV) at an angle of incidence of 70.1°. For all the films, the empirical Cauchy dispersion formula has been adopted to model the optical properties and the thicknesses.

4.3. Properties of the TiO_2 Film

Figure 4a shows the SEM image of a ALD-grown TiO_2 film deposited on Si substrate after 4000 ALD cycles. The conformal coating of the Si substrate by the ALD TiO_2 film can be clearly seen.

Spectroscopic ellipsometry (SE) measurements were carried out to evaluate the TiO_2 film thickness as well, and for this specific sample, a thickness of 82 ± 2 nm has been obtained.

The crystallinity study that we carried out showed that the ALD films prepared were amorphous. In fact, grazing-incidence XRD measurements have been realized and the absence of peaks in the spectra obtained suggested that the as-deposited TiO_2 film at 120 °C was amorphous. The formation the amorphous TiO_2 phase was further confirmed by Raman spectroscopy (Figure 4b), since the Raman spectra of the TiO_2 films deposited did not show any peaks either.

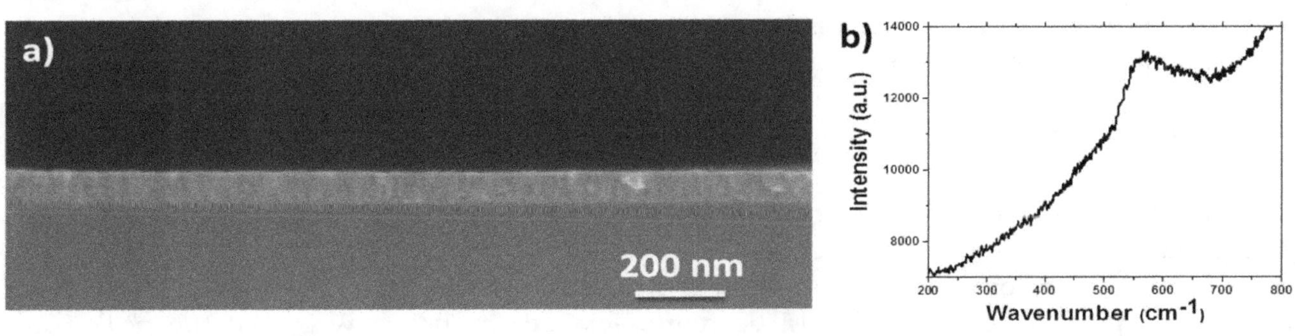

Figure 4. (**a**) SEM cross section image of TiO_2 films deposited by ALD on Si substrates and (**b**) Raman spectrum of TiO_2 films deposited by ALD.

This result is in agreement with previous studies that showed that TiO_2 films deposited by ALD below 200 °C are amorphous, and that annealing at temperatures above 300 °C are typically required to obtain the crystallization of the films. Crystalline TiO_2 typically exhibits the anatase phase, but the rutile phase can also be achieved by ALD, using ozone or plasmas as coreactants [33,35,36]. The relative density of the ALD TiO_2 has been reported elsewhere to be 3.6 g/cm^3 [37].

5. Measurements

After the deposition of an 80 nm TiO_2 film on SMF-28 optical fibers (Thorlabs, Newton, MA, USA) has been carried out, the performance of the this ALD film in a Fabry-Pérot interferometer has been tested. For this purpose, a low-coherence interferometric sensor has been used (the design of this experimental sensor is depicted in Figure 5). The sensor consists of a Fabry-Pérot interferometer working in reflective mode, an optical spectrum analyzer (Ando AQ6319, Tokyo, Japan), broadband NIR-radiation sources (S1300-G-I-20: λ = 1290 nm, $\Delta\lambda_{FWHM}$ = 50 nm and S-1550-G-I-20: λ = 1550 nm, $\Delta\lambda_{FWHM}$ = 45 nm Superlum), and a single-mode 2 × 2 coupler with 50: 50 power splitting ratio. The standard telecommunication single-mode optical fiber (SMF-28, Thorlabs) coated by ALD is used to connect all components of the setup.

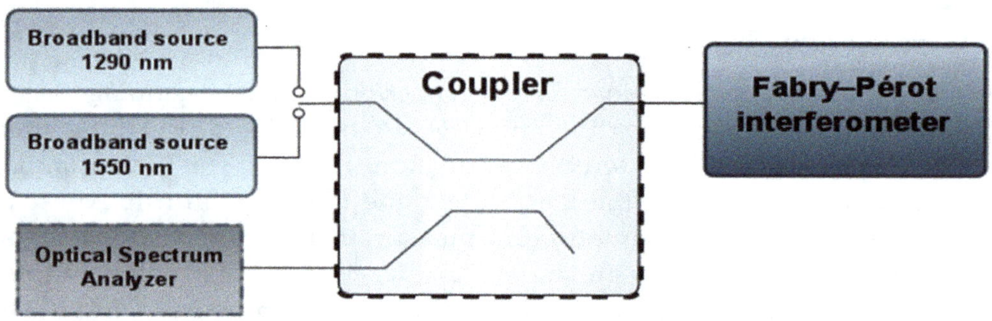

Figure 5. Design of the experimental sensor.

In our study, two Fabry-Pérot interferometers working in reflective mode and having a tunable cavity length were used. The first one had an 80 nm TiO_2 thin film deposited on the fiber end face, as shown in Figure 1b. The second FPI had no film deposited and was used as the reference. The measurement was performed in two steps. First, the cavity of the FPI was set to a known length. Then, the spectrum of the light reflected from the FPI was recorded. The measurements were performed for cavity lengths ranging from 50 μm to 500 μm, yielding a series of spectra for each interferometer.

6. Results

In this study, the influence of TiO_2 thin films on the quality of the spectrum reflected from the Fabry-Pérot interferometers was investigated. As the optimization function, the visibility V of the measured signal was used. V was defined as:

$$V = \frac{I_{max} - I_{min}}{I_{max} + I_{min}} \tag{7}$$

where I_{max} is the maximum intensity of the optical signal, I_{min} the minimum intensity of the optical signal.

This choice of the optimization function is dictated by the fact that FPI used in low-coherence sensors with spectral detection should be manufactured in such a way that the peaks on the spectral characteristics recorded by the detection setup have the maximum amplitude, i.e., maximum visibility V defined by (7) (in an ideal case V should be equal to 1.0). This contributes to the maximum accuracy of data processing algorithms in these sensors. When V decreases, the accuracy of these algorithms may degrade, although not significantly, as long as V is above 0.7–0.8. Values of V corresponding to optimal cavity length l_{opt} and to 50% and 200% of l_{opt} are shown in Table 2, for each interferometer and each wavelength.

It is important to note that the optimal length l_{opt} of the cavity of the Fabry-Pérot interferometer with TiO_2 thin film is around 100 μm and for the Fabry-Pérot interferometer with no film is around 200 μm. The corresponding visibility values are at least 0.95 for both light sources.

Table 2. Visibility of the measured signal in the Fabry-Pérot interferometer.

Fabry-Pérot Interferometer Made by	Length of the Fabry-Pérot Cavity	Central Wavelength of Light Source 1290 nm	Central Wavelength of Light Source 1550 nm
Optical fiber	100 μm	0.75	0.70
	200 μm	0.96	0.95
	400 μm	0.77	0.87
Optical fiber with TiO_2 thin film	50 μm	0.89	0.84
	100 μm	0.99	0.98
	200 μm	0.8	0.88

It can be seen that the visibility does not fall steeply. In particular, the visibility for 0.5 l_{opt} and 2.0 l_{opt} does not decrease below 0.7 for any investigated Fabry-Pérot interferometer. This indicates that the cavity length of such an interferometer can be varied in a relatively broad range, up to 4:1, without significant degradation of the performance of the sensor. The measured spectra obtained with the cavity length equal to 100 μm and 200 um are presented in Figures 6 and 7.

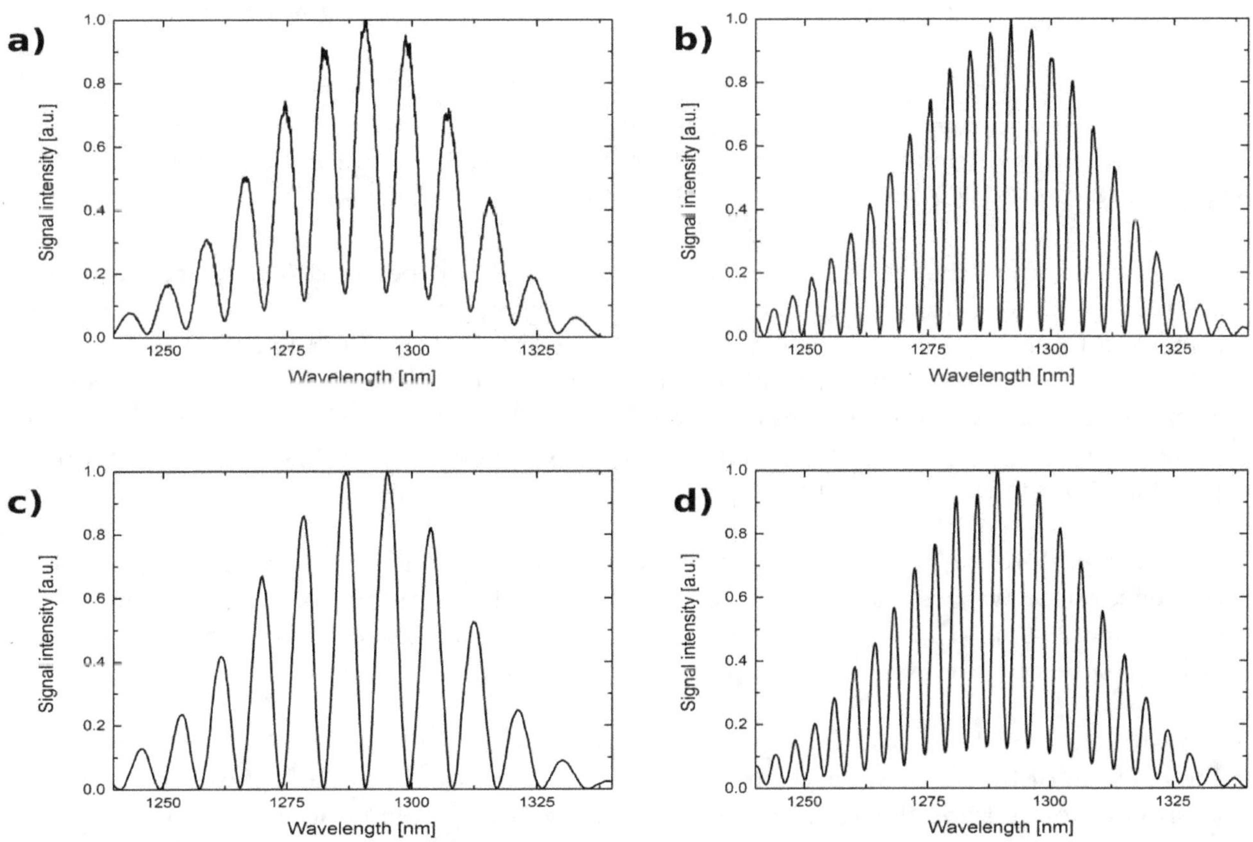

Figure 6. The measurement signal for the 1290 nm source. The Fabry-Pérot interferometer made by: optical fiber and cavity length: (**a**) 100 μm; (**b**) 200 μm; optical fiber with TiO_2 thin film and cavity length: (**c**) 100 μm; (**d**) 200 μm.

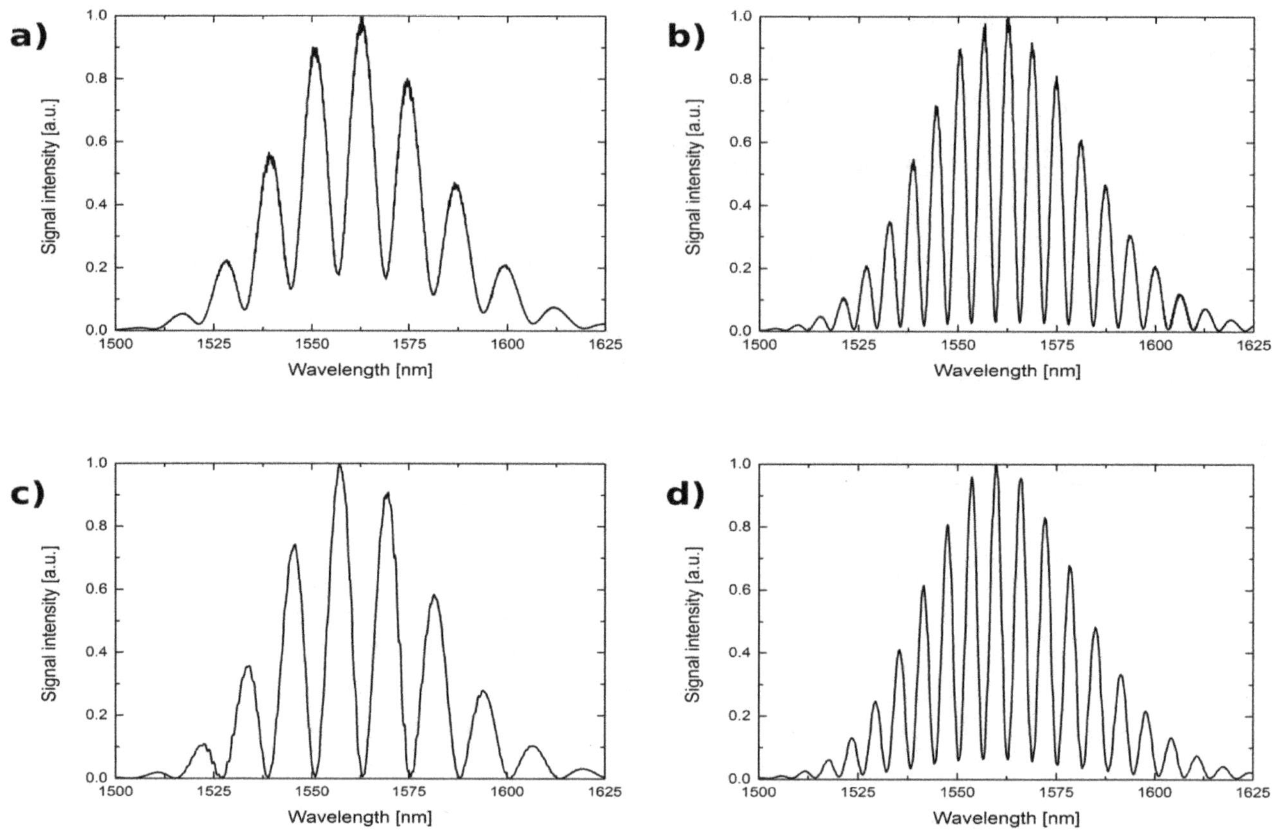

Figure 7. The measurement signal for the 1550 nm source. The Fabry-Pérot interferometer made by: optical fiber and cavity length: (**a**) 100 μm; (**b**) 200 μm; optical fiber with TiO_2 thin film and cavity length: (**c**) 100 μm; (**d**) 200 μm.

In order to confirm that proposed ALD-enhanced FPI can be used for measurements of the materials with refractive index close to that of silica glass, sensor response was examined for measurements of benzene (refractive index equal 1.4769 at 1550 nm, while for the core of SMF-28 optical fiber it is 1.468). The calculated value of refractive index obtained from recorded spectra and the reference data are shown to be in good agreement, with difference below 0.029. Following, the measurements were performed for pure water. The value of refractive index measured by our sensor was within 0.032 of the reference value.

To further explore the potential of presented construction in the biosensing applications, the fabricated sensor head was tested with sample of glucose and hemoglobin solution, obtaining refractive index values of 1.3940 and 1.2958, respectively. All of the measurements were performed with the 1550 nm source, the obtained spectra are presented in Figure 8.

The visibility V of the measured signals has decreased in all cases, which was expected as the cavity length was optimized for mediums with a refractive index of 1.0. However, this reduced visibility should not degrade the accuracy of the refractive index calculations.

For each sample, the measurements were performed during a 7-h period. The spectra recorded for each liquid remained stable during this time period. This initial stability test indicated that there was no degradation in the sensing properties of the TiO_2 film.

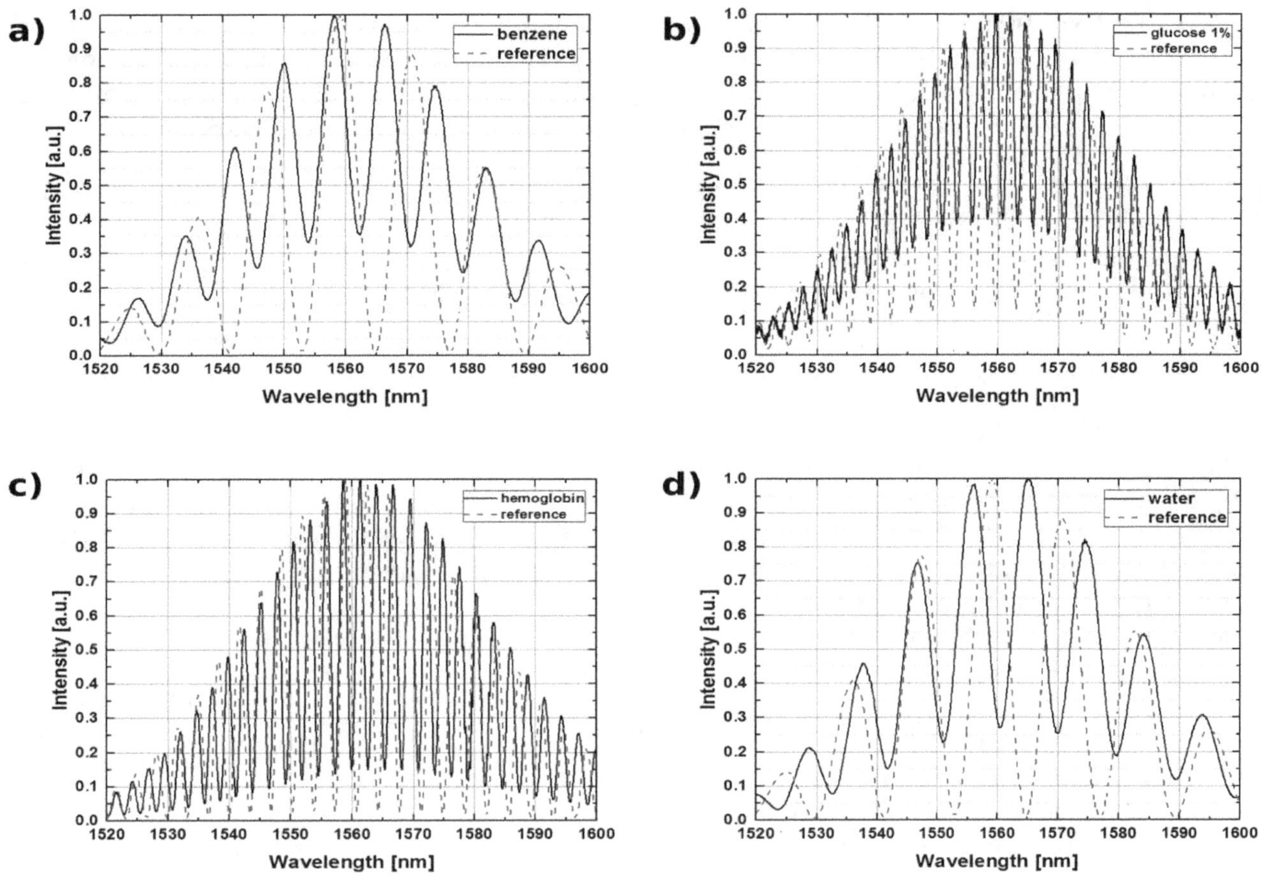

Figure 8. Measurements of Fabry-Pérot interferometer carried out with an optical fiber coated with TiO_2 layer when the cavity is filled with: (**a**) benzene; (**b**) glucose (1% solution); (**c**) hemoglobin (13.4 g/dL); and (**d**) water.

7. Conclusions

In the present study, the application of oxide ultrathin films in low coherence fiber-optic Fabry-Pérot sensing interferometers was investigated. The thin films on the tip of SM fibers were aimed to tune the reflectivity of the FPI cavity. The reflectance and transmission spectra were modelled for TiO_2 and Al_2O_3 films of various thicknesses. The obtained results indicate that it is possible to use thin TiO_2 film of a thickness around 200–300 nm as active medium in a Fabry-Pérot interferometer. However, the measurements require either an extremely broadband source or a specific adapted signal processing technique. TiO_2 and Al_2O_3 thin films of 100–200 nm deposited on the tip of the optical fiber can also be used as semi-reflective surfaces in order to improve the performance of extrinsic Fabry-Pérot interferometers.

Experiments with a Fabry-Pérot interferometer working in reflective mode were performed in order to illustrate and to verify the modelling presented. The cavity of the interferometer was delimited by an 80 nm TiO_2 film deposited by ALD on the fiber end face and by a silver mirror. The cavity length of the interferometer corresponding to the maximum fringe visibility was 100 μm. The reference interferometer (without the TiO_2 film) presented an optimal length of 200 μm. Moreover, the level of the signal reflected from the coated interferometer was two times higher than the one from the reference interferometer.

The measurement of refractive index of benzene, which is close to that of silica glass fiber, did not result in any appreciable signal deterioration and yielded a result within 0.029 from the reference value. This confirms the ability of the presented sensor to operate in the refractive index range close to that of silica glass, where sensors without reflective films do not work. Based on the measurement results of refractive index of air and water it can be concluded that the measurement range of our sensor extends from 1.0 to at least 1.5, which gives the sensor good application prospects in biosensing. These prospects were further enhanced by measuring the refractive index of hemoglobin and glucose, during which no degradation in the sensing properties of the TiO_2 film was observed.

Acknowledgments: This study was partially supported by the DS Programs of the Faculty of Electronics, Telecommunications and Informatics of the Gdańsk University of Technology.

Author Contributions: M.H. and M.J.-S. conceived and designed the experiments; D.M. and M.H. performed the experiments; P.W. and M.J.-S. analyzed the data; M.B. and M.W. contributed TiO_2 layers; M.J.-S., D.M., M.H., P.W., M.B. and M.W. wrote the paper.

References

1. Tuchin, V.V. *Handbook of Optical Biomedical Diagnostics*; SPIE Press: Bellingham, WA, USA, 2002.
2. Jakovels, D.; Kuzmina, I.; Berzina, A.; Valeine, L.; Spigulis, J. Noncontact monitoring of vascular lesion phototherapy efficiency by RGB multispectral imaging. *J. Biomed. Opt.* **2013**, *18*, 126019. [CrossRef] [PubMed]
3. Pandey, R.; Paidi, S.K.; Kang, J.W.; Spegazzini, N.; Dasari, R.R.; Valdez, T.A.; Barman, I. Discerning the differential molecular pathology of proliferative middle ear lesions using Raman spectroscopy. *Sci. Rep.* **2015**, *5*, 13305. [CrossRef] [PubMed]
4. Pandey, R.; Dingari, N.C.; Spegazzini, N.; Dasari, R.R.; Horowitz, G.L.; Barman, I. Emerging trends in optical sensing of glycemic markers for diabetes monitoring. *TrAC Trends Anal. Chem.* **2015**, *64*, 100–108. [CrossRef] [PubMed]
5. Głowacki, M.J.; Gnyba, M.; Strąkowska, P.; Gardas, M.; Kraszewski, M.; Trojanowski, M.; Strąkowski, M.R. OCT and Raman spectroscopic investigation of sol-gel derived hydroxyapatite enhaced with silver nanoparticles. *Metrol. Meas. Syst.* **2017**, in press.
6. Brezinski, M.E. *Optical Coherence Tomography*, 1st ed.; Academic Press: Cambridge, MA, USA, 2006.
7. Rao, Y.-J. Recent progress in fiber-optic extrinsic Fabry–Perot interferometric sensors. *Opt. Fiber Technol.* **2006**, *12*, 227–237. [CrossRef]
8. Kirkendall, C.K.; Dandridge, A. Overview of high performance fibre-optic sensing. *J. Phys. Appl. Phys.* **2004**, *37*, R197–R216. [CrossRef]
9. Grattan, K.T.; Meggitt, B.T. *Optical Fiber Sensor Technology*; Kluwer Academic Publisher: Boston, MA, USA, 2000.
10. Islam, M.R.; Ali, M.M.; Lai, M.-H.; Lim, K.-S.; Ahmad, H. Chronology of Fabry-Perot interferometer fiber-optic sensors and their applications: A review. *Sensors* **2014**, *14*, 7451–7488. [CrossRef] [PubMed]
11. Wierzba, P.; Jedrzejewska-Szczerska, M. Optimization of a Fabry-Perot Sensing Interferometer Design for an Optical Fiber Sensor of Hematocrit Level. *Acta Phys. Pol. A* **2013**, *124*, 586–588. [CrossRef]
12. Jędrzejewska-Szczerska, M. Response of a New Low-Coherence Fabry-Perot Sensor to Hematocrit Levels in Human Blood. *Sensors* **2014**, *14*, 6965–6976. [CrossRef] [PubMed]
13. Milewska, D.; Karpienko, K.; Jędrzejewska-Szczerska, M. Application of thin diamond films in low-coherence fiber-optic Fabry Pérot displacement sensor. *Diam. Relat. Mater.* **2016**, *64*, 169–176. [CrossRef]
14. Majchrowicz, D.; Hirsch, M.; Wierzba, P.; Bechelany, M.; Viter, R.; Jędrzejewska-Szczerska, M. Application of Thin ZnO ALD Layers in Fiber-Optic Fabry-Pérot Sensing Interferometers. *Sensors* **2016**, *16*, 416. [CrossRef] [PubMed]
15. Majchrowicz, D.; Hirsch, M. Fiber optic low-coherence Fabry-Pérot interferometer with ZnO layers in transmission and reflective mode: Comparative study. *Proc. SPIE* **2016**, *9917*, 99171C.
16. Leskelä, M.; Ritala, M. Atomic Layer Deposition Chemistry: Recent Developments and Future Challenges. *Angew. Chem. Int. Ed.* **2003**, *42*, 5548–5554. [CrossRef] [PubMed]
17. Auth, C.; Allen, C.; Blattner, A.; Bergstrom, D.; Brazier, M.; Bost, M.; Buehler, M.; Chikarmane, V.; Ghani, T.; Glassman, T.; et al. A 22nm high performance and low-power CMOS technology featuring fully-depleted tri-gate transistors, self-aligned contacts and high density MIM capacitors. In Proceedings of the 2012 Symposium on VLSI Technology (VLSIT), Honolulu, HI, USA, 12–14 June 2012; pp. 131–132.
18. Dingemans, G.; Kessels, W.M.M. Status and prospects of Al2O3-based surface passivation schemes for silicon solar cells. *J. Vac. Sci. Technol. A* **2012**, *30*, 40802. [CrossRef]

19. Jędrzejewska-Szczerska, M.; Wierzba, P.; Chaaya, A.A.; Bechelany, M.; Miele, P.; Viter, R.; Mazikowski, A.; Karpienko, K.; Wróbel, M. ALD thin ZnO layer as an active medium in a fiber-optic Fabry–Perot interferometer. *Sens. Actuators A Phys.* **2015**, *221*, 88–94. [CrossRef]
20. George, S.M. Atomic Layer Deposition: An Overview. *Chem. Rev.* **2010**, *110*, 111–131. [CrossRef] [PubMed]
21. Weber, M.J.; Verheijen, M.A.; Bol, A.A.; Kessels, W.M.M. Sub-nanometer dimensions control of core/shell nanoparticles prepared by atomic layer deposition. *Nanotechnology* **2015**, *26*, 94002. [CrossRef] [PubMed]
22. Weber, M.J.; Mackus, A.J.M.; Verheijen, M.A.; van der Marel, C.; Kessels, W.M.M. Supported Core/Shell Bimetallic Nanoparticles Synthesis by Atomic Layer Deposition. *Chem. Mater.* **2012**, *24*, 2973–2977. [CrossRef]
23. Chaaya, A.A.; Viter, R.; Baleviciute, I.; Bechelany, M.; Ramanavicius, A.; Gertnere, Z.; Erts, D.; Smyntyna, V.; Miele, P. Tuning Optical Properties of Al_2O_3/ZnO Nanolaminates Synthesized by Atomic Layer Deposition. *J. Phys. Chem. C* **2014**, *118*, 3811–3819. [CrossRef]
24. Snure, M.; Paduano, Q.; Hamilton, M.; Shoaf, J.; Mann, J.M. Optical characterization of nanocrystalline boron nitride thin films grown by atomic layer deposition. *Thin Solid Films* **2014**, *571*, 51–55. [CrossRef]
25. Boudiombo, J.; Boudrioua, A.; Loulergue, J.C.; Malhouitre, S.; Machet, J. Optical waveguiding properties and refractive index analysis of boron nitride (BN) thin films prepared by reactive ion plating. *Opt. Mater.* **1998**, *10*, 143–153. [CrossRef]
26. López, J.; Martínez, J.; Abundiz, N.; Domínguez, D.; Murillo, E.; Castillón, F.F.; Machorro, R.; Farías, M.H.; Tiznado, H. Thickness effect on the optical and morphological properties in Al_2O_3/ZnO nanolaminate thin films prepared by atomic layer deposition. *Superlattices Microstruct.* **2016**, *90*, 265–273. [CrossRef]
27. Wierzba, P.; Jędrzejewska-Szczerska, M. Spectral reflectance modeling of ZnO layers made with Atomic Layer Deposition for application in optical fiber Fabry-Perot interferometric sensors. *Proc. SPIE* **2015**, *9448*, 944819.
28. Wang, Z.-Y.; Zhang, R.-J.; Lu, H.-L.; Chen, X.; Sun, Y.; Zhang, Y.; Wei, Y.-F.; Xu, J.-P.; Wang, S.-Y.; Zheng, Y.-X.; et al. The impact of thickness and thermal annealing on refractive index for aluminum oxide thin films deposited by atomic layer deposition. *Nanoscale Res. Lett.* **2015**, *10*, 46. [CrossRef] [PubMed]
29. Kumar, P.; Wiedmann, M.K.; Winter, C.H.; Avrutsky, I. Optical properties of Al_2O_3 thin films grown by atomic layer deposition. *Appl. Opt.* **2009**, *48*, 5407–5412. [CrossRef] [PubMed]
30. Kasikov, A.; Aarik, J.; Mändar, H.; Moppel, M.; Pärs, M.; Uustare, T. Refractive index gradients in TiO_2 thin films grown by atomic layer deposition. *J. Phys. Appl. Phys.* **2006**, *39*, 54–60. [CrossRef]
31. Refractive Index of Al_2O_3 (Aluminium Oxide, Sapphire)—Kischkat. Available online: http://refractiveindex.info/?shelf=main&book=Al2O3&page=Kischkat (accessed on 23 September 2016).
32. Refractive Index of TiO_2 (Titanium Dioxide)—Devore-o. Available online: http://refractiveindex.info/?shelf=main&book=TiO2&page=Devore-o (accessed on 23 September 2016).
33. Schlicht, S.; Assaud, L.; Hansen, M.; Licklederer, M.; Bechelany, M.; Perner, M.; Bachmann, J. An electrochemically functional layer of hydrogenase extract on an electrode of large and tunable specific surface area. *J. Mater. Chem. A* **2016**, *4*, 6487–6494. [CrossRef]
34. Profijt, H.B.; van de Sanden, M.C.M.; Kessels, W.M.M. Substrate Biasing during Plasma-Assisted ALD for Crystalline Phase-Control of TiO_2 Thin Films. *Electrochem. Solid-State Lett.* **2011**, *15*, G1–G3. [CrossRef]
35. Xie, Q.; Jiang, Y.-L.; Detavernier, C.; Deduytsche, D.; Van Meirhaeghe, R.L.; Ru, G.-P.; Li, B.-Z.; Qu, X.-P. Atomic layer deposition of TiO_2 from tetrakis-dimethyl-amido titanium or Ti isopropoxide precursors and H_2O. *J. Appl. Phys.* **2007**, *102*, 83521. [CrossRef]
36. Kim, S.K.; Kim, W.-D.; Kim, K.-M.; Hwang, C.S.; Jeong, J. High dielectric constant TiO_2 thin films on a Ru electrode grown at 250 °C by atomic-layer deposition. *Appl. Phys. Lett.* **2004**, *85*, 4112–4114. [CrossRef]
37. Triani, G.; Evans, P.J.; Mitchell, D.R.G.; Attard, D.J.; Finnie, K.S.; James, M.; Hanley, T.; Latella, B.; Prince, K.E.; Bartlett, J. Atomic layer deposition of TiO_2/Al_2O_3 films for optical applications. *Proc. SPIE* **2005**, *5870*, 587009.

5

Machine Learning Aided Photonic Diagnostic System for Minimally Invasive Optically Guided Surgery in the Hepatoduodenal Area

Evgeny Zherebtsov [1,2,*], Marina Zajnulina [3], Ksenia Kandurova [1], Elena Potapova [1], Viktor Dremin [1,3], Andrian Mamoshin [1,4], Sergei Sokolovski [3], Andrey Dunaev [1] and Edik U. Rafailov [3]

1 Research and Development Center of Biomedical Photonics, Orel State University, 302026 Orel, Russia; kandkseniya@gmail.com (K.K.); e.potapova@oreluniver.ru (E.P.); v.dremin1@aston.ac.uk (V.D.); dr.mamoshin@mail.ru (A.M.); dunaev@bmecenter.ru (A.D.)
2 Faculty of Information Technology and Electrical Engineering, University of Oulu, Optoelectronics and Measurement Techniques Unit, 90570 Oulu, Finland
3 Aston Institute of Photonic Technologies, Aston University, Birmingham B4 7ET, UK; MZArea@hotmail.com (M.Z.); s.sokolovsky@aston.ac.uk (S.S.); e.rafailov@aston.ac.uk (E.U.R.)
4 Department of X-ray Surgical Methods of Diagnosis and Treatment, Orel Regional Clinical Hospital, 302028 Orel, Russia
* Correspondence: evgenii.zherebtsov@oulu.fi

Abstract: Abdominal cancer is a widely prevalent group of tumours with a high level of mortality if diagnosed at a late stage. Although the cancer death rates have in general declined over the past few decades, the mortality from tumours in the hepatoduodenal area has significantly increased in recent years. The broader use of minimal access surgery (MAS) for diagnostics and treatment can significantly improve the survival rate and quality of life of patients after surgery. This work aims to develop and characterise an appropriate technical implementation for tissue endogenous fluorescence (TEF) and assess the efficiency of machine learning methods for the real-time diagnosis of tumours in the hepatoduodenal area. In this paper, we present the results of the machine learning approach applied to the optically guided MAS. We have elaborated tissue fluorescence approach with a fibre-optic probe to record the TEF and blood perfusion parameters during MAS in patients with cancers in the hepatoduodenal area. The measurements from the laser Doppler flowmetry (LDF) channel were used as a sensor of the tissue vitality to reduce variability in TEF data. Also, we evaluated how the blood perfusion oscillations are changed in the tumour tissue. The evaluated amplitudes of the cardiac (0.6–1.6 Hz) and respiratory (0.2–0.6 Hz) oscillations was significantly higher in intact tissues ($p < 0.001$) compared to the cancerous ones, while the myogenic (0.2–0.06 Hz) oscillation did not demonstrate any statistically significant difference. Our results demonstrate that a fibre-optic TEF probe accompanied with ML algorithms such as k-Nearest Neighbours or AdaBoost is highly promising for the real-time in situ differentiation between cancerous and healthy tissues by detecting the information about the tissue type that is encoded in the fluorescence spectrum. Also, we show that the detection can be supplemented and enhanced by parallel collection and classification of blood perfusion oscillations.

Keywords: liver cancer; endogenous fluorescence; laser Doppler flowmetry; blood perfusion; minimally invasive interventions; machine learning

---

1. Introduction

Abdominal cancer is a widely prevalent group of tumours with a high level of mortality if diagnosed at a late stage. Although the cancer death rates have in general declined over the past few decades, the mortality from tumours in the hepatoduodenal area specifically has increased in recent years [1]. Moving towards the broader use of minimally invasive techniques for diagnosis and treatment is promising to significantly improve the survival rate and quality of life of patients after surgery. Minimally invasive techniques require the use of reliable tools for real-time feedback to assist the surgeon. Usually, the manipulations in the operation field are conducted under ultrasound or X-ray control and visualisation. While the methods can provide an exceptional accuracy of the tool positioning, they hardly give sufficient information on the tissue type and, specifically, on the tumour borders. Various approaches have been put forward to solve this issue. The optical methods have been widely investigated in that respect and demonstrated high diagnostic potential in many applications [2–5]. Despite the gradual transition from the in vivo single-point measurements towards the in vivo imaging techniques, the use of fibre optical probes for the surgical guidance has great potential to compete with the costly techniques and to significantly improve the outcome of the routine procedures for cancer eradication. Most imaging approaches still need to address major issues concerning the motion artefacts, real time imaging processing and the trade-off between the parameters of resolution, frame rate and aperture diameter [6]. In particular, this set of limitations affects the minimally invasive surgical interventions as one deals with the tools of low outer diameters being applied in confined space of the abdominal cavity [7].

In recent years, there has been considerable interest in the measurements of the fluorescence parameters to be applied for the diagnostics in minimally invasive surgery [8]. The methods are based on the recording of the endogenous fluorescence. However, they often require the intravenous injection of fluorescence dyes or molecular fluorescence probes specifically binding to tumour cells [9,10]. The association between TEF emission and changes in tissue metabolism as well as the blood circulation and histological architecture offers a powerful diagnostic tool for direct monitoring of the malignancy of studied biotissues. TEF, based on autofluorescence spectra registration, can provide comprehensive information about the physiological or altered morphofunctional properties of cells and tissues, including ones caused by oncology [11]. Due to high proliferation, tumour cells have increased metabolic needs compared to normal ones [12], and tumour metabolism is associated with changes in relative concentrations of NADH and FAD [13]. These endogenous fluorophores of cells and tissues can serve as biomarkers for studying differences between tumour and non-tumour areas [14–18].

In the traditional approach, the TEF measurements were used to evaluate the changes in tissues based on the comparison of the absolute values of the related emission parameters in tumour and non-tumour areas. Nowadays, research tends to focus on machine learning (ML) approaches that combine input feature sets in one or several diagnostic classifiers [19]. One promising application of ML is MAS as the medical procedure commonly requires a high speed of the onsite decision making for the surgeon. More recent evidence shows that the diagnostic techniques based on the measurements of the intrinsic fluorescence aided with the machine learning algorithms can be used for distinguishing malignant and benign colorectal tissue [20].

To the best of our knowledge, the applicability of ML in fluorescence liver cancer diagnostics has not yet been studied thoroughly. The available published results in this research area either focus on the MRI or CT studies [21], are limited using tumour-targeting fluorescent labels [22] or reported results obtained ex vivo [23].

Recently, authors have published data on the evaluation of the liver tumours with the needle optical probe combining TEF and diffuse reflectance measurements [24]. Except for that, despite high interest and potential outcome, no one, to the best of our knowledge, has demonstrated results of the ML application for cancer diagnosis that deploys data obtained by optical probe in vivo and in situ in the hepatoduodenal area.

In this work, we present results of the ML techniques to facilitate optically guided surgery on tumours by the detection and classification of cancerous and healthy tissues. The data that we use in our studies was obtained in vivo and *in situ*. In particular, we focus on cancers of the liver and bile duct and collect and classify the data for TEF and blood perfusion. The focus on two types of data has the following reason: it is known that in vivo recorded fluorescence spectra are influenced by many factors such as the absorption by blood in the living tissue [25]. This blood-induced absorption attenuates and changes the shape of the fluorescence signal [26]. To mitigate this problem, we additionally analyse the parameters of the blood perfusion measured in living intact tissue (cf. [27]). For this, we deploy laser Doppler flowmetry (LDF). LDF provides a powerful tool for the blood perfusion measurements and analysis of rhythmic oscillations in the fine structure of microvascular blood flow. It was demonstrated that LDF is a highly informative method across a range of medical conditions and general physiological health monitoring applications. To record TEF and LDF blood perfusion parameters during MAS in patients with cancers of liver and bile duct, we implemented a flexible optical fibre probe capable of measurements in the hepatoduodenal area. We used ML techniques to detect the tumour borders by classification of healthy and cancerous tissues using the TEF and LDF data. The general aim of this work was to develop an appropriate technical implementation for TEF and LDF measurements and to assess the efficiency of ML methods for real-time diagnosis of liver cancer and tumours in the hepatoduodenal area.

2. Materials and Methods

2.1. Setup and In Situ Data Collection

The setup to collect data on TEF and LDF consists of a custom-built, flexible fibre-optical probe, two LED sources for fluorescence excitation (at 365 nm and 450 nm), a set of fluorescent filters, a CCD-based spectrometer and a laser Doppler flowmetry channel for blood perfusion measurements that utilises a single-mode laser at 1064 nm. The prototype of the fibre-optical probe (Figure 1) has two emitting fibres to excite TEF at wavelengths of 365 nm and 450 nm and a fibre to collect the fluorescence emission (all fibres are of 400 μm in diameter). Moreover, the probe is equipped with one emitting single-mode optical fibre and two multimode collecting fibres for the LDF channel. This configuration enables to register the fluorescence of all major endogenous fluorophores in living tissue, as well as to record the level of blood perfusion in the area of interest (Figure 2).

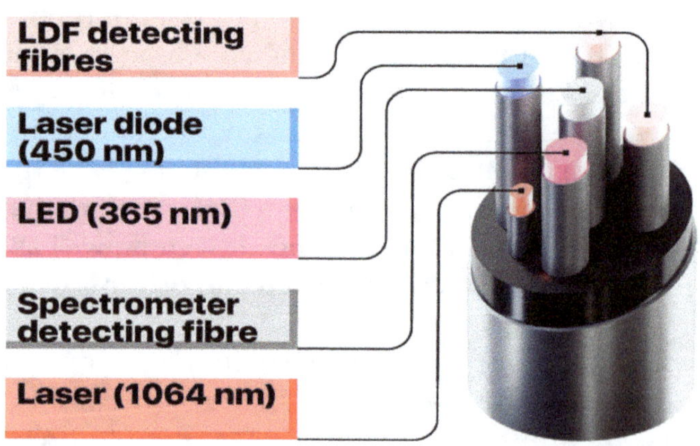

Figure 1. The configuration and measuring channels of the used fibre-optic probe.

The proposed setup was validated in the framework of limited tests in patients with obstructive jaundice caused by liver cancer. The patient cohort comprised of 27 volunteers. The measurements from the LDF channel were used as a sensor of the tissue vitality. The TEF spectra were recorded primarily in the areas of interest demonstrated a stable level of blood perfusion of about 15 a.u. Figure 3 (top panel) shows the exemplary records of blood perfusion registered in the intact bile duct and in the cancer block. This procedure allowed us to avoid areas of necrosis and to decrease the TEF data variation associated with the variable blood volume fraction in the tissue. The measurements were performed during planned diagnostic and therapeutic interventions under ultrasound and X-ray examination. For every patient, 8–10 spectra were taken at the excitation wavelength of 365 nm and 450 nm. They were equally split between cancerous and intact tissues. In that way, 4–5 spectra were measured for each class in a patient. The measurement points were evenly distributed over the area of interest except for places with low blood perfusion prominent necrosis or covered with blood. Also, two 1 min long LDF recordings were made for places with apparent tumour and normal tissues respectively. The studies were conducted at the department of interventional radiology of Orel Regional Clinical Hospital (Orel, Russia) and were approved by the local Committee for Human Biomedical Research Ethics (record of the meeting No. 10 of 16.11.2017).

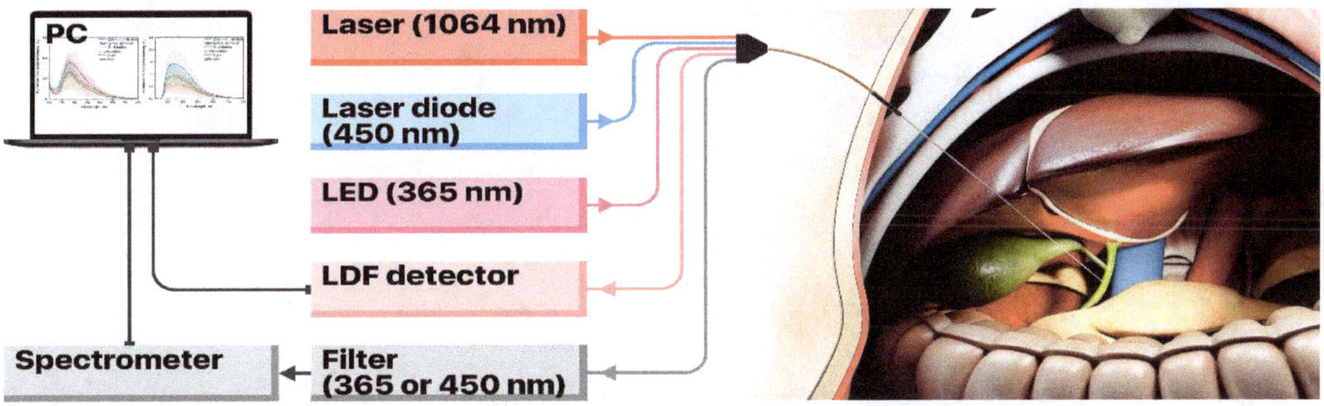

Figure 2. The components of measuring setup and probe placement in the region of interest.

2.2. *Data Collection*

The main challenge of the proposed technique lies in the collection of TEF data under the X-ray control directly during a surgical procedure. The imaging procedure, being realised with a radiopaque substance that fills the cavity of the bile duct, allows the surgeon to visualise the contour of the walls and the tumour block. In this case, the 2D radiological control is the only piece of feedback information about the probe position with respect to the bile duct and the tumour itself. Actually, this indirect approach might be sufficient for MAS as such. However, from the point of view of the data collection quality for ML, the indirect control might be insufficient for a precise localisation of the sampling point and, as a result, for a right labelling of the TEF spectrum. Thus, a spectrum coming from a healthy tissue can be falsely labelled as cancerous and vice versa. When used for training and testing of ML models, such spectra contribute towards a high value of the intrinsic lowest possible error (LPE) in classification and make it difficult to evaluate the performance of the ML models and to interpret their prediction results.

Besides the difficulty of the probe positioning due to the limitations of the available 2D X-ray visualisation (i), we identify three other sources of possible data mislabelling: (ii) the lack of ability to reliably visualise blood and bile in the field of view of the fibre-optical probe which significantly affects the quality of the collected fluorescence spectra; (iii) the uncertainty of the distribution of the cancer cells over the mucous surface; and (iv) the effects of the probe pressure on the tissues that manifests itself in the variable blood volume fraction in the tissue.

In the presented study, all patients were diagnosed with cancer and their samples were verified morphologically by biopsy. Nevertheless, regarding the challenges (i) and (iii), it should be noted that the allocation of the areas with cancer tissue significantly varies between the patients. The X-ray visualisation helps to identify the tumour block and the position of the probe. At the same time, in the vicinity of the tumour block, the malignant cells can belong to the primary tumour originated from the epithelial tissues of the bile duct or cells proliferated from the surrounding organs. Also, in some cases, the cancer cells can be absent on the surface of the cancerous tissues. This happens when the tumour block compresses the healthy tissue where the probe is placed but does not permeate through the wall of the organ. These aspects further contribute to the increase of the system's LPE by leading to false labelling of spectra used for the training and testing of ML models.

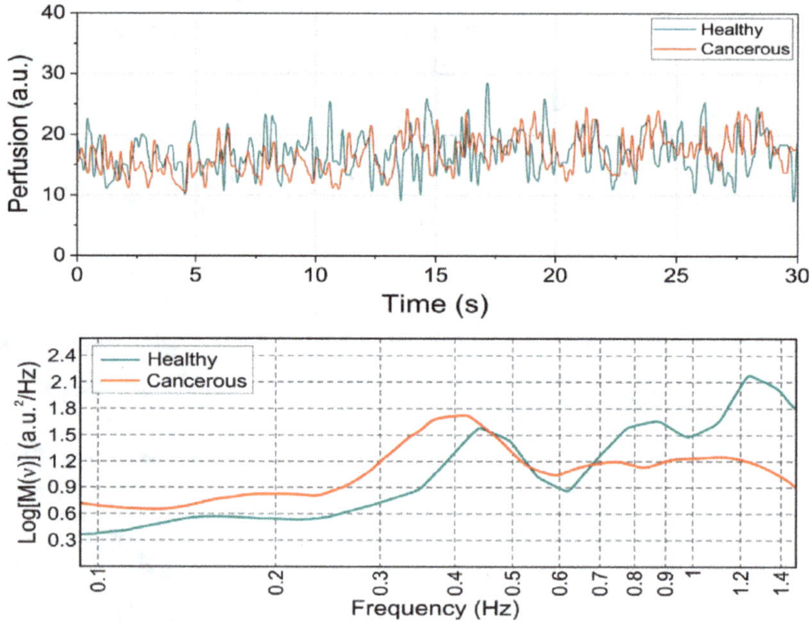

Figure 3. Exemplary blood perfusion records (upper panel) from the intact bile duct wall and the tumour located in the bile duct and the corresponding integrated wavelet spectra (IWS; bottom panel).

2.3. *Machine Learning Method*

In our experiments, the spectrometer for the TEF measurements covers the range between 346 nm and 816 nm sampled with 2100 pixels. To build and determine suitable machine learning models for classification of healthy and cancerous tissues, we consider the intensity spectra taken at 365 nm and 450 nm separately. For the purposes of classification, the following labels were used to label the spectra: "C" for cancerous tissues and "N" for healthy tissues. Figure 4 shows 5 arbitrary spectra and their labels for each channel. On the left side of each spectrum, we see a sharp excitation peak and to its right, a broad fluorescence spectrum. The information on whether a tissue is healthy or cancerous is encoded in the intensity of the fluorescence peak, its position in the spectrum and its shape. We use a Python-based library called Scikit-learn to pre-process and to classify the spectra automatically by ML methods.

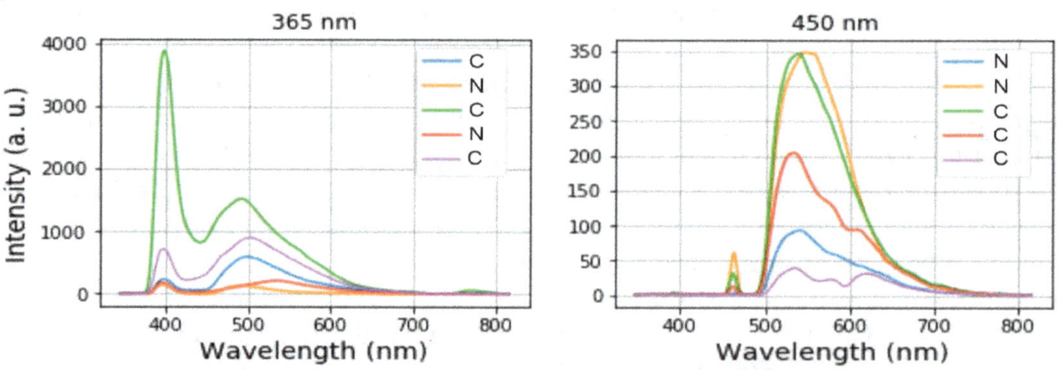

Figure 4. 5 arbitrary fluorescence spectra and their labels obtained at the excitation channel of 365 nm (**left**) and 450 nm (**right**). In these graphs, the label "N" denotes a normal tissue whereas "C" a cancerous tissue.

In terms of data pre-processing, we first removed the data samples where the noise floor overlapped with the actual fluorescence spectra. To further reduce the influence of noise, the remaining spectra were smoothed using a FIR filter. In the next step, noisy, not informative sections at the beginning (blue sides) of the spectra as well as at their (red) ends were cut off. This resulted in the reduced dimensionality of each spectrum of (1, 1920) instead of the initial dimension of (1, 2100) that was determined by the spectrometer pixel number.

The training and test sets were randomly split as follows: 199 samples for training and 40 samples for testing in the case of the 356 nm channel and 120 samples for training and 40 samples for testing in the case of the 450 nm channel. To increase the performance of our ML models, the data was standardised by subtracting the data mean value and dividing the result by the standard deviation.

To further reduce the dimensionality of our training and test data, we applied the principal component analysis (PCA) with 5 principal components. As Figure 5 shows, 5 principal components retain more than 90% of the information stored in the spectra. The first two components having the highest values carry the biggest part of this information. We interpret the first two components as the indicators of the fluorescence peak intensity and its position in the spectrum. After the PCA is performed, the dimension of each spectrum is only (1, 5). In our statistical experiments, we observe a variation of the first two PCA components values by ±3% and much smaller variation in other components. However, this variability does not prevent us from seeing a clear difference between the first and the second component.

Five classification models and their performance in differentiating between the healthy and cancerous tissues were considered for the TEF spectra of each channel as well as for the LDF blood flow oscillations. Those are the k-Nearest-Neighbours (KNN) algorithm [28], a Decision Tree (DT) [29], Support Vector Machines (SVM) [30] and such ensemble methods as the Random Forest (RF) [31] and AdaBoost [32]. In the blood perfusion analysis, the logistic regression model was applied instead of AdaBoost. A 10-fold validation was applied to evaluate the accuracy of each method. The accuracy denotes the ratio between the rightly classified values, and all considered ones and measures how close the predicted value of the class is to the true class label. Two further metrics that we used to evaluate the classifiers' performance are the sensitivity and the specificity. The sensitivity is the ratio between the true positives and the sum of true positives and false negatives, i.e., the portion of actual positives that are correctly predicted. The specificity measures the number of true negatives put into relation to the sum of true negatives and false positives, it is the portion of actual negatives that are correctly predicted [33]. The sensitivity is an important measure to accurately diagnose the cancerous tissues, whereas the specificity determines how well the system detects healthy tissues. In an ideal case, both sensitivity and specificity tend towards 100%. In the following, all three metrics (accuracy, sensitivity and specificity) are evaluated as an average of 10 statistical experiments for which the data was randomly shuffled each time.

When looking at Figure 3, we can assume that the information of the tissue type is encoded in the frequency components of the blood perfusion time series. The oscillations in the cancerous tissue are slower whereas the time series collected from healthy tissue exhibits more high-frequency components. To validate the assumption and extract this information, we pre-process the LDF data by means of the wavelet analysis with the Morlet wavelet taken as a mother function. We calculated the integrated wavelet spectra (IWS) using the signal analysis technique in the frequency domain. Examples of representative IWS for cancerous and normal tissues are presented in Figure 3 (bottom panel). The length of the recordings allowed us to calculate 3 spectral ranges of the oscillations in the fine structure of capillary blood flow corresponding to the cardiac (0.6–1.6 Hz), respiratory (0.2–0.6 Hz) and myogenic activities (0.2–0.06 Hz) [34]. The maximal amplitude of the oscillations in every spectral range was taken as a diagnostic parameter. One-Way ANOVA with Tukey's post hoc test was used to check the significance of the statistical variation between blood perfusion parameters measured in the tumour and the intact tissue. Only demonstrated statistically significant difference parameters of blood perfusion oscillations were used as the feature space for the ML methods.

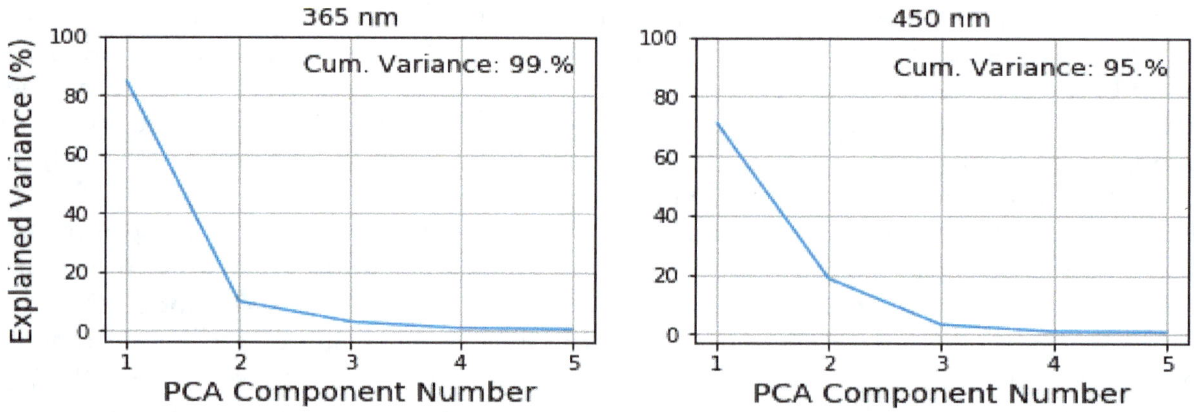

Figure 5. Example of percentage of explained variance at the excitation channel of 365 nm (**left**) and 450 nm (**right**) achieved by PCA.

3. Results

As in the case with data pre-processing, the data evaluation for TEF was done using the Scikit-learn library. The considered ML models underwent initial tuning in terms of the best prediction accuracy to pick the best possible hyperparameters. The resulting KNN classifier had 4 neighbours with distance weighting for both channels; also for both channels, the best maximum depth of the decision tree turned out to be only 1; the SVM model had a regularisation parameter of $Z = 0.1$ and a linear kernel for both 365 nm and 450 nm; the RF classifier for the 365 nm channel consisted of 5 estimators with a depth of 3; whereas the RF model for the 450 nm channel had 7 estimators with a depth of 3; the AdaBoost model consisted of 5 sub-estimators for each channel.

Tables 1 and 2 summarise the results for accuracy, sensitivity and specificity we achieved for 10 statistical experiments where the data used for training and testing was randomly shuffled each time. The results are presented as a mean value ± standard deviation in percent.

As Table 1 shows, the results of the TEF classification exhibit higher values for the 450 nm channel than for the 365 nm channel for all considered metrics. This suggests dropping the 365 nm channel in future which might considerably simplify the setup. Additionally, the dropping of the 365 nm channel would increase the in-field practicability of the suggested method. This is because the excitation radiation of 365 nm lying within the UV spectrum induces higher phototoxicity for living tissues than the light at 450 nm [35]. For TEF, the accuracy varies between 60% and 67% for the 365 nm channel and between 62% and 72% for the 450 nm channel.

Table 1. Achieved results of Accuracy and Specificity in % for each classifier and each excitation channel for TEF measurements.

Channel		*365 nm*			*450 nm*	
Model	**Accuracy**	**Sensitivity**	**Specificity**	**Accuracy**	**Sensitivity**	**Specificity**
KNN	60 ± 8	41 ± 21	73 ± 12	62 ± 6	46 ± 21	78 ± 8
Decision Tree	67 ± 7	28 ± 25	89 ± 9	67 ± 8	27 ± 37	94 ± 13
SVM	67 ± 8	15 ± 28	96 ± 6	72 ± 6	28 ± 35	99 ± 2
Random Forest	65 ± 8	27 ± 27	86 ± 11	64 ± 7	28 ± 28	88 ± 8
AdaBoost	65 ± 6	26 ± 26	87 ± 7	64 ± 5	37 ± 37	86 ± 16

As discussed in Section 2.2, we assume a high LPE implicating that several spectra were falsely labelled right at the beginning. We assume an LPE of around 15%. In this case, the accuracy is limited by this value, meaning that even a perfect classifier would not be able to achieve better accuracy results than around 85%. From this point of view, to achieve accuracy values up to 72% is highly promising.

In detail, from all considered values of accuracy, the SVM algorithm for the TEF data provides the best performance. Moreover, in terms of specificity, SVM shows the best results, going to 96–99%

well predicting the negative cases, i.e., the cases of healthy tissues. The second-best result is shown by the DT model. However, if you consider the sensitivity values, both SVM and DT perform poorly on the prediction of cancerous tissues, which is the most important aspect for in situ diagnosis. Taking into account the value of sensitivity, the best performance is shown by KNN for both channels and AdaBoost, specifically for the 450 nm channel. The considered Random Forest performs poorly in terms of all three metrics.

In general, we observe a high variety in sensitivity values that manifests itself in high values of standard deviation. This occurs due to the difficulties of the data collection described in Section 2.2 and poses the requirement to improve the data collection and labelling in further stages of the approach development.

As for LDF, the evaluated amplitudes of the cardiac and respiratory oscillation were significantly higher in intact tissues ($p < 0.001$) compared to the cancerous ones, while the myogenic oscillation did not demonstrate any statistically significant difference. The results on the statistical analysis of the differences in the oscillations in normal intact and cancerous tissues are presented in Figure 6. The reason for the observed distinction of the amplitude values in the healthy and cancerous tissues can lie in the mechanical properties of the tumour resulting in the dimming of the amplitude of the pulse that propagates through the microvessels within the cancerous tissue.

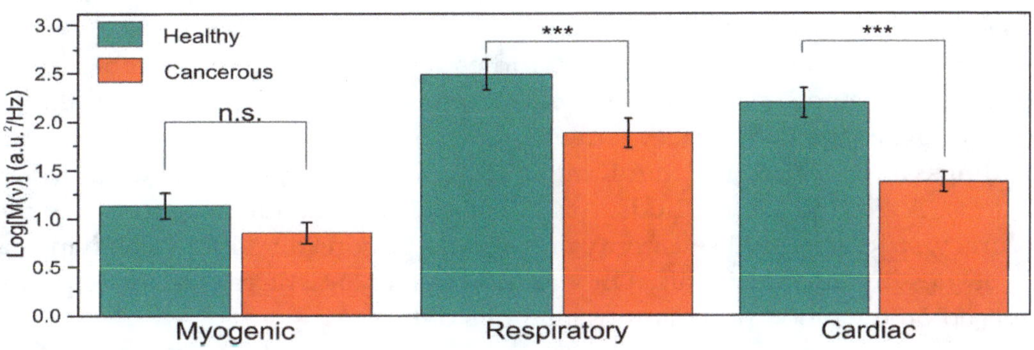

Figure 6. Results on the statistical analysis (One-Way ANOVA with Tukey's post hoc test, *** $p < 0.001$, n.s.: not significant, Mean ± SE) of the differences in the oscillations in normal intact and cancerous tissues in the hepatoduodenal area.

The results obtained by the ML models applied to the values of blood perfusion oscillations obtained from wavelet transform (Table 2) suggest that the parameters especially of the cardiac oscillations are of high a diagnostic value and can effectively supplement the TEF analysis and classification. However, more clinical research and better feature extraction as well as the fine-tuning of the ML models are needed to produce better prediction results and to correctly interpret them.

Table 2. Results of Accuracy and Specificity in % for each classifier for blood perfusion rhythmic oscillations.

Channel	*Cardiac Oscillations*			*Respiratory Oscillations*		
Model	**Accuracy**	**Sensitivity**	**Specificity**	**Accuracy**	**Sensitivity**	**Specificity**
KNN	58 ± 7	34 ± 26	82 ± 16	56 ± 10	35 ± 10	77 ± 18
Decision Tree	62 ± 7	61 ± 22	65 ± 24	55 ± 6	37 ± 20	72 ± 18
SVM	60 ± 9	26 ± 20	93 ± 8	59 ± 8	36 ± 19	81 ± 13
Random Forest	54 ± 15	57 ± 17	51 ± 30	58 ± 6	42 ± 14	73 ± 13
Logistic Regression	70 ± 7	52 ± 9	87 ± 9	64 ± 8	49 ± 11	79 ± 12

As Table 2 presents, the best results are achieved by logistic regression applied to classify the cardiac oscillations. This suggests focussing only on the data obtained for cardiac oscillations and to use logistic regression to evaluate it in future. Further, reliable evaluation of the blood perfusion pulsations associated with the heart activity requires as much as twice shorter LDF recording duration than the one required for the respiratory oscillations. As a result, the duration of the LDF recording can be shortened.

4. Discussion

The challenge of more accurate data collection to significantly minimise the LPE still requires an appropriate solution. Further development of the proposed multimodal approach by equipping it with additional optical methods (e.g., diffuse reflectance spectroscopy or optical proximity sensor) can be an option to improve the accuracy of the probe placement. An approach based on the diffuse reflectance measurements might allow for a significant decrease in the influence of blood absorption on the recorded TEF spectra.

A non-contact proximity sensor embedded in the probe combined with the subsequent automation of the data collection at a fixed optimal distance might eliminate the negative effects of the sensor tip pressure on the soft tissues under study. Moreover, the saline delivery subsystem for the pus, mucus and blood removal from the tissue surface and optical probe cleaning during the procedure are also considered to be promising for the improvement of the quality of the data collection.

Based on the achieved results, we believe that the use of the 365 nm channel can be dropped in the further design development of the fibre-optic probe since it does not contribute to the overall performance. We see that TEF analysis and classification can be assisted by the analysis of the LDF data for cardiac oscillations. However, deeper-going studies with respect to the suitable feature extraction and ML model hyper-parameters are needed to effectively supplement the TEF classification with LDF classification. To improve the data quality and efficiency for the LDF analysis, the length of the blood perfusion recordings can be shortened from 1 min to 30 s as it is enough for the suggested analysis of the cardiac oscillations. As for the ML methods, AdaBoost and KNN models demonstrate the best results in terms of accuracy, specificity, and sensitivity and should be considered for classifying cancerous and noncancerous tissues in real-time in situ TEF diagnosis. The logistic regression is preferable for the classification based on the blood perfusion oscillations data.

5. Conclusions

Our results clearly demonstrate that a fibre-optic TEF probe accompanied with ML algorithms such as k-Nearest Neighbours or AdaBoost is highly promising for real-time in situ differentiation between cancerous and healthy tissues by detection the information about the tissue type that is encoded in the fluorescence spectrum. This detection can be supplemented and enhanced by parallel collection and classification of blood perfusion rhythmic data, especially the one that denote cardiac oscillations. Clearly, the data collection procedure as well as the design of the proposed fibre-optic probe have to be improved. Once it is done, we are convinced that the proposed fibre probe together with the elaborated ML techniques constitutes a highly promising device for a prompt and precise in situ decision-making and would allow to choose the optimal surgical tactics during the tumour resection.

As a next step, we will elaborate a procedure for the collection of data with much higher quality as well as improve the design of the fibre-optic probe by, for instance, dropping the 365 nm excitation channel and introducing a non-contact proximity sensor.

Author Contributions: Original draft preparation, data curation and processing, data acquisition software, E.Z.; data processing, draft preparation, M.Z.; measurements, methodology, data curation, E.P.; measurements, K.K.; data acquisition setup, methodology, V.D.; experiments at the Orel Regional Clinical Hospital, conceptualisation, A.M.; conceptualisation, S.S.; initiated and supervised the work, project administration, E.U.R.; funding acquisition, supervision, project administration, A.D.; all authors edited the manuscript. All authors have read and agreed to the published version of the manuscript.

Acknowledgments: This study was supported by the Russian Science Foundation under project No. 18-15-00201 (development of experimental setup and data acquisition). Special thanks are extended to the patients of the Orel Regional Clinical Hospital who kindly agreed to take part in the studies in the framework of their planned minimally invasive surgical intervention. M.Z. would like to acknowledge the funding received within the H2020-MSCA-IF-2017 scheme (grant No. 792421). E.Z. acknowledges the support of the Academy of Finland (grant No. 318281). V.D. acknowledges the funding received within the H2020-MSCA-IF-2018 scheme (grant No. 839888).

References

1. Siegel, R.L.; Miller, K.D.; Jemal, A. Cancer statistics, 2019. *CA Cancer J. Clin.* **2019**, *69*, 7–34. [CrossRef] [PubMed]
2. Tearney, G.; Brezinski, M.; Bouma, B.; Boppart, S.; Pitris, C.; Southern, J.; Fujimoto, J. In vivo endoscopic optical biopsy with optical coherence tomography. *Science* **1997**, *276*, 2037–2039. [CrossRef] [PubMed]
3. Sonn, G.A.; Jones, S.N.E.; Tarin, T.V.; Du, C.B.; Mach, K.E.; Jensen, K.C.; Liao, J.C. Optical biopsy of human bladder neoplasia with in vivo confocal laser endomicroscopy. *J. Urol.* **2009**, *182*, 1299–1305. [CrossRef] [PubMed]
4. Ladabaum, U.; Fioritto, A.; Mitani, A.; Desai, M.; Kim, J.P.; Rex, D.K.; Imperiale, T.; Gunaratnam, N. Real-time optical biopsy of colon polyps with narrow band imaging in community practice does not yet meet key thresholds for clinical decisions. *Gastroenterology* **2013**, *144*, 81–91. [CrossRef]
5. Wang, T.D.; Van Dam, J. Optical biopsy: A new frontier in endoscopic detection and diagnosis. *Clin. Gastroenterol. Hepatol.* **2004**, *2*, 744–753. [CrossRef]
6. Soulet, D.; Lamontagne-Proulx, J.; Aube, B.; Davalos, D. Multiphoton intravital microscopy in small animals: Motion artefact challenges and technical solutions. *J. Microsc.* **2020**, *278*, 3–17. [CrossRef]
7. Tonutti, M.; Elson, D.S.; Yang, G.Z.; Darzi, A.W.; Sodergren, M.H. The role of technology in minimally invasive surgery: State of the art, recent developments and future directions. *Postgrad. Med. J.* **2017**, *93*, 159–167. [CrossRef]
8. Nazeer, S.S.; Saraswathy, A.; Shenoy, S.J.; Jayasree, R.S. Fluorescence spectroscopy as an efficient tool for staging the degree of liver fibrosis: An in vivo comparison with MRI. *Sci. Rep.* **2018**, *8*, 10967. [CrossRef]
9. Zhao, M.; Dong, L.; Liu, Z.; Yang, S.; Wu, W.; Lin, J. In vivo fluorescence imaging of hepatocellular carcinoma using a novel GPC3-specific aptamer probe. *Quant. Imaging Med. Surg.* **2018**, *8*, 151–160. [CrossRef]
10. Sun, H.; Tan, W.; Zu, Y. Aptamers: Versatile molecular recognition probes for cancer detection. *Analyst* **2016**, *141*, 403–415. [CrossRef]
11. Buttemere, C.; Chari, R.; Anderson, C.; Washington, M.; Mahadevan-Jansen, A.; Lin, W. In vivo assessment of thermal damage in the liver using optical spectroscopy. *J. Biomed. Opt.* **2004**, *9*, 1018–1027. [CrossRef]
12. Gulledge, C.; Dewhirst, M. Tumor oxygenation: A matter of supply and demand. *Anticancer Res.* **1996**, *16*, 741.
13. Druzhkova, I.N.; Shirmanova, M.V.; Lukina, M.M.; Dudenkova, V.V.; Mishina, N.M.; Zagaynova, E.V. The metabolic interaction of cancer cells and fibroblasts–coupling between NAD (P) H and FAD, intracellular pH and hydrogen peroxide. *Cell Cycle* **2016**, *15*, 1257–1266. [CrossRef]
14. Liu, Q.; Grant, G.; Li, S.; Wilson, C.; Li, J.; Bigner, D.; Zhang, Y.; Hu, F.; Vo-Dinh, T.; Chen, K. Compact point-detection fluorescence spectroscopy system for quantifying intrinsic fluorescence redox ratio in brain cancer diagnostics. *J. Biomed. Opt.* **2011**, *16*, 037004. [CrossRef]
15. Palmer, S.; Litvinova, K.S.; Rafailov, E.U.; Nabi, G. Detection of urinary bladder cancer cells using redox 35ratio and double excitation wavelengths autofluorescence. *Biomed. Opt. Express* **2015**, *6*, 977–986. [CrossRef]
16. Awasthi, K.; Moriya, D.; Nakabayashi, T.; Li, L.; Ohta, N. Sensitive detection of intracellular environment of normal and cancer cells by autofluorescence lifetime imaging. *J. Photochem. Photobiol. B Biol.* **2016**, *165*, 256–265. [CrossRef] [PubMed]
17. Wang, M.; Long, F.; Tang, F.; Jing, Y.; Wang, X.; Yao, L.; Ma, J.; Fei, Y.; Chen, L.; Wang, G.; et al. Autofluorescence imaging and spectroscopy of human lung cancer. *Appl. Sci.* **2017**, *7*, 32. [CrossRef]
18. Kandurova, K.; Dremin, V.; Zherebtsov, E.; Potapova, E.; Alyanov, A.; Mamoshin, A.; Ivanov, Y.; Borsukov, A.; Dunaev, A. Fiber-optic system for intraoperative study of abdominal organs during minimally invasive surgical interventions. *Appl. Sci.* **2019**, *9*, 217. [CrossRef]
19. Zherebtsov, E.; Dremin, V.; Popov, A.; Doronin, A.; Kurakina, D.; Kirillin, M.; Meglinski, I.; Bykov, A. Hyperspectral imaging of human skin aided by artificial neural networks. *Biomed. Opt. Express* **2019**, *10*, 3545–3559. [CrossRef]

21. Zhen, S.H.; Cheng, M.; Tao, Y.B.; Wang, Y.F.; Juengpanich, S.; Jiang, Z.Y.; Jiang, Y.K.; Yan, Y.Y.; Lu, W.; Lue, J.M.; et al. Deep learning for accurate diagnosis of liver tumor based on magnetic resonance imaging and clinical data. *Front. Oncol.* **2020**, *10*, 680. [CrossRef] [PubMed]
22. Pan, C.; Schoppe, O.; Parra-Damas, A.; Cai, R.; Todorov, M.I.; Gondi, G.; von Neubeck, B.; Bögürcü-Seidel, N.; Seidel, S.; Sleiman, K.; et al. Deep learning reveals cancer metastasis and therapeutic antibody targeting in the entire body. *Cell* **2019**, *179*, 1661–1676.e19. [CrossRef]
23. Lin, H.; Wei, C.; Wang, G.; Chen, H.; Lin, L.; Ni, M.; Chen, J.; Zhuo, S. Automated classification of hepatocellular carcinoma differentiation using multiphoton microscopy and deep learning. *J. Biophotonics* **2019**, *12*, e201800435. [CrossRef] [PubMed]
24. Dremin, V.; Potapova, E.; Zherebtsov, E.; Kandurova, K.; Shupletsov, V.; Alekseyev, A.; Mamoshin, A.; Dunaev, A. Optical percutaneous needle biopsy of the liver: A pilot animal and clinical study. *Sci. Rep.* **2020**, *10*, 14200. [CrossRef] [PubMed]
25. Dunaev, A.V.; Drernin, V.V.; Zherebtsov, E.A.; Rafailov, I.E.; Litvinova, K.S.; Palmer, S.G.; Stewart, N.A.; Sokolovski, S.G.; Rafailov, E.U. Individual variability analysis of fluorescence parameters measured in skin with different levels of nutritive blood flow. *Med. Eng. Phys.* **2015**, *37*, 574–583. [CrossRef]
26. Zherebtsov, E.; Dremin, V.; Zharkikh, E.; Zherebtsova, A.; Rafailov, I.; Dunaev, A.; Bazieva, N.; Rafailov, E. Fibre-Optic Probe for Fluorescence Diagnostics with Blood Influence Compensation. In Proceedings of the SPIE Conference on Dynamics and Fluctuations in Biomedical Photonics XV, San Francisco, CA, USA, 28–29 January 2018; Tuchin, V.V., Larin, K.V., Leahy, M.J., Wang, R.K., Eds.; SPIE: Bellingham, WA, USA, 2018; Volume 10493.
27. Lancaster, G.; Stefanovska, A.; Pesce, M.; Vezzoni, G.M.; Loggini, B.; Pingitore, R.; Ghiara, F.; Barachini, P.; Cervadoro, G.; Romanelli, M.; et al. Dynamic markers based on blood perfusion fluctuations for selecting skin melanocytic lesions for biopsy. *Sci. Rep.* **2015**, *5*, 12825. [CrossRef] [PubMed]
28. Cover, T.; Hart, P. Nearest neighbor pattern classification. *IEEE Trans. Inf. Theory* **1967**, *13*, 21–27. [CrossRef]
29. Podgorelec, V.; Kokol, P.; Stiglic, B.; Rozman, I. Decision trees: An overview and their use in medicine. *J. Med. Syst.* **2002**, *26*, 445–463. [CrossRef]
30. Vapnik, V.N. *Statistical Learning Theory*; Wiley-Interscience: Hoboken, NJ, USA, 1998.
31. Breiman, L. Random Forests. *Mach. Learn.* **2001**, *45*, 5–32. [CrossRef]
32. Freund, Y.; Schapire, R.; Abe, N.A. Short Introduction to Boosting. *J. Jpn. Soc. Artif. Intell.* **1999**, *14*, 1612.
33. Loong, T. Understanding sensitivity and specificity with the right side of the brain. *BMJ Br. Med. J.* **2003**, *327*, 716–719. [CrossRef] [PubMed]
34. Dremin, V.; Kozlov, I.; Volkov, M.; Margaryants, N.; Potemkin, A.; Zherebtsov, E.; Dunaev, A.; Gurov, I. Dynamic evaluation of blood flow microcirculation by combined use of the laser Doppler flowmetry and high-speed videocapillaroscopy methods. *J. Biophotonics* **2019**, *12*, e201800317. [CrossRef] [PubMed]
35. McKinlay, A.; Bernhardt, J.; Ahlbom, A.; Cesarini, J.; de Gruijl, F.; Hietanen, M.; Owen, R.; Sliney, D.; Soderberg, P.; Swerdlow, A.; et al. Guidelines on limits of exposure to ultraviolet radiation of wavelengths between 180 nm and 400 nm (incoherent optical radiation). *Health Phys.* **2004**, *87*, 171–186.

6

Neuron Stimulation Device Integrated with Silicon Nanowire-Based Photodetection Circuit on a Flexible Substrate

Suk Won Jung [1,2], Jong Yoon Shin [1], Kilwha Pi [1], Yong Sook Goo [3] and Dong-il "Dan" Cho [1,*]

[1] ISRC/ASRI, Department of Electrical and Computer Engineering, Seoul National University, 1 Gwanak-ro, Gwanak-gu, Seoul 08826, Korea; jungsw@keti.re.kr (S.W.J.); jshin33@snu.ac.kr (J.Y.S.); khpi1@snu.ac.kr (K.P.)

[2] Human Care System Research Center, Convergence System R&D Division, Korea Electronics Technology Institute, 25 Saenari-ro, Bundang-gu, Seongnam-si, Gyeonggi-do 13509, Korea

[3] Department of Physiology, College of Medicine, Chungbuk National University, 1 Chungdae-ro, Seowon-gu, Cheongju, Chungbuk 28644, Korea; ysgoo@chungbuk.ac.kr

* Correspondence: dicho@snu.ac.kr

Academic Editors: Dragan Indjin, Željka Cvejić and Małgorzata Jędrzejewska-Szczerska

Abstract: This paper proposes a neural stimulation device integrated with a silicon nanowire (SiNW)-based photodetection circuit for the activation of neurons with light. The proposed device is comprised of a voltage divider and a current driver in which SiNWs are used as photodetector and field-effect transistors; it has the functions of detecting light, generating a stimulation signal in proportion to the light intensity, and transmitting the signal to a micro electrode. To show the applicability of the proposed neural stimulation device as a high-resolution retinal prosthesis system, a high-density neural stimulation device with a unit cell size of 110 × 110 μm and a resolution of 32 × 32 was fabricated on a flexible film with a thickness of approximately 50 μm. Its effectiveness as a retinal stimulation device was then evaluated using a unit cell in an in vitro animal experiment involving the retinal tissue of retinal Degeneration 1 (*rd1*) mice. Experiments wherein stimulation pulses were applied to the retinal tissues successfully demonstrate that the number of spikes in neural response signals increases in proportion to light intensity.

Keywords: neuron stimulation; silicon nanowire; photodetector; micro electrode; retinal prosthesis

---

1. Introduction

Impaired connectivity or functional disorders in the neural system hinder the activation of cells or the proper transmission of information. Neural stimulation methods have been extensively investigated as potential cures for a wide range of neurological disorders, such as mental disorders, dementia, motor disabilities, and visual impairment owing to retinal degeneration [1–4]. In such investigations, electrical stimulation using extracellular electrodes is extensively used as the method for activating neurons [5–7]. In conjunction with the use of extracellular electrodes, methods for the activation of neurons using light are also being studied. In these methods, light-sensitive devices are used for generating electrical stimulation signals [8–10]. For instance, in a retinal prosthetic system, image data are acquired from external cameras connected to intraocular micro electrodes through wires [11–14] or from internal photodetectors integrated with intraocular micro electrodes [15–18]. The modulated electrical signals are then transmitted to a micro electrode array (MEA) mounted into retinal cells.

In retinal prostheses, a high-resolution system is required to provide high-quality image perception ability to a visually handicapped patient. A key to successfully developing high-resolution systems is that the stimulation signals generated from image information are individually transmitted to a large number of stimulating electrodes [19]. In the case of retinal prosthesis systems that use external cameras, such an electrical interface becomes very complicated and difficult to implement because a camera and MEA are physically distinct and separate from each other. In fact, many commercialized retinal prostheses that use an external camera, such as the Argus II system [14] from Second Sight Medical Products Inc. (Sylmar, CA, USA) or EpiRet3 [13] of EpiRet GmbH, have a low resolution; these systems have only 60 and 25 stimulating electrodes integrated into the implant device, respectively. On the other hand, in the case of retinal prostheses with embedded photodetectors for image perception within their retinal implant devices instead of using externally worn cameras, the photodetector, the signal processing circuit, and stimulating electrodes are collocated at each cell of retinal implant devices. Much research on this topic is also underway. The US Optobionics Corporation manufactured a subretinal implant device called an 'artificial silicon retina' (ASR) [18] and conducted clinical experiments. The ASR device comprises 5000 cells, where micro photodiodes and stimulating electrodes are integrated on a silicon substrate of approximately 25 μm in thickness. The German Retina Implant AG developed a subretinal implant device using a silicon chip, in which 1500 cells with TiN electrodes are integrated with photodiodes and amplifying circuits fabricated by a CMOS process [15]. It was also reported that, by using the above subretinal implants, patients could recognize things or letters. Furthermore, it has been found from the existing research cases that photodetectors embedded in a device can easily solve the problem of signal line connection to high-density stimulating electrodes, and thus this method is advantageous for the implementation of a high-resolution retinal prosthesis system for a high-level image perception function. Despite the recent results of various studies on the development of a high-resolution retinal prosthesis system, there still remain problems that should be solved to implement a safer and more reliable retinal prosthesis system, such as low flexibility in a retinal stimulator device, the possibility of cell necrosis due to the overheating of a retinal stimulator chip [20], and low biocompatibility of the device material [21].

As a method for light-based activation of neurons that can be applied to high-resolution retinal prosthesis systems by solving the above-described problems, this paper proposes a novel neural stimulation method as well as a flexible neural stimulation device integrated with a silicon nanowire (SiNW)-based photodetection circuit. The SiNW-based photodetection circuit comprises a voltage divider and a current driver that uses a SiNW PD [22], SiNW FETs [19], and micro electrodes. The SiNW FET and the SiNW PD are connected in series via the voltage divider, making a large resistance variation in the SiNW PD desirable because the output voltage changes when the resistance varies when light detection occurs. In the fabricated SiNW PD, the resistance is approximately 5.6 GΩ in a dark environment and approximately 2.9 MΩ at 4040 lux, corresponding to a resistance ratio of approximately 1930, which is sufficiently large and useful over a high dynamic range. Thus, the output voltage of the voltage divider at the supply voltage is 5 V and the illuminance range is 0–10,000 lux, corresponding to a very large swing range of 0.1 V (dark)–4.8 V (10,000 lux). In the current driver, where the SiNW FET and micro electrodes are connected in series, the SiNW FET is driven by the output voltage of the voltage divider and the maximum on-current at the 5 V supply voltage was found to be approximately 480 μA with an on–off ratio of 5×10^4. Thus, the current driver has a sufficient on-current level and on–off characteristics to stimulate neurons via micro electrodes. Based on this preliminary analysis, the proposed process—stimulation signal modulation proportional to light intensity using a neuron stimulation device with a voltage divider and the current driver—could then be validated.

To demonstrate the applicability of the proposed neural stimulation method in high-resolution retinal prosthesis systems, a high-density neural stimulation device with a unit cell size of 110 × 110 μm and a resolution of 32 × 32 was fabricated on a flexible film approximately 50 μm thick. Its effectiveness as a light-based retinal stimulation device was evaluated by testing the unit cell in an in vitro animal experiment using the retinal tissue of *rd1* mice. Application of retinal stimulation pulses to the retinal tissue demonstrated that the number of spikes in neural response signals increase in proportion to light intensity.

2. Experimental

2.1. Device Design and Configuration

This paper proposes a neural stimulation device and a method to evoke neural signals through the use of light. Figure 1a shows a block diagram of the unit cell of the proposed neural stimulation device and the process of neural stimulation resulting from the modulation of a stimulation signal according to the intensity of light irradiated onto the neural stimulation device. Figure 1b shows the configuration of the unit cell. The neural stimulation device comprises a SiNW PD, SiNW FETs, and micro electrodes (a stimulation electrode and a ground electrode). The resistance of the SiNW PD decreases as the light illumination intensity increases and the device can be classified as a sort of variable resistor. Thus, the neural stimulation device in Figure 1b can be expressed as the equivalent circuit in Figure 1c, which can functionally be divided into two parts: the voltage divider circuit on the left, and the current driver circuit on the right.

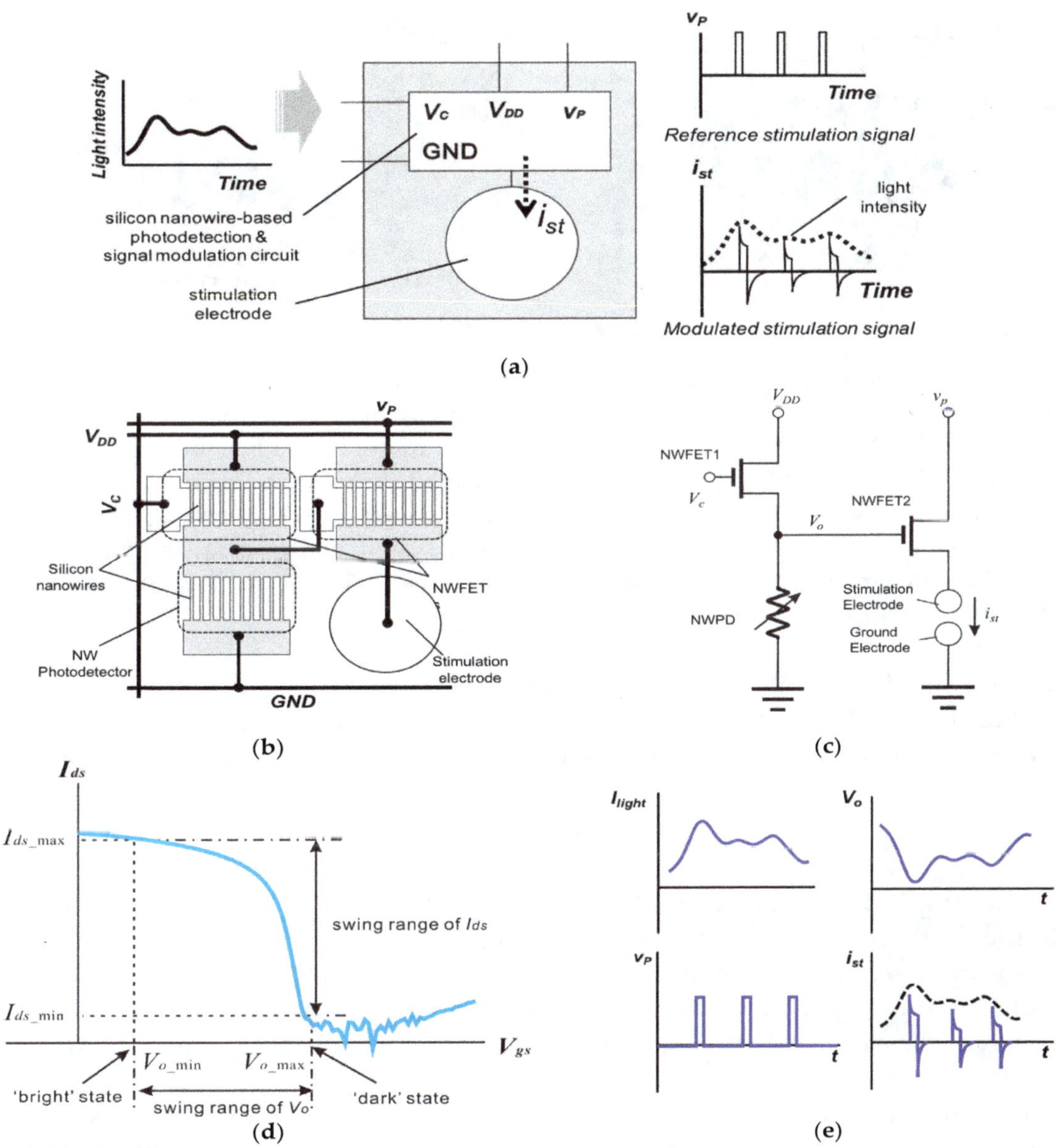

Figure 1. *Cont.*

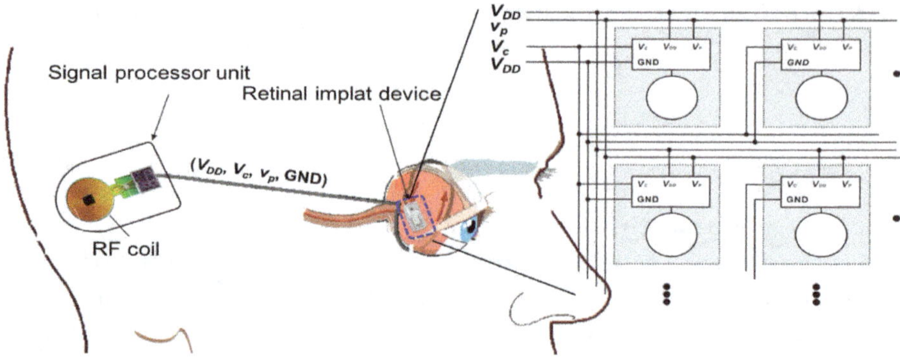

(f)

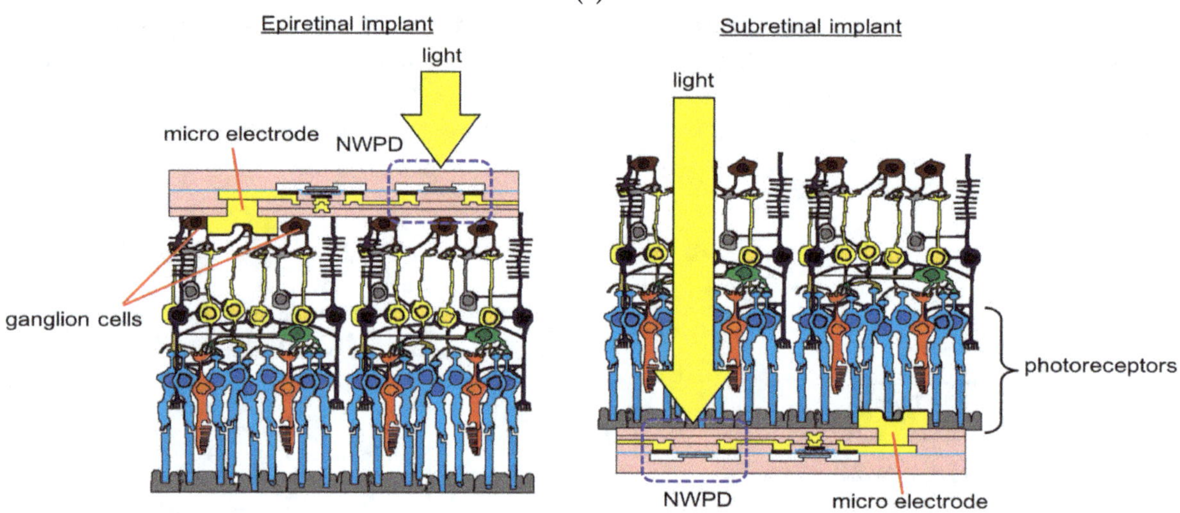

(g)

Figure 1. (**a**) Configuration and a block diagram of unit cell of the proposed neuron stimulation device and a modulation procedure of stimulation signal by light detection; (**b**) Configuration of device composed of SiNW FETs, a SiNW PD, and micro electrodes; (**c**) Equivalent circuit of the device; (**d**) V_{gs}-I_{ds} curve of the SiNW FET2 (NWFET2) and the relation between the V_o's swing range and the current swing range of the NWFET2; (**e**) Waveforms of the signals I_{light}, V_o, v_p and i_{st}; (**f**) Configuration of proposed device for a high resolution retinal prosthetic system and internal electrical connection diagram of the retinal prosthetic device; (**g**) Epiretinal and subretinal implantation of the proposed neural stimulation device in an eye ball.

In the voltage divider circuit on the left, the resistance of SiNW FET1 (NWFET1) is controlled by the control voltage (V_c), and the resistance of SiNW PD (NWPD) varies with light illumination intensity. Therefore, the output voltage (V_o) of the voltage divider can be expressed by the following equation:

$$V_o = \frac{R_{NWPD}}{R_{NWFET1} + R_{NWPD}} \cdot V_{DD}, \quad (1)$$

where V_{DD} is the supply voltage, R_{NWFET1} is the resistance of NWFET1, and R_{NWPD} is the resistance of NWPD. In the 'dark' condition with no light illumination, V_o becomes maximum because R_{NWPD} becomes maximum. As the intensity of light irradiated onto NWPD increases, both R_{NWPD} and V_o gradually decrease. If the intensity of light irradiated onto the neural stimulation device varies over time, V_o will have a waveform with a shape inverse to the waveform of light intensity, as shown in Figure 1e.

In the current driver circuit on the right side of the equivalent circuit, NWFET2 is driven by V_o. If NWFET2 has the gate-source voltage to drain-source current (V_{gs}-I_{ds}) characteristics shown in Figure 1d, I_{ds} becomes minimum ($I_{ds} = I_{ds\_min}$) when V_o is maximum ($V_o = V_{o\_max}$, at the dark state), and I_{ds} becomes maximum ($I_{ds} = I_{ds\_max}$) when V_o is minimum ($V_o = V_{o\_min}$, when light intensity is the greatest). Figure 1e illustrates one example of the waveform of v_p. The reference stimulation signal of a unipolar pulse signal with fixed amplitude and frequency is applied to the drain of NWFET2. If NWFET2 is driven by V_o with the wave waveform shown in Figure 1e, the pattern of the stimulation signal that is transmitted to the micro electrodes and neurons has the shape i_{st}, as shown in Figure 1e. It is seen that each pulse of the reference stimulation signal is modulated to have an amplitude proportional to light intensity; in this way, the proposed neural stimulation detects light intensity and can perform stimulation signal modulation in proportion to light intensity.

The proposed neural stimulation device can most effectively be used in retinal prosthetic systems. To do so, it is necessary to fabricate a retinal implant unit integrated with high-density cells. Figure 1f shows a method for high-density integration of the proposed neural stimulation device for application to a high-resolution retinal prosthetic system. The block diagram shows the arrangement of the device's cells in a 2D matrix pattern and the method for the connection of signal lines for each cell. As each unit cell can modulate stimulation signals through the independent detection of light intensity, it is only necessary to connect the four signal lines V_{DD}, v_p, V_c, and a ground (GND) electrode. The retinal implant unit integrated with these high-density neural stimulation cells is connected to a separately fabricated signal processor. The retinal implant unit is easily implantable into the eyeball as it is fabricated in a flexible form that can be bent to fit the curvature of the eye; the signal processor unit, on the other hand, is implanted remotely. An RF coil for communication with external devices and a wireless electric power supply and a signal processing chip for controlling the implant device are embedded into the processor unit. An electrostatic discharge (ESD) protection circuit is required for a practical implementation and it can be integrated in the signal processing chip. The proposed retinal implant unit can be applied to both epiretinal and subretinal implant methods as shown in Figure 1g. In epiretinal implants, the micro electrodes are in contact with ganglion cells and the light is incident on the opposite side where the micro electrodes are formed and reaches the NWPDs. In subretinal implants, the micro electrodes are in contact with photoreceptors and the light is incident on the same side where the micro electrodes are formed and reaches the NWPDs.

2.2. Fabrication and Results

Figure 2 shows the process for fabricating the proposed neural stimulation device into a flexible form and the process for fabrication of the current driver component, in which the silicon nanowire FET and micro electrodes are connected in series. In the first step, silicon nanowires are formed using the top-down method (Figure 2a–e) [23]. Subsequently, polysilicon gates and source and drain electrodes are fabricated (Figure 2f–j). The electric signal lines (V_{DD}, v_p, V_c and GND) are then formed via a multi-layer metallization process (Figure 2k,l). A 5 μm-thick polyimide layer is patterned and Au micro electrodes are then formed via an Au electroplating process (Figure 2m). For biocompatibility, a Pt-black layer can be formed on the surface of the Au electrodes by a successive Pt electroplating process after the Au electroplating process [24]. Theoretically, TiN micro electrodes can be fabricated by TiN sputtering and RIE (Reactive Ion Etching) processes instead of electroplating. In this paper, Pt-black micro electrodes are fabricated and are used for the following in vitro experiments. After the micro electrodes are fabricated, the device wafer is bonded with a dummy wafer using a bonding wax, BGL-7160 (AI Technology Inc., Princeton, NJ, USA), and the device wafer is thinned to approximately 30 μm via a chemical-mechanical planarization (CMP) process (Figure 2n,o). Photoresist (PR) patterning is performed and the silicon is etched by using a deep reactive ion etch (DRIE) process (Figure 2p). The bonding wax is melted by heating the substrate to 160 °C, and the fabrication of the flexible neural stimulation device is completed by separating the neural stimulation device from the dummy substrate (Figure 2q–s).

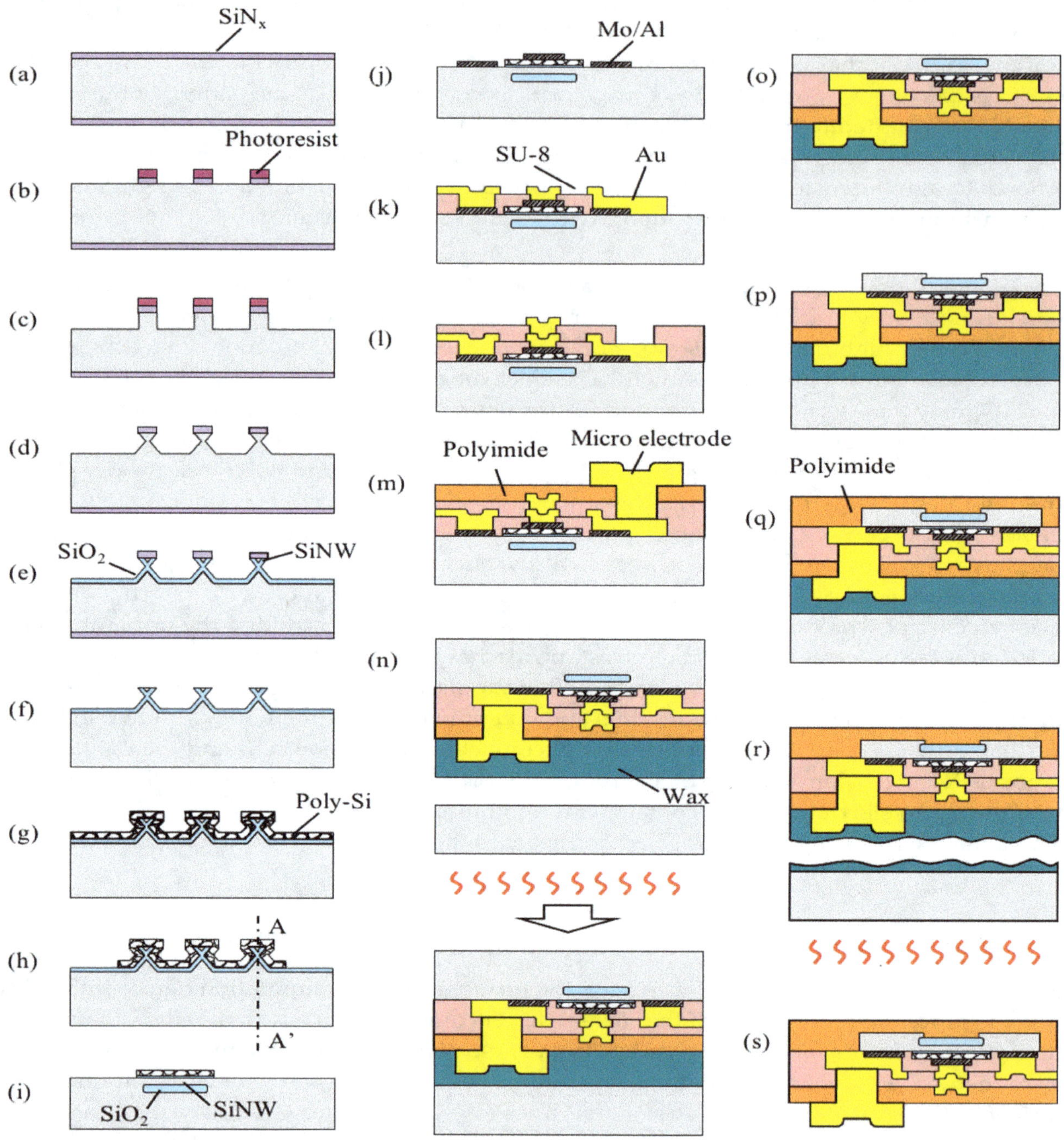

Figure 2. Fabrication process of the proposed high resolution neural stimulation devices integrated with SiNW-based photodetection circuit. (**a**) SiN deposition by low pressure chemical vapor deposition (LPCVD); (**b**) SiN dry etch; (**c**) Si dry etch; (**d**) Si wet etch using tetra-methyl-ammonium-hydroxide (TMAH) solution; (**e**) SiNW formation by wet oxidation process; (**f**) SiN strip by the use of H_3PO_4 solution; (**g**) Gate oxide and Poly-Si formation; (**h**) Poly-Si dry etch; (**i**) Cross-sectional view of A-A′ of Figure 2h; (**j**) Source, drain, gate electrodes formation; (**k**) First dielectric layer (SU-8) and electrical lines (V_{DD}, GND) formation; (**l**) Second dielectric layer and electrical lines (V_c, v_p) formation; (**m**) Third dielectric layer (polyimide) and micro electrodes formation; (**n**) Device wafer bonding on a dummy wafer; (**o**) Device wafer thinning by chemical-mechanical polishing (CMP); (**p**) Si dry etch; (**q**) Cover polyimide coating; (**r**) Separating fabricated devices from the dummy wafer; (**s**) Device cleaning by residual wax removal.

Figure 3a shows the shape of the column structure after the dry etching of silicon in Figure 2c: scallops formed on the sidewall of the structure are seen, as the Si DRIE process is used. As seen in Figure 3b, following wet etching using tetra-methyl-ammonium-hydroxide (TMAH) solution, the scallops disappear as the sidewall of the column structure is etched. Figure 3c shows the triangular shape of a silicon nanowire formed following the wet oxidation process. It is seen that the top of the silicon nanowire has formed with a width of approximately 450 nm. Figure 4 shows the 32 × 32 neural stimulation device fabricated using the process in Figure 2. Figure 4a–c show the device after the Si DRIE process in Figure 2p has been completed. The size of the unit cell is 110 × 110 μm and it used 10 SiNWs with a length of 20 μm each to compose NWFET1, NWFEET2, and NWPD. A center microelectrode 30 μm in diameter with a surrounding ground electrode is also present. Figure 4d shows the neural stimulation device separated from the substrate after the process has been completed. The device is approximately 50 μm thick and it is very flexible.

The characteristics of NWPD and NWFET depend on the thickness and doping concentration of the silicon nanowires. In this paper, the thickness of silicon nanowires is controlled by a photolithography process, RIE processes, a Si TMAH wet etching process, and an oxidation process. In the case of TMAH silicon wet etching process, even though there is a slight difference in the wet etching time, an etch stop condition is formed by the hourglass silicon structure so that the deviation of the top width of the silicon structure is insignificant. In the remaining processes, the process deviations are controlled to within approximately 5%, and therefore, the effects on the thickness of the nanowire are not significant. The doping concentration of the silicon nanowires can also be precisely controlled by an ion implantation process. Therefore, the influences of the process variation on the characteristics of NWPD and NWFET are not significant.

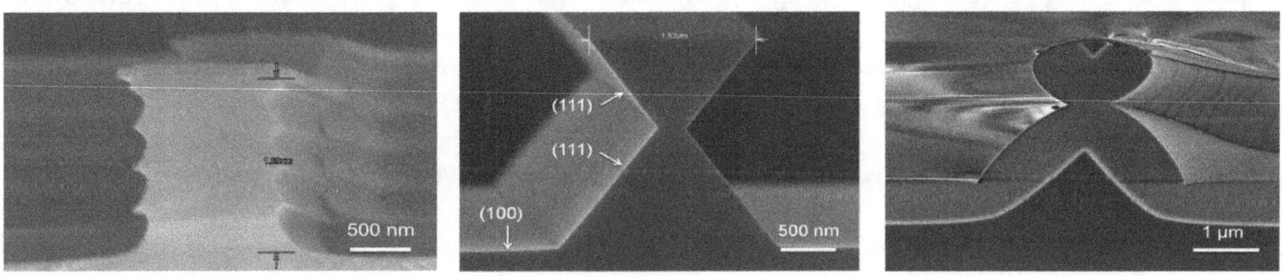

(a) (b) (c)

Figure 3. Fabricated SiNWs. (**a**) Formation of column structures by Si deep RIE process; (**b**) Formation of hourglass shaped structures by Si anisotropic wet etch process; (**c**) SiNW formation by wet oxidation process.

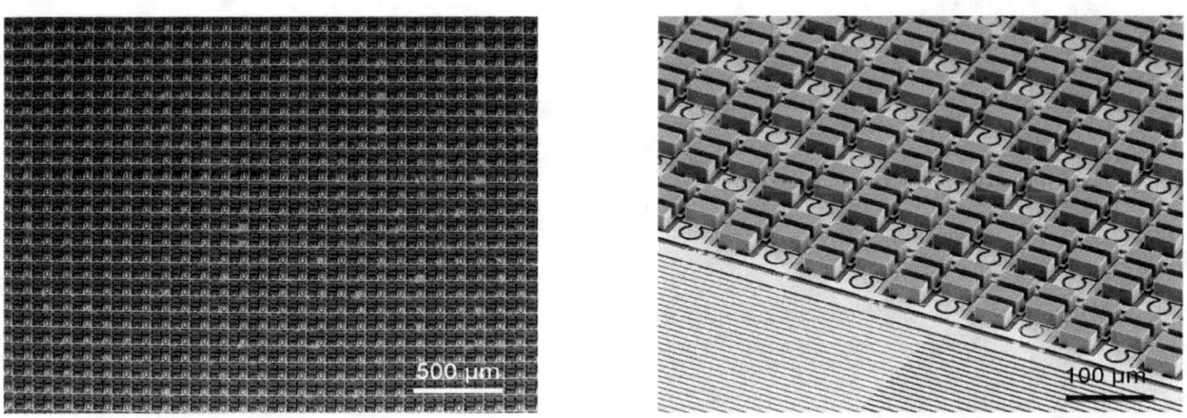

(a) (b)

Figure 4. *Cont.*

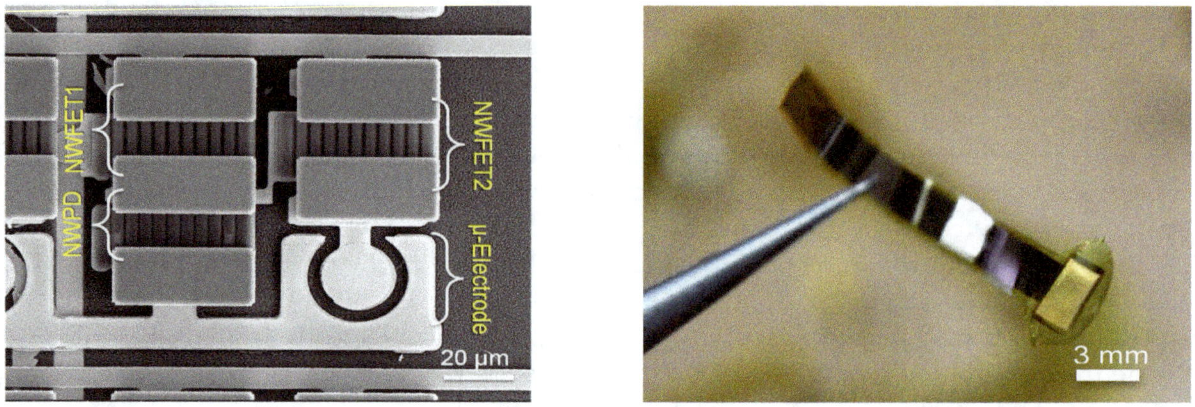

(c) (d)

Figure 4. Fabricated high-resolution neural stimulation device. (**a**) Top view of the fabricated device after Si deep RIE process of Figure 2p; (**b**) Perspective view of Figure 4a; (**c**) Unit cell of the device; (**d**) Flexible neural stimulation device with 32 × 32 resolution.

3. Results and Discussions

3.1. Device Characterization

SiNW PDs and SiNW FETs, the basic devices composing the neural stimulation device, were fabricated using the process shown in Figure 2, following which the characteristics of each device were examined. To investigate the resistance variation of an SiNW PD as a function of light intensity, the photo-induced output ($I_{ds} \sim V_{ds}$) characteristics of the SiNW PD were measured at varying halogen lamp-produced light intensities (I_{light}), as shown in Figure 5a. Figure 5b shows the results of calculating the photocurrent (I_{ph}) and resistance (R_{NWPD}) of the SiNW PD against light intensity for V_{ds} = 1 V using the *I–V* graph in Figure 5a. The graph shows that both I_{ph} and R_{NWPD} abruptly change within an illuminance range of low light intensity, above which the change is more gradual. R_{NWPD} shows a high value of approximately 5.6 GΩ in a dark environment and approximately 2.9 MΩ in a bright environment of 4040 lux. Thus, the resistance change rate is so great that the ratio between the two resistance values, $R_{NWPD(dark)}/R_{NWPD(bright)}$, goes as high as 1930. In particular, it is apparent from the graph that the SiNW PD shows high sensitivity in a low illuminance range.

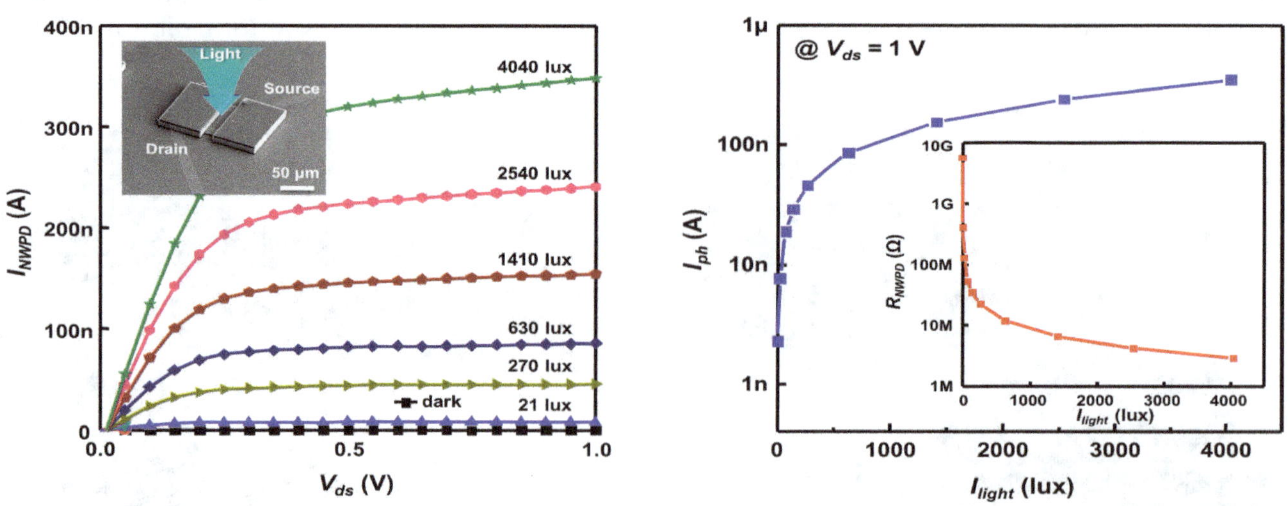

(a) (b)

Figure 5. *Cont.*

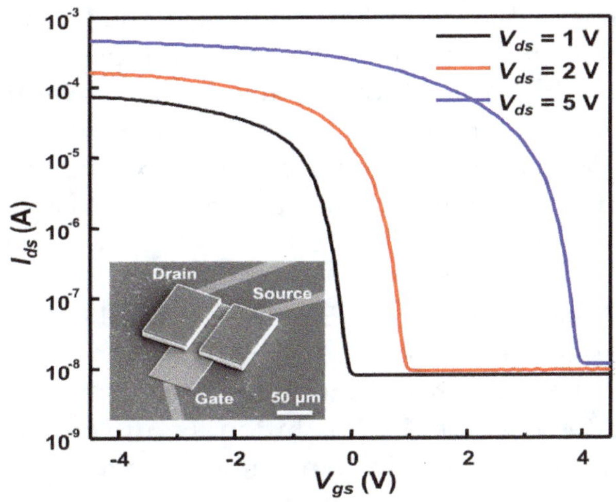

(c)

Figure 5. (**a**) *I-V* curves of the fabricated SiNW PD against varying light illumination intensity; (**b**) Photocurrent and resistance values of the SiNW PD against light intensity; (**c**) V_{gs}-I_{ds} curves of the SiNW FET for several bias voltages.

The relative resistance of the SiNW FET used in the voltage divider circuit to that of the SiNW PD is important. The resistance of the SiNW FET (R_{NWFET}) is controlled by the gate-source voltage (V_{gs}), and the value that it can obtain is shown in Figure 5c, which shows the transfer ($I_{ds} \sim V_{gs}$) characteristics of a fabricated SiNW FET. If the conditions of $R_{NWPD(dark)} \gg R_{NWFET}$ in a dark environment and $R_{NWPD(bright)} \ll R_{NWFET}$ in a bright environment are satisfied, the voltage range V_o of the voltage divider is found according to Equation (1) to be V_{DD} (dark)–0 V (bright), resulting in the maximum swing range. For this, V_{gs} must be set so that $R_{NWPD(dark)} \gg R_{NWFET} \gg R_{NWPD(bright)}$. On the other hand, the threshold voltage (V_{th}), maximum on-current (I_{ON_max}), and on–off ratio are important parameters for the SiNW FET used in the current driver circuit. In Figure 5c, the threshold voltage moves from approximately 0 V (when V_{ds} is 1 V) to 4 V (when V_{ds} is 5 V). I_{ON_max} is approximately 480 μA when V_{ds} is 5 V, and the on–off ratio of SiNW FET is approximately 5×10^4 when V_{ds} is 5 V. Thus, it is found that the SiNW FET has sufficient on-current level and on–off characteristics for use as the current driver circuit.

Figure 6 shows the results of an experiment evaluating the characteristics of both the voltage divider and current driver (which together form the proposed neural stimulation device) and verifying the previously discussed process of stimulation signal modulation. Figure 6a shows the fabricated neural stimulation device. Figure 6b shows the measurement results obtained from the voltage divider, in which V_o was measured against V_c by varying the intensity of light irradiated onto the SiNW PD. In Figure 6b, it is seen that if $V_c < 3.4$ V (Region I in Figure 6b), V_o remains at close to V_{DD} = 5 V despite the variations in R_{NWPD} induced by variations in light intensity. This occurs because the value of V_c that determines that R_{NWFET1} always remains much smaller than R_{NWFET1} even though R_{NWPD} is lowered under a bright environment: that is, $R_{NWFET1} \ll R_{NWPD}$. Under this condition, Equation (1) gives $V_o \approx V_{DD}$ regardless of the light intensity. By contrast, if $V_c > 4.1$ V (Region III in Figure 6b), V_o remains in the very low range of 0–0.6 V despite variations in light intensity. This is a case that falls under the condition in which $R_{NWFET1} \gg R_{NWPD}$, under which Equation (1) gives $V_o \approx 0$ V regardless of the light intensity. For the region 3.4 V $< V_c <$ 4.1 V (Region II in Figure 6b), the output characteristics of V_o are shown in the graph in Figure 6c, in which the *x*-axis is replaced by light intensity. If V_c is set close to 3.8 V, the ideal condition of the voltage divider, $R_{NWPD(dark)} \gg R_{NWFET} \gg R_{NWPD(bright)}$, is satisfied. Therefore, when V_c is 3.8 V, V_o has the maximum output range of 4.8 V (dark) to 0.1 V (10,000 lux). From the graph, it is apparent that for V_c = 3.8 V and above, the voltage divider works sensitively in the range of low illuminance below 100 lux and is increasingly insensitive as illuminance increases.

By contrast, for $V_c = 3.8$ V and below, it is seen that the voltage divider is rather insensitive in the range of low illuminance and works sensitively in the range of high illuminance above 100 lux. In addition, as V_o acts as the gate voltage of the NWFET2 of the current driver circuit that determines the output current level, it is necessary to consider the light intensity range and the level of concomitant output current in the selection of the value of V_c. Figure 6d shows an experimental setup for investigating the output characteristics of the current driver circuit. The drain of NWFET2 is connected to a reference stimulation signal generated by a function generator having an amplitude of 5 V and a duration of 20 ms. The reference stimulation signal used in the experiment is monophasic, but a biphasic pulse signal can also be used. The drain of NWFET2 is connected to the reference stimulation signal generated by a function generator. The reference stimulation signal has an amplitude of 5 V and a duration of 20 ms. The source of NWFET2 is connected to the Au test electrode, and the test electrode is immersed in phosphate buffered saline (PBS) solution. Figure 6e shows the waveform of current transmitted to the micro electrode measured against gate voltage (V_o). The maximum peak current for V_o is approximately 123 μA when V_o is 0 V, and when $V_o > 4$ V, NWFET2 is off and therefore the current signal is no longer transmitted. Figure 6f shows the waveform of a stimulation current signal (i_{st}) transmitted to test electrodes after randomly varying the intensity of light illuminated onto a neural stimulation device employing a voltage divider and a current driver. The illuminance waveform (I_{light}) and the concomitant stimulation current waveform are simultaneously depicted on the graph. It is seen that each pulse of the reference stimulation signal is modulated to have an amplitude that is relatively proportional to light intensity. The above results show that the proposed neural stimulation device detects light intensity and can perform stimulation signal modulation in proportion to the light intensity.

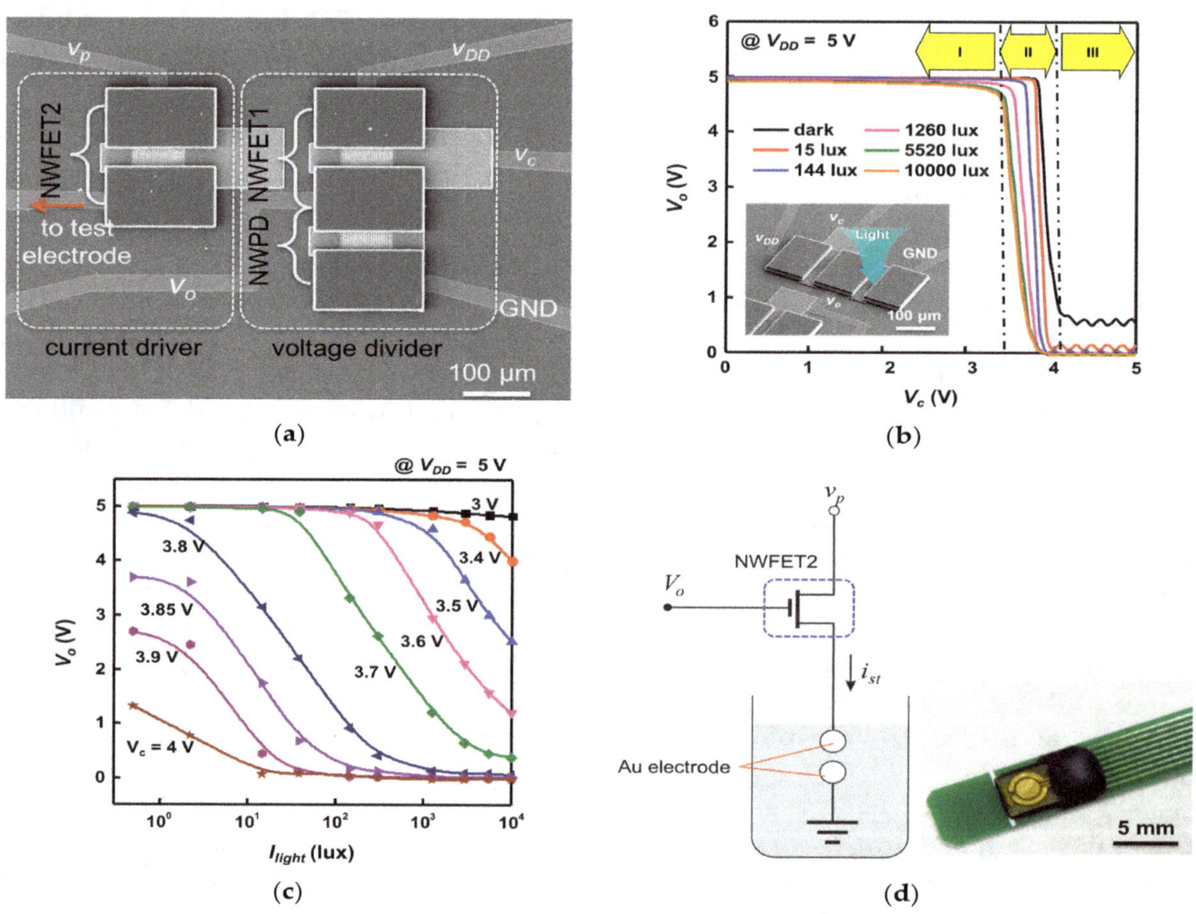

Figure 6. *Cont.*

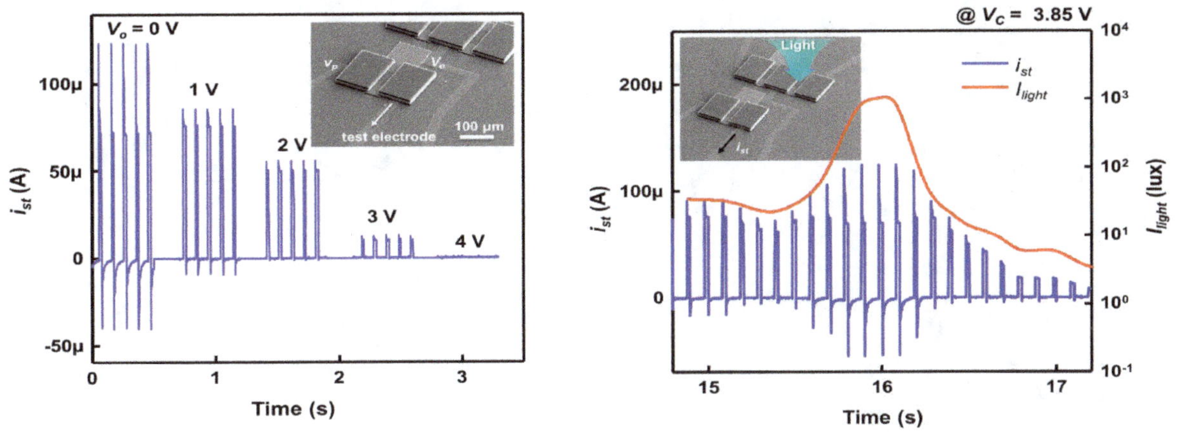

(e) (f)

Figure 6. (**a**) Fabricated neural stimulation device; (**b**) Output voltage curve of the voltage divider against control voltage by light intensity; (**c**) Output voltage curve of the voltage divider against light intensity by control voltage; (**d**) Measurement setup of the current driver; (**e**) Waveform of current is transmitted to the micro electrode against gate voltage V_o when V_c = 3.85 V; (**f**) Modulation waveform of stimulation signal for the neural stimulation device, which is proportional to light intensity.

3.2. *In Vitro Experiment*

An in vitro animal experiment was performed in order to evaluate the effectiveness of activating neurons using the fabricated neural stimulation device. The experimental setup was configured as shown in Figure 7a. A drain voltage (V_{DD}) of 10 V was applied to the voltage divider of the neural stimulation device, and a uniform rectangular pulse v_{st}, with amplitude 12 V, pulse width (duration) 1 ms, and frequency 1 Hz, was generated using a field programmable gate array (FPGA). The source side of NWFET2 was connected to one of the MEA electrodes, as shown in Figure 7a. The MEA, which is shown in Figure 7b, comprised 60 micro electrodes and a reference electrode. The micro electrode was a circular electrode 50 μm in diameter and was fabricated by forming an Au (~2 μm) layer and a Pt-black layer (~4 μm) via successive electroforming processes. The Pt-black layer of the micro electrode had a wide surface area owing to its nano-porous structure and had the effects of lowering the interface impedance between the micro electrodes and the retinal cells and enlarging the injection charge capacity [24]. One MEA electrode connected to the current driver was used to stimulate the retinal nerve, and the remaining electrodes were used to record neural response signals. The retinal cell for the in vitro experiment was extirpated from an *rd1* mouse. As shown in Figure 7c, the separated retinal cell was stuck closely to the MEA chip so that the ganglion cell could come into contact with the MEA. A well structure was formed around the retinal cell and then filled with cerebrospinal fluid (CSF) so that the retinal cell could maintain its function for a long time.

Figure 8a–d shows the neural response signals produced in the in vitro experiment using the neural stimulation device. Figure 8a shows an example of the neural response signals at 60 channels and represents the locations of a stimulating electrode and of a reference electrode. The effectiveness of stimulation can be evaluated by observing significant changes in the number of spikes after the stimulation signal is applied. Figure 8b shows the results of analyzing the neural response signals of two channels. The histogram graph represents the total number of spikes in neural signals in an interval of 10 ms before and after the application of 100 stimulation pulses. In Figure 8b, a distinctive increase in the number of spikes can be identified within about 0.2 s after application of the stimulation pulses. Figure 8c is a color map that represents the number of spikes per pulse (spikes/pulse) obtained from the histogram of Figure 8b against light intensity for 60 channels. As is seen in Figure 8c, the number of spikes increase prominently as the light intensity increases. The neural response against intensity of stimulus can be quantified using the normalized response defined by Equation (2).

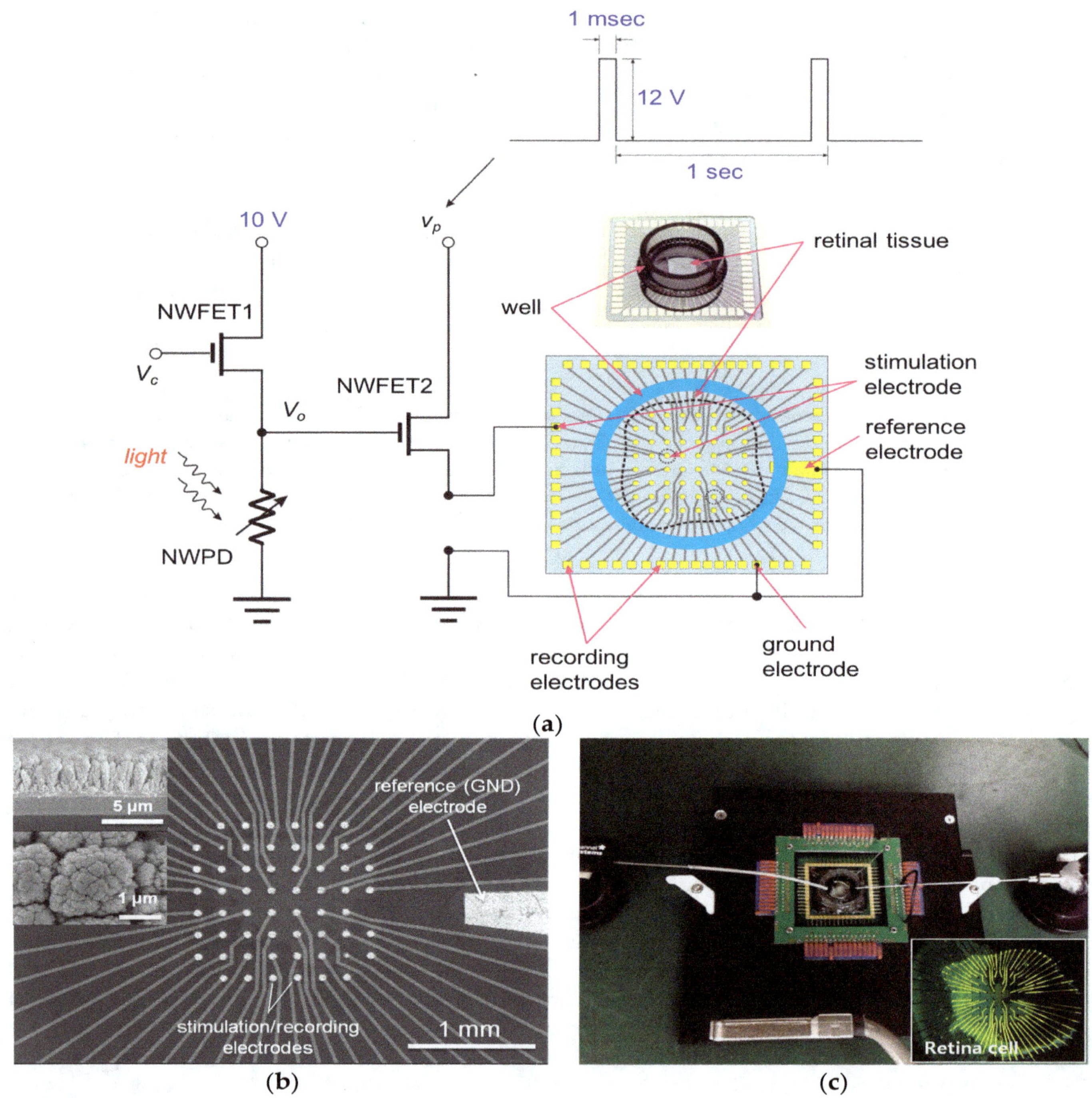

Figure 7. (**a**) Circuit diagram of in vitro animal experimental setup; (**b**) Micro electrode array for recording multi-channel neural signals; (**c**) Arrangement of micro electrode array and retinal tissue using multi-channel probing system (in vitro MEA-Systems of Multi Channel Systems).

$$\text{normalized response} = \frac{\sum_{\text{ch}} \text{spikes per pulse after stimulation}}{\sum_{\text{ch}} \text{spikes per pulse before stimulation}}, \quad (2)$$

Figure 8d shows the normalized response curves for four patches of retinal tissue extirpated from *rd1* mice. It is seen that the retinal neurons tend to respond in proportion to the amplitude of the stimulation pulse (i.e., the intensity of light) although there exist some differences in level and shape among the normalized response curves.

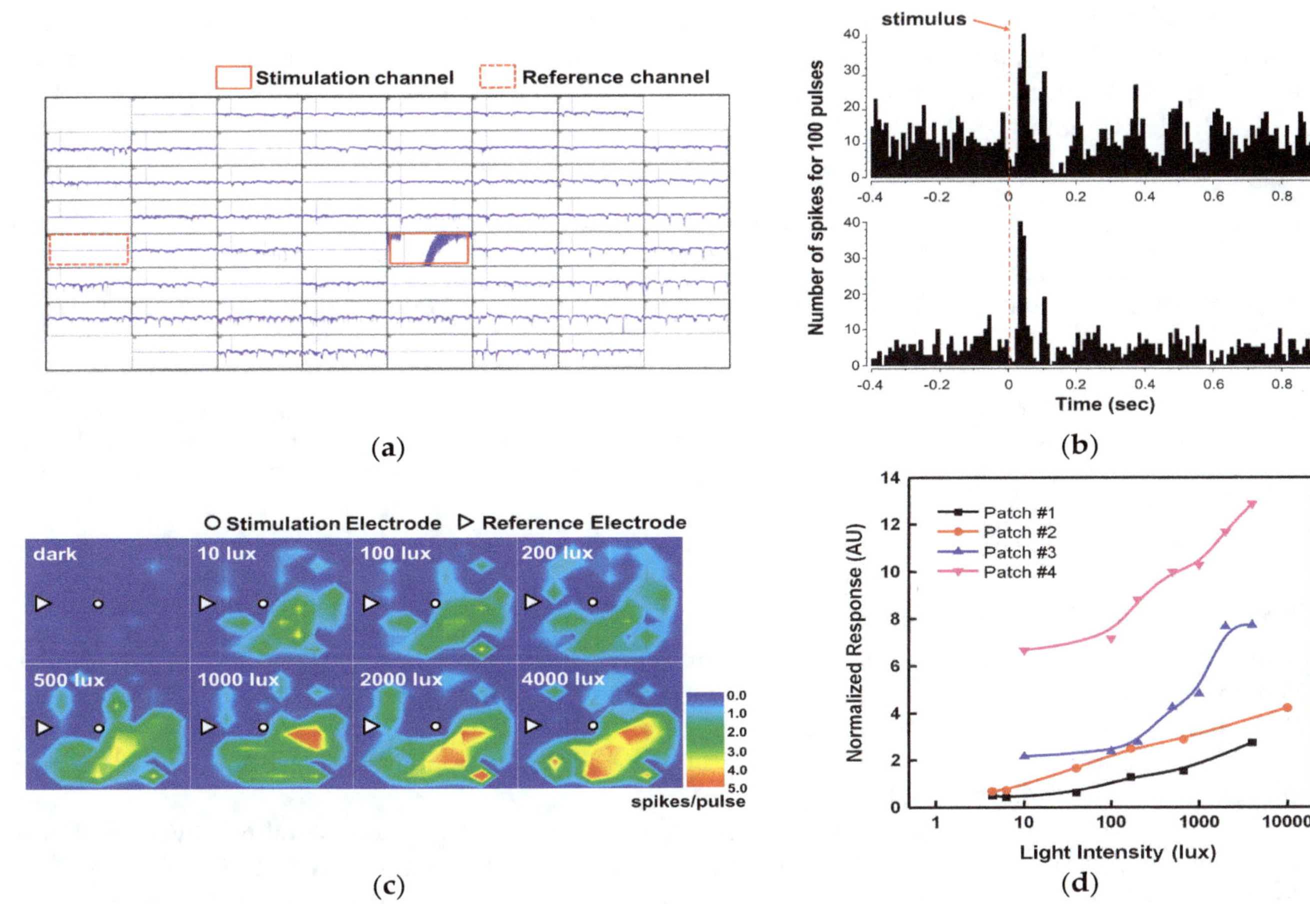

Figure 8. (**a**) Neural response signals recorded at 60 channels; (**b**) Changes in the number of spikes during, before, and after the application of stimulation signals; (**c**) Number of spikes per pulse at each channel against light intensity; (**d**) Normalized response by light intensity as a result of stimulation experiment using four retinal tissues.

4. Conclusions

This paper proposed a method for neural stimulation and a neural stimulation device integrated with an SiNW-based photodetection circuit. The SiNW-based photodetection circuit is designed to have the functions of detecting light and generating a stimulation signal in proportion to light intensity that is then transmitted to a micro electrode. Large resistance variation in the SiNW PD of the voltage divider circuit of a neuron stimulation device is desirable, and the fabricated SiNW PD produces a very large ratio $R_{NWPD(dark)}/R_{NWPD(bright)}$ of 1930. Owing to the large resistance variation of the SiNW PD, the voltage divider exhibits a very large swing range of output voltage. In the current driver circuit of the neuron stimulation device, the SiNW FET, which is driven by the output voltage of the voltage divider, produces a maximum on-current of approximately 480 μA and an on–off ratio of 5×10^4. It was determined that the current driver has a high enough current value and sufficient on–off characteristics to stimulate neurons via micro electrodes. The proposed neuron stimulation device can be applied to a high-resolution retinal prosthesis system, as was demonstrated by fabricating a high-density neural stimulation device with a unit cell size of 110 × 110 μm and a resolution of 32 × 32 in the form of a flexible film about 50 μm thick. Its effectiveness as a retinal stimulation device was evaluated by utilizing a unit cell of the neural stimulation device in an in vitro animal experiment involving the retinal tissue of *rd1* mice. A reference stimulation signal of uniform rectangular pulses modulated by the neural stimulation device into a stimulation signal proportional to light intensity was produced and transmitted into micro electrodes to stimulate the retinal nerve. Application of the retinal stimulation pulses to the retinal tissues demonstrated that the number of spikes in neural response signals increase in proportion to light intensity. These results address new challenges in developing neuron stimulation devices using SiNW-based circuits and are a promising step in the development of high-resolution retinal prosthetic systems.

Acknowledgments: This research was partially supported by a grant to Bio-Mimetic Robot Research Center Funded by Defense Acquisition Program Administration and by Agency for Defense Development (UD160027ID). In addition, this research was partially supported by the Public Welfare and Safety Research Program through the National Research Foundation of Korea (NRF) funded by the Ministry of Education, Science and Technology (2012-0008611). The English proofreading service was also supported by the Brain Korea 21 Plus Project in 2016.

Author Contributions: S.W. Jung fabricated SiNW devices and analyzed experimental results. J.Y. Shin and K. Pi conducted in vitro experiments and analyzed the experimental results. Y.S. Goo enucleated the eye from the *rd1* mice, detached retinal tissues from the eye, and set up the in vitro experiments. D.D. Cho supervised all of the SiNW fabrication and experiments.

References

1. Laxton, A.W.; Tang-Wai, D.F.; Mcandrews, M.P.; Zumsteg, D.; Wennberg, R.; Keren, R.; Wherrett, J.; Naglie, G.; Hamani, C.; Smith, G.S.; et al. A phase I trial of deep brain stimulation of memory circuits in Alzheimer's disease. *Ann. Neurol.* **2010**, *68*, 521–534. [CrossRef] [PubMed]
2. Jackson, A.; Zimmermann, J.B. Neural interfaces for the brain and spinal cord-restoring motor function. *Nat. Rev. Neurol.* **2012**, *8*, 690–699. [CrossRef] [PubMed]
3. O'Brien, E.E.; Greferath, U.; Vessey, K.A.; Jobling, A.I.; Fletcher, E.L. Electronic restoration of vision in those with photoreceptor degenerations. *Clin. Exp. Optim.* **2012**, *95*, 473–483. [CrossRef] [PubMed]
4. Koo, K.I.; Lee, S.M.; Yee, J.H.; Ryu, S.B.; Kim, K.H.; Goo, Y.S.; Cho, D.I. A novel in vitro sensing configuration for retinal physiology analysis of a sub-retinal prosthesis. *Sensors* **2012**, *12*, 3131–3144. [CrossRef] [PubMed]
5. Koo, K.I.; Lee, S.M.; Bae, S.H.; Seo, J.M.; Chung, H.; Cho, D.I. Arrowhead-shaped microelectrodes fabricated on a flexible substrate for enhancing the spherical conformity of retinal prostheses. *J. Microelectromech. Syst.* **2011**, *20*, 251–259. [CrossRef]
6. Seo, J.M.; Kim, K.H.; Goo, Y.S.; Park, K.S.; Kim, S.J.; Cho, D.I.; Chung, H. Vision rehabilitation by electrical retinal stimulation: Review of microelectrode approaches. *Sens. Mater.* **2012**, *24*, 153–164.
7. Lee, S.M.; Ahn, J.H.; Seo, S.M.; Chung, H.; Cho, D.I. Electrical characterization of 3D Au microelectrodes for use in retinal prostheses. *Sensors* **2015**, *15*, 14345–14355. [CrossRef] [PubMed]
8. Hirase, H.; Nikolenko, V.; Goldberg, J.H.; Yuste, R. Multiphoton stimulation of neurons. *J. Neurobiol.* **2002**, *51*, 237–247. [CrossRef] [PubMed]
9. Zemelman, B.V.; Lee, G.A.; Ng, M.; Miesenböck, G. Selective photostimulation of genetically ChARGed neurons. *Neuron* **2002**, *33*, 15–22. [CrossRef]
10. Oh, S.J.; Ahn, J.H.; Lee, S.M.; Ko, H.H.; Seo, J.M.; Goo, Y.S.; Cho, D.I. Light-controlled biphasic current stimulator IC using CMOS image sensors for high-resolution retinal prosthesis and in vitro experimental results with rd1 mouse. *IEEE Trans. Biomed.* **2015**, *62*, 70–79. [CrossRef] [PubMed]
11. Wilke, R.; Gabel, V.P.; Sachs, H.; Schmidt, K.U.B.; Gekeler, F.; Besch, D.; Szurman, P.; Stett, A.; Wilhelm, B.; Peters, T.; et al. Spatial resolution and perception of patterns mediated by a subretinal 16-electrode array in patients blinded by hereditary retinal dystrophies. *Investig. Ophthalmol. Vis. Sci.* **2011**, *52*, 5995–6003. [CrossRef] [PubMed]
12. Fujikado, T.; Kamei, M.; Sakaguchi, H.; Kanda, H.; Morimoto, T.; Ikuno, Y.; Nishida, K.; Kishima, H.; Maruo, T.; Konoma, K.; et al. Testing of semichronically implanted retinal prosthesis by suprachoroidal-transretinal stimulation in patients with retinitis pigmentosa. *Investig. Ophthalmol. Vis. Sci.* **2011**, *52*, 4726–4733. [CrossRef] [PubMed]
13. Klauke, S.; Goertz, M.; Rein, S.; Hoehl, D.; Thomas, U.; Eckhorn, R.; Bremmer, F.; Wachtler, T. Stimulation with a wireless intraocular epiretinal implant elicits visual percepts in blind humans. *Investig. Ophthalmol. Vis. Sci.* **2011**, *52*, 449–455. [CrossRef] [PubMed]

14. Humayun, M.S.; Dorn, J.D.; da Cruz, L.; Gagnelle, G.; Sahel, J.A.; Stanga, P.E.; Cideciyan, A.V.; Duncan, J.L.; Eliott, D.; Filley, E.; et al. Interim results from the international trial of Second Sight's visual prosthesis. *Ophthalmology* **2012**, *119*, 779–788. [CrossRef] [PubMed]
15. Zrenner, E.; Bartz-Schmidt, K.U.; Benav, H.; Besch, D.; Bruckmann, A.; Gabel, V.P.; Gekeler, F.; Greppmaier, U.; Harscher, A.; Kibbel, S.; et al. Subretinal electronic chips allow blind patients to read letters and combine them to words. *Proc. Biol. Sci.* **2011**, *278*, 1489–1497. [CrossRef] [PubMed]
16. Palanker, D.; Vankov, A.; Huie, P.; Baccus, S. Design of a high-resolution optoelectronic retinal prosthesis. *J. Neural Eng.* **2005**, *2*, S105–S120. [CrossRef] [PubMed]
17. DeMarco, P.J.; Yarbrough, G.L.; Yee, C.W.; McLean, G.Y.; Sagdullaev, B.T.; Ball, S.L.; McCall, M.A. Stimulation via a subretinally placed prosthetic elicits central activity and induces a trophic effect on visual responses. *Investig. Ophthalmol. Vis. Sci.* **2007**, *48*, 916–926. [CrossRef] [PubMed]
18. Chow, A.Y.; Bittner, A.K. The artificial silicon retina in retinitis pigmentosa aatients (An American Ophthalmological Association Thesis). *Trans. Am. Ophthalmol. Soc.* **2010**, *108*, 120–154. [PubMed]
19. Lee, S.M.; Jung, S.W.; Ahn, J.H.; Yoo, H.J.; Oh, S.J.; Cho, D.I. Microelectrode array with integrated nanowire FET switches for high-resolution retinal prosthetic systems. *J. Microelectromech. Syst.* **2014**, *24*, 075018. [CrossRef]
20. Ahn, J.H.; Lee, S.M.; Hong, S.J.; Yoo, H.J.; Jung, S.W.; Park, S.K.; Ko, H.H.; Cho, D.I. Multi-channel stimulator IC using a channel sharing method for retinal prosthesis. *J. Biomed. Nanotechnol.* **2013**, *9*, 621–625. [CrossRef] [PubMed]
21. Bae, S.H.; Che, J.H.; Seo, J.M.; Jeong, J.; Kim, E.T.; Lee, S.W.; Koo, K.I.; Suaing, G.J.; Lovell, N.H.; Cho, D.I.; et al. In vitro biocompatibility of various polymer-based microelectrode arrays for retinal prosthesis. *Investig. Ophthalmol. Vis. Sci.* **2012**, *53*, 2653–2657. [CrossRef] [PubMed]
22. Lee, S.M.; Jung, S.W.; Park, S.K.; Ahn, J.H.; Hong, S.J.; Yoo, H.J.; Lee, M.H.; Cho, D.I. Fabrication and evaluation of silicon nanowire photodetectors on a flexible substrate for retinal prosthetic system. *Sens. Mater.* **2012**, *24*, 205–220.
23. Lee, K.N.; Jung, S.W.; Shin, K.S.; Kim, W.H.; Lee, M.H.; Seong, W.K. Fabrication of suspended silicon nanowire arrays. *Small* **2008**, *4*, 642–648. [CrossRef] [PubMed]
24. Pi, K.; Shin, J.Y.; Jung, S.W.; Lee, S.; Cho, D.I. Electrical characterization of nanostructured 3D microelectrodes for retinal neuron stimulation. In Proceedings of the 2015 IEEE Sensors, Busan, Korea, 1–4 November 2015.

7

Cataract Surgery Performed by High Frequency LDV Z8 Femtosecond Laser: Safety, Efficacy and its Physical Properties

Bojan Pajic [1,2,3,4,*], **Zeljka Cvejic** [2] **and Brigitte Pajic-Eggspuehler** [1]

1 Eye Clinic Orasis, Swiss Eye Research Foundation, 5734 Reinach AG, Switzerland; brigitte.pajic@orasis.ch
2 Department of Physics, Faculty of Sciences, University of Novi Sad, Trg Dositeja Obradovica 4, 21000 Novi Sad, Serbia; zeljkac@uns.ac.rs
3 Division of Ophthalmology, Department of Clinical Neurosciences, Geneva University Hospitals, Rue Gabrielle-Perret-Gentil 4, 1205 Genève, Switzerland
4 Faculty of Medicine of the Military Medical academy, University of Defense, 11000 Belgrade, Serbia
* Correspondence: bpajic@datacomm.ch

Abstract: Background: The aim of our study was to investigate the safety and efficacy of the LDV Z8 femtosecond laser in cataract surgery compared to the conventional procedure. Methods: This prospective study was performed at the Swiss Eye Research Foundation, Eye Clinic ORASIS, Reinach, Switzerland. The study included 130 eyes from 130 patients: 68 treated with femtosecond laser-assisted cataract surgery (FLACS) using the FEMTO LDV Z8 and 62 treated with conventional phacoemulsification. Capsulotomy and lens fragmentation in the laser group were performed with the FEMTO LDV Z8 femtosecond laser system, which employs a new, low-energy, high repetition rate laser process for cataract surgery. In the conventional group, the capsulotomy was performed by a cystotome, and lens fragmentation was achieved by the stop-and-chop. Results: Ease of phacoemulsification (on a 4-point scale), the completeness of capsulotomy (on a 10-point scale), effective phacoemulsification time (seconds), uncorrected distance visual acuity (UCVA), best spectacle-corrected distance visual acuity (BSCVA), spherical equivalent (SE), and safety of the procedure were evaluated. The total follow-up time was three months. Conclusions: FLACS with the FEMTO LDV Z8 system was characterized by complete and reproducible capsulotomy and highly effective lens fragmentation. Postoperative visual outcomes were excellent, and the safety of the procedure was optimal.

Keywords: femtosecond laser; physical properties; cataract surgery; clinical outcomes; complications

1. Introduction

Femtosecond laser technology was first introduced in corneal refractive surgery for performing LASIK flaps. Compared to the microkeratome, an increase in precision and safety was observed [1,2]. Femtosecond technology was soon expanded to cataract surgery where its application introduced a higher predictability, safety, and potentially improved refractive outcome. Femtosecond laser systems are designed to perform anterior capsulotomy, lens fragmentation using different patterns, clear corneal incisions, and arcuate incisions. In the past few years, a significant amount of research investigating the advantages of femtosecond laser-assisted cataract surgery compared to conventional ultrasound phacoemulsification cataract surgery has been conducted. These studies have demonstrated that femtosecond laser-assisted capsulotomies have a higher precision regarding circularity and placement versus achieved diameter than those created by manual continuous curvilinear capsulorhexis. The femtosecond laser lens fragmentation results in a significant decrease in phacoemulsification energy exposure to the eye [3–8]. In the literature, it has been shown that the cut quality of clear corneal incisions done by femtosecond laser improves the tunnel morphology with less tissue damage compared with the conventional procedure. Due to its high precision and excellent surgical planning, femtosecond use in cataract surgery has also reduced the occurrence of high-order aberrations [9–11]. Femtosecond laser technology is, at the moment, more expensive compared to conventional cataract surgery but offers several advantages. A slightly greater amount of time is necessary for the femtosecond laser procedure compared with conventional phacoemulsification.

Femtosecond Laser

The Femto LDV Z8 (Ziemer Ophthalmic Systems AG, Port, Switzerland) is a high frequency femtosecond laser system for corneal surgery, corneal-refractive surgery, and cataract surgery. Unique among cataract laser systems, the Z8 applies the concept of overlapping low-energy near-infrared (1030 nm) femtosecond laser pulses in the nano-Joule range. This concept was originally developed by Ziemer Ophthalmic Systems for corneal surgery but was later adapted for cataract surgery applications such as lens fragmentation, capsulotomy, clear corneal incisions, and arcuate incisions. In order to shorten surgery time because small spots with large numerical aperture are used (Figure 1a), the laser system runs in the MHz range applying up to 1 billion pulses per surgery. Conventional femtosecond lasers with small numerical apertures (Figure 1b) that run in the kHz range, leads to a larger spot with a higher pulse energy and more gas creation.

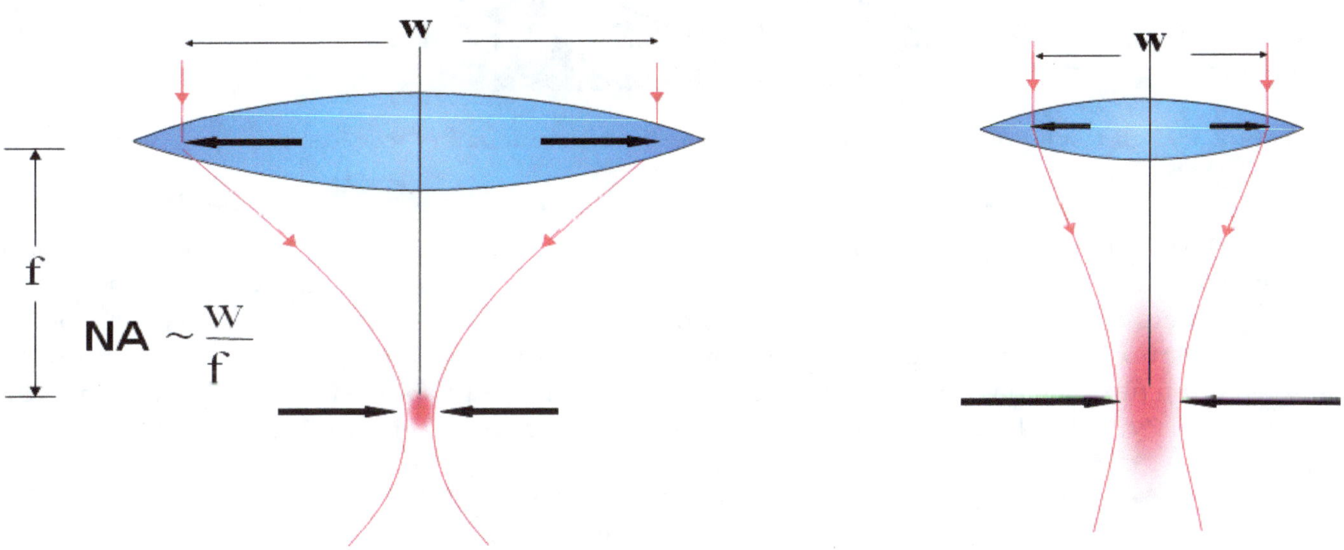

(a) (b)

Figure 1. (**a**) The large numerical aperture is the key for minimizing the focal volume which leads to low pulse energy and less bubbles (LDV Z8 femtosecond laser). (**b**) The small numerical aperture leads to higher pulse energy and more bubbles (conventional laser systems).

Each pulse creates a cavitation bubble approximately a few microns wide, which gently separates tissue. The handpiece (Figure 2) is the size of a compact camera and integrates all required electronics, optics, and actuators to perform visualization and resection in the anterior chamber of the eye. Visual esolution is possible down to 5 microns and is performed with a combination of a color camera and spectral-domain optical coherence tomography (OCT) operated at 840 nm (Figure 3).

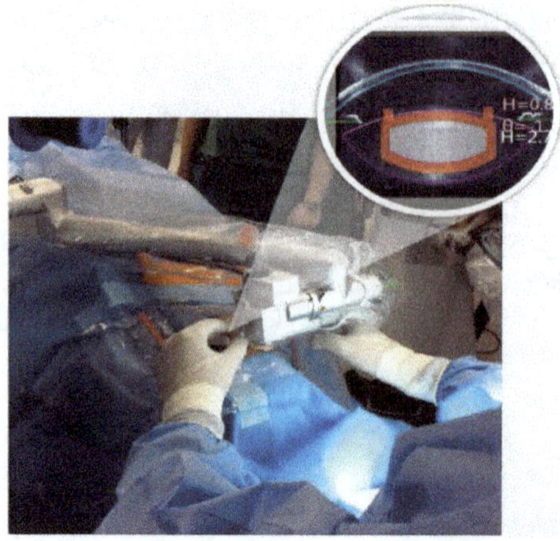

Figure 2. Femtosecond laser handpiece of the LDV Z8.

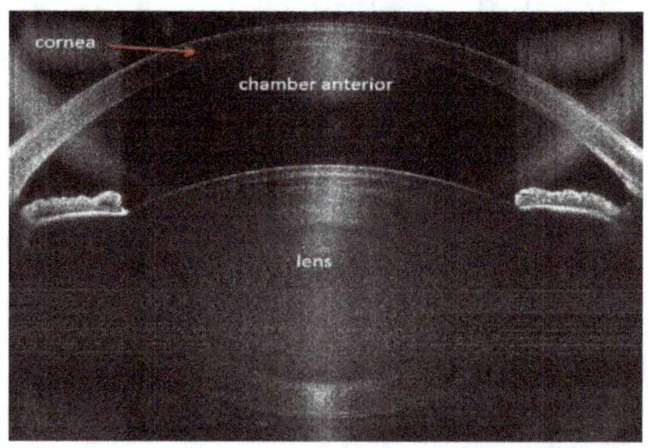

Figure 3. High-resolution OCT at a wavelength of 840 nm is mandatory for receiving a precise cut in the right position.

The FEMTO LDV Z8 uses a high focusing power microscope lens integrated in the handpiece to achieve focusing to a small spot size (<2 µm), which enables cuts to be made with nJ pulse energy. Low pulse energy with high-frequency applications is very precise and allows a spot diameter of less than 2 µm (Figure 4a). Conventional femtosecond lasers with a small numerical aperture and pulse energies in the µJ range has spot diameters greater than 5 µm and spot separation greater than the spot diameter (typically 10–20 µm), which can lead to tissue bridges (Figure 4b).

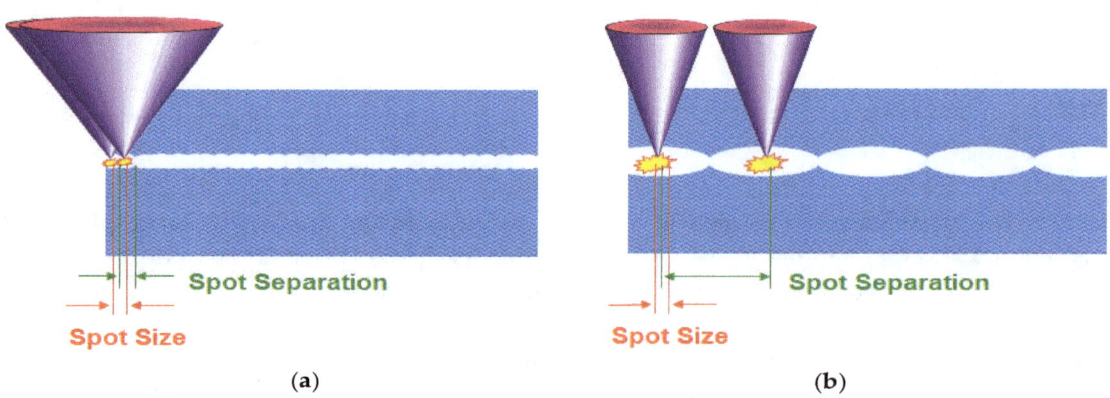

Figure 4. (**a**) The cutting process is limited to the focal spot size. Many pulses are needed to cut the tissue, so a high frequency repetition rate is needed. (**b**) The cutting process is mainly performed by mechanical forces of the expanding gas bubbles). Fewer pluses are needed but stress is generated in the tissue.

Given this unique combination of technical parameters, FLACS is able to create a more precise and circular capsulorhexis that could improve phacoemulsification and IOL centration, so a more precise refractive outcome after surgery could be expected [4,11–15].

2. Materials and Methods

This prospective randomized operative-interventional case–control study compares the performance and safety of femtosecond laser-assisted cataract procedures with those of conventional phacoemulsification cataract surgery.

The inclusion criteria required eligibility to undergo lens extraction by phacoemulsification followed by IOL implantation, an ability to complete patient interface docking with the femtosecond laser, an age of 50 years of older, willingness and ability to return for scheduled follow-up examination, and no current infections. Exclusion criteria consisted of minimal and maximal K-values of the central 3 mm zone that differ by more than 5D on topographic map of the cornea, a maximum K-value that exceeds 50D, a minimum K-value of less than 37D, corneal disease or pathology, such as corneal scaring or opacity, that precludes the transmission of laser wavelength or that distorts laser light, poorly dilating pupils of less than 6 mm or any other defect of the pupil that prevents the iris from adequate refraction peripherally, manifest glaucoma and ocular hypertension, and pseudoexfoliation. Additionally, any systemic or ocular pathology or previous ocular surgery was also excluded. All surgery procedures were performed by an experienced surgeon (BP) at the Eye Clinic ORASIS between January 2015 and September 2016.

The Z8 is a mobile femtosecond laser system that can be used in a sterile environment of the operating theatre. The hand-held patient interface allows for surgery to be performed without making significant alterations to the operation room layout in terms of space and equipment, thus preserving existing workflows. In the current study, all femtosecond laser cataract surgeries and conventional cataract surgeries were performed under the surgeon's microscope, and no patients were moved into or out of the operating room during the procedure. All surgeries were performed under topical anesthesia rapidocain intracameral. Preoperative the pupil dilation was achieved by application of Mydriasert (combination of phenylephrine hydrochlorid (5.4 mg) and Tropicamide (0.28 mg)).

2.1. Femtosecond Laser-Assisted Cataract Surgery Technique

The suction ring of a disposable liquid–patient interface was applied to the eye with centration over the limbus. The system contains a liquid interface (no applanation), which prevents posterior corneal descemet folds, ensuring an unhindered laser beam transmission. As soon as the suction vacuum reached 400 mbar, the suction ring was filled with a balanced salt solution (BSS). The handpiece, which is attached to an articulating arm of the laser system, was docked over the corneal apex. In the handpiece, there is a color camera and an integrated ocular coherence tomography (OCT) system that images the ocular structures. Treatment parameters were customized to accommodate each individual patient. Custom surgical planning is performed by the precise placement of surgical incisions based on OCT images that identify ocular structures and automatically determine and display safety margins and suggested cut locations. Via a touchscreen, the surgeon has the ability to reposition treatment patterns. Laser treatment begins with lens fragmentation (an eight-piece pie-cut pattern) followed by anterior capsulotomy (5.0 mm in diameter). Unlike other FLACS systems, lens fragmentation before anterior capsulotomy is possible with the Z8, as the low energy results in minimal gas production, which significantly reduces the risk of intra-operative complications. As shown in Figure 5, the capsular button in the OCT image can be seen free-floating, while the fragmented lens shows no accumulation of gas.

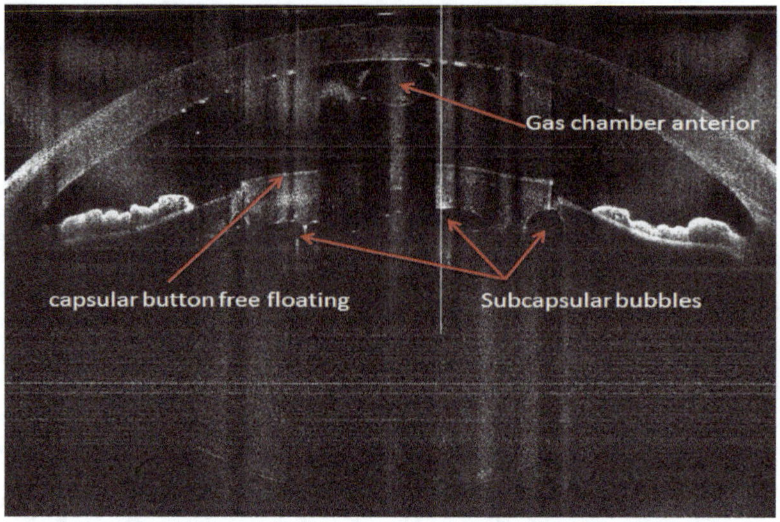

Figure 5. A complete capsulotomy is seen with the capsular button free floating in the anterior chamber, while there is nearly no accumulation of gas in the fragmented lens. There are minimal subcapsular bubbles in the anterior chamber.

2.2. *Conventional Cataract Surgery Technique*

Two paracentesis 0.8 mm in diameter were performed. Intracameral anesthesia was administered (Lidocaine hydrochlorid and Epinephrine, 0.005 mg). A capsulorhexis 5 mm in diameter was attempted. For phacoemulsification, the stop-and-chop technique was applied. The remainder of the surgical steps required to complete the operation were identical between FLACS and conventional groups.

Minimal gas accumulation was visible at the posterior surface of the cornea, which was observed in the OCT through the creation of shadows seen on the lower part of the image. For all patients, the phacoemulsification device Catharex 3 system (Oertli Instrumente AG, Berneck, Switzerland) was used. By using the bimanual irrigation/aspiration system, residual cortex was removed. In all cases, an IOL was implanted in the capsular bag. Patients were scheduled for postoperative examination at Day 1, Day 12, and 4, 8, and 12 weeks after surgery. The main outcome measures evaluated in this study were best corrected visual acuity (BCVA), effective phacoemulsification time (EPT, seconds), and complications. Cataract severity was graded according to nuclear opalescence on the Lens Opacities Classification System III [16] with Grades 1–4.

Statistical analysis was computed with IBM SPSS Statistics version 20.0 (IBM Corp., Armonk, NY, USA). Normal distribution of data was determined by the Shapiro–Wilk test (data was considered normal if $p > 0.05$). Normal values were shown as mean $\pm$ standard deviation, whereas the median value was shown as non-parametric data. The level of significance was set at $p < 0.05$. BCVA was measured with Snellen projector charts, and data were converted to logarithm of the minimum angle of resolution (logMAR) units for statistical analysis. Related-samples Wilcoxon signed rank test was used to compare preoperative and postoperative BCVA and intended versus measured capsulotomy diameters.

3. Results

There were 33 males (48.5%) and 35 females (51.5%) in the FLACS group and 25 (40.3%) males and 37 females (59.7%) in the conventional cataract surgery group enrolled in the study.

The ethics committee of Northwest and Central Switzerland (EKNZ) approved the study. A total of 130 eyes from 130 patients were recruited for cataract treatment, with 68 patients recruited to the FLACS group (Group 1) and 62 patients recruited to the conventional cataract surgery group (Group 2). The mean age of patients in the FLACS group was 70.4 ± 8.4 years (range: 50–83 years) and 69.6 ± 8.2 years (range: 50–85 years) for the conventional cataract surgery group. There was no statistically significant difference in age ($p = 0.25$) between the two groups. Regarding the preoperative BCVA, there were no significant differences between the groups ($p = 0.49$). According to the Lens Opacities Classification System III, the preoperative cataract grade density in the femtosecond laser cataract surgery group was 2.57 ± 0.58 and the conventional cataract surgery group was 2.23 ± 0.42, which is highly significant ($p < 0.001$).

All patients in both groups underwent a successful operation. The intended capsulotomy diameter was set at 5.0 mm in all cases. The achieved capsulotomy diameter in the FLACS group was 5.0 ± 0.12 mm (range: 4.6–5.4 mm), median 5.0 mm, and in the conventional cataract surgery group 4.7 ± 0.36 mm (range: 4.0–5.6 mm), median 4.7 mm, which is highly significant ($p < 0.001$). The mean phacoemulsification time in Group 1 was 1.9 ± 2.25 s (range: 0–11 s), median 1.0 s, and in Group 2, 2.3 ± 2.41 s (range: 0.3–14 s), median 1.7 s, which is significant ($p = 0.042$). The effective phacoemulsification time (EPT) in Group 1 was found to be 1.48 ± 1.80 s (range: 0–8.8 s), median 0.8 s, and in Group 2 1.81 ± 1.93 s (range: 0.24–11.2 s), median 1.36 s, which is significant ($p = 0.044$) (Table 1).

Table 1. Mean phacoemulsification time/effective phacoemulsification time for Groups 1 and 2.

	Group 1	Group 2	*p*-Value
mean phacoemulsification time (s)	1.9 ± 2.25	2.3 ± 2.41	0.042
effective phacoemulsification time (EPT)	1.48 ± 1.80	1.81 ± 1.93	0.044

Overall surgery time in Group 1 was 7.5 ± 1.22 min (range: 5–12 min) and 6.6 ± 1.76 min (range: 4.6–12 min) in Group 2, that is slightly significant ($p = 0.048$).

The mean preoperative BCVA was 0.29 logMAR (range 1.30–0.01 logMAR) in Group 1 and 0.30 logMAR (range 1.30–0.01 logMAR) in Group 2 ($p = 0.50$). There is no difference between the groups. The mean BCVA, 1 day post-operation, was 0.16 logMAR (range 1.30–0 logMAR) in Group 1 and 0.22 logMAR (range 1.30–0 logMAR) ($p = 0.038$) in Group 2; 12 days post-operation, 0.06 logMAR (range 0.49–0 logMAR) in Group 1 and 0.06 logMAR (range 0.60–(−0.10) logMAR) in Group 2 ($p = 0.48$); 4 weeks post-operation, 0.03 logMAR (range 0.49–(−0.10) logMAR) in Group 1 and 0.06 logMAR (range 0.30–(−0.10) logMAR) in Group 2 ($p = 0.31$); 8 weeks post-operation, 0.03 logMAR (range 0.40–(−0.10) logMAR) in Group 1 and 0.06 logMAR (range 0.49–(−0.10) logMAR) in Group 2 ($p = 0.41$); 12 weeks post-operation, 0.01 logMAR (range 0.30–(−0.10) logMAR) in Group 1 and 0.02 logMAR (range 0.49–(−0.10) logMAR) in Group 2 ($p = 0.37$). Only the value at 1 day is significant, whereas at any later follow-up there are no significant differences between the groups (Table 2).

Table 2. Mean BCA for Group 1 and Group 2 in the follow-up.

Mean BCVA	Group 1	Group 2	
preoperative	0.29 logMAR (range 1.30–0.01)	0.30 logMAR (range 1.30–0.01)	$p = 0.50$
1 day post-operation	0.16 logMAR (range 1.30–0)	0.22 logMAR (range 1.30–0)	$p = 0.038$
12 days post-operation	0.06 logMAR (range 0.49–0)	0.06 logMAR (range 0.60–(−0.10))	$p = 0.48$
4 weeks post-operation	0.03 logMAR (range 0.49–(−0.10))	0.06 logMAR (range 0.30–(−0.10))	$p = 0.31$
8 weeks post-operation	0.03 logMAR (range 0.40–(−0.10))	0.06 logMAR (range 0.49–(−0.10))	$p = 0.41$
12 weeks post-operation	0.01 logMAR (range 0.30–(−0.10))	0.02 logMAR (range 0.49–(−0.10))	$p = 0.37$

The vacuum time for FLACS patients 139 ± 26 s.

Follow-up was 3 months for all patients. No intraoperative complications were recorded.

4. Discussion

Numerous studies have reported advantages of femtosecond laser over conventional phacoemulsification cataract surgery [3,4,6,8,13,14,17–23]. Our study shows that a targeted 5 mm capsulotomy could be achieved very precisely with the femtosecond laser treatment, demonstrating only small variance in reproducibility, whereas the manual capsulorhexis differed significantly. Other studies have demonstrated very similar results, where the capsulotomies created using the femtosecond laser were more accurate in size than those created by manual continuous curvilinear capsulorhexis [4,8,13,14,22]. The accuracy of the capsulotomy is very important because it provides the surgeon access to the capsular bag for fragmentation and removal of natural lens and placement of the IOL. The diameter of the capsulotomy should allow overlap between the capsul rim and the IOL optic and haptic for correct IOL positioning. In special IOL, like toric IOL, the alignment is particularly important. Thus, the diameter, shape, and centration of the capsulorhexis can influence IOL position and may have an impact on refractive outcomes.

According of Lens Opacities Classification System III, the preoperative cataract grade density in the femtosecond laser-assisted cataract surgery group (Group 1) was significantly higher ($p < 0.001$) than in the conventional cataract surgery group (Group 2) in our study. Despite this potential disadvantage, we needed significantly less phacoemulsification time and effective phacoemulsification time in the femtosecond laser group (Group 1) compared with the conventional phacoemulsification surgery group (Group 2). Other studies have shown that the reduction of ultrasound energy from phacoemulsification can reduce the risk of capsule complication. Phacoemulsification time and effective phacoemulsification time are known to increase with nuclear density, but other groups have reported similar findings regarding FLACS and EPT [4] as we have observed. In our study, it was seen that, even with a low-energy laser application, the lens fragmentation was perfectly cut. Low energy creates smaller gas bubbles, which reduces the tension on the capsular bag during the procedure. Thus, the Femto LDV Z8 femtosecond laser is able to perform the optimal procedure algorithm, where the cut procedure begins with the lens fragmentation followed by capsulotomy and clear corneal incisions. We did not observe any bubbles during any of the stages of the laser procedure, which could disturb the optimal cut quality.

In our study, we detected an improvement in visual acuity one day post-operation, an improvement that was significantly greater with the femtosecond laser compared with the conventional procedure. This may reveal that the rehabilitation time in the first postoperative day is faster. In all other follow-up times after 12 days, no significant differences regarding the visual acuity were observed.

FLACS with the LDV Z8, a low-energy high frequency femtosecond laser, shows very high precision, with a significant decrease in effective phacoemulsification time (EPT) compared to the conventional procedure, even when the lens density was higher. Our results indicate that the healing time involved in visual acuity is faster in the first postoperative days, demonstrating the clinical advantages of a gentle technique with the femtosecond laser. However, regarding the overall surgery time, we report that slightly more time is needed to perform femtosecond laser treatment, but the potential to optimize workflow further and eliminate this difference is a future aim.

5. Conclusions

One of the main goals is providing repeatable and precise outcomes, with an aim to offer customized medical solutions for patients. The low-energy LDV Z8 with its advanced OCT visualization allows the best placement of the capsulotomy and optimizes surgical planning. All of this influences the strength of capsulotomy and significantly improves refractive outcomes due to reduced IOL tilt [14,24]. A high-frequency device with low pulse energy enables minimal gas creation during lens fragmentation. This sets it apart from other cataract laser devices with higher energy and low frequency, where larger bubbles and tissue bridges are created.

Acknowledgments: A special thanks goes to Holger Lubatschowski, Hannover, Germany, for distributing the images (Figures 1 and 4).

Author Contributions: Bojan Pajic and Brigitte Pajic-Eggspuehler conceived and designed the experiments; Bojan Pajic performed the experiments; Zeljka Cvejic contributed analysis tools; all authors wrote the paper.

References

1. Ratkay-Traub, I.; Juhasz, T.; Horvath, C.; Suarez, C.; Kiss, K.; Ferincz, I.; Kurtz, R. Ultra-short puls (femtosecond) laser surgery: Initial use in LASIK flap creation. *Ophthalmol. Clin. N. Am.* **2001**, *14*, 347–355.
2. Kim, P.; Sutton, G.L.; Rootman, D.S. Applications of femtosecond laser in corneal refractive surgery. *Curr. Opin.* **2011**, *22*, 238–244. [CrossRef] [PubMed]
3. Conrad-Hengerer, I.; Al Juburi, M.; Schultz, T.; Hengerer, F.H.; Dick, H.B. Corneal endothelial cell loss and corneal thickness in conventional compared with femtosecond laser-assisted cataract surgery: Three-month follow-up. *J. Cataract Refract. Surg.* **2013**, *39*, 1307–1313. [CrossRef] [PubMed]
4. Conrad-Hengerer, I.; Hengerer, F.H.; Schultz, T.; Dick, H.B. Effect of femtosecond laser fragmentation on effective phacoemulsification time in cataract surgery. *J. Refract. Surg.* **2012**, *28*, 879–883. [CrossRef] [PubMed]
5. Abell, R.G.; Kerr, N.M.; Vote, B.J. Toward zero effective phacoemulsification time using femtosecond laser pretreatment. *Ophthalmology* **2013**, *120*, 942–948. [CrossRef] [PubMed]
6. Abell, R.G.; Kerr, N.M.; Vote, B.J. Femtosecond laser-assisted cataract surgery compared with conventional cataract surgery. *Clin. Exp. Ophthalmol.* **2013**, *41*, 455–462. [CrossRef] [PubMed]
7. Reddy, K.P.; Kandulla, J.; Auffarth, G.U. Effectiveness and safety of femtosecond laser-assisted lens fragmentation and anterior capsulotomy versus the manual technique in cataract surgery. *J. Cataract Refract. Surg.* **2013**, *39*, 1297–1306. [CrossRef] [PubMed]
8. Nagy, Z.Z.; Kranitz, K.; Takacs, A.I.; Mihaltz, K.; Kovacs, I.; Knorz, M.C. Comparison of intraocular lens decentration parameters after femtosecond and manual capsulotomies. *J. Refract. Surg.* **2011**, *27*, 564–569. [CrossRef] [PubMed]
9. Grewal, D.S.; Basti, S. Comparison of morphologic features of clear corneal incisions created with a femtosecond laser or a keratome. *J. Cataract Refract. Surg.* **2014**, *40*, 521–530. [CrossRef] [PubMed]
10. Alió, J.L.; Abdou, A.A.; Soria, F.; Javaloy, J.; Fernández-Buenaga, R.; Nagy, Z.Z.; Filkorn, T. Femtosecond laser cataract incision morphology and corneal higher-order aberration analysis. *J. Refract. Surg.* **2013**, *29*, 590–595. [CrossRef] [PubMed]
11. Mastropasqua, L.; Toto, L.; Mastropasqua, A.; Vecchiarino, L.; Mastropasqua, R.; Pedrotti, E.; Di Nicola, M. Femtosecond laser versus manual clear corneal incision in cataract surgery. *J. Refract. Surg.* **2014**, *30*, 27–33. [CrossRef] [PubMed]
12. Moshirfar, M.; Churgin, D.S.; Hsu, M. Femtosecond laser-assisted cataract surgery: A current review. *Middle East Afr. J. Ophthalmol.* **2011**, *18*, 285–291. [CrossRef] [PubMed]
13. Friedman, N.J.; Palanker, D.V.; Schuele, G.; Andersen, D.; Marcellino, G.; Seibel, B.S.; Batlle, J.; Feliz, R.; Talamo, J.H.; Blumenkranz, M.S.; et al. Femtosecond laser capsulotomy. *J. Cataract Refract. Surg.* **2011**, *37*, 1189–1198. [CrossRef] [PubMed]
14. Kranitz, K.; Takacs, A.; Mihaltz, K.; Kovacs, I.; Knorz, M.C.; Nagy, Z.Z. Femtosecond laser capsulotomy and manual continuous curvilinear capsulorrhexis parameters and their effects on intraocular lens centration. *J. Refract. Surg.* **2011**, *27*, 558–563. [CrossRef] [PubMed]
15. Assia, E.I.; Apple, D.J.; Tsai, J.C.; Morgan, R.C. Mechanism of radial tear formation and extension after anterior capsulectomy. *Ophthalmology* **1991**, *98*, 432–437. [CrossRef]
16. Chylack, L.T., Jr.; Wolfe, J.K.; Singer, D.M.; Leske, M.C.; Bullimore, M.A.; Bailey, I.L.; Friend, J.; McCarthy, D.; Wu, S.Y. The Longitudinal Study of Cataract Study Group The Lens Opacities Classification System III. *Arch. Ophthalmol.* **1993**, *111*, 831–836. [CrossRef] [PubMed]
17. Takács, A.I.; Kovács, I.; Miháltz, K.; Filkorn, T.; Knorz, M.C.; Nagy, Z.Z. Central corneal volume and endothelial cell count following femtosecond laser-assisted refractive cataract surgery compared to conventional phacoemulsification. *J. Refract. Surg.* **2012**, *28*, 387–391. [CrossRef] [PubMed]
18. Filkorn, T.; Kovács, I.; Takács, A.; Horváth, E.; Knorz, M.C.; Nagy, Z.Z. Comparison of IOL power calculation and refractive outcome after laser refractive cataract surgery with a femtosecond laser versus conventional phacoemulsification. *J. Refract. Surg.* **2012**, *28*, 540–544. [CrossRef] [PubMed]
19. Nagy, Z.; Takacs, A.; Filkorn, T.; Sarayba, M. Initial clinical evaluation of an intraocular femtosecond laser in cataract surgery. *J. Refract. Surg.* **2009**, *25*, 1053–1060. [CrossRef] [PubMed]
20. Conrad-Hengerer, I.; Hengerer, F.H.; Joachim, S.C.; Schultz, T.; Dick, H.B. Femtosecond laser-assisted cataract surgery in intumescent white cataracts. *J. Cataract Refract. Surg.* **2014**, *40*, 44–50. [CrossRef] [PubMed]

21. Conrad-Hengerer, I.; Dick, H.B.; Schultz, T.; Hengerer, F.H. Femtosecond laser-assisted capsulotomy after penetrating injury of the cornea and lens capsule. *J. Cataract Refract. Surg.* **2014**, *40*, 153–156. [CrossRef] [PubMed]
22. Palanker, D.V.; Blumenkranz, M.S.; Andersen, D.; Wiltberger, M.; Marcellino, G.; Gooding, P.; Angeley, D.; Schuele, G.; Woodley, B.; Simoneau, M.; et al. Femtosecond laser-assisted cataract surgery with integrated optical coherence tomography. *Sci. Trans. Med.* **2010**, *2*, 58ra85. [CrossRef] [PubMed]
23. Naranjo-Tackman, R. How a femtosecond laser increases safety and precision in cataract surgery? *Curr. Opin. Ophthalmol.* **2011**, *22*, 53–57. [CrossRef] [PubMed]
24. Packer, M.; Teuma, E.V.; Glasser, A.; Bott, S. Defining the ideal femtosecond laser capsulotomy. *Br. J. Ophthalmol.* **2015**, *99*, 1137–1142. [CrossRef] [PubMed]

8

Multispectral, Fluorescent and Photoplethysmographic Imaging for Remote Skin Assessment

Janis Spigulis

Biophotonics Laboratory, Institute of Atomic Physics and Spectroscopy, University of Latvia, Riga, LV-1586, Latvia; janis.spigulis@lu.lv

Academic Editors: Dragan Indjin, Željka Cvejić and Małgorzata Jędrzejewska-Szczerska

Abstract: Optical tissue imaging has several advantages over the routine clinical imaging methods, including non-invasiveness (it does not change the structure of tissues), remote operation (it avoids infections) and the ability to quantify the tissue condition by means of specific image parameters. Dermatologists and other skin experts need compact (preferably pocket-size), self-sustaining and easy-to-use imaging devices. The operational principles and designs of ten portable in-vivo skin imaging prototypes developed at the Biophotonics Laboratory of Institute of Atomic Physics and Spectroscopy, University of Latvia during the recent five years are presented in this paper. Four groups of imaging devices are considered. Multi-spectral imagers offer possibilities for distant mapping of specific skin parameters, thus facilitating better diagnostics of skin malformations. Autofluorescence intensity and photobleaching rate imagers show a promising potential for skin tumor identification and margin delineation. Photoplethysmography video-imagers ensure remote detection of cutaneous blood pulsations and can provide real-time information on cardiovascular parameters and anesthesia efficiency. Multimodal skin imagers perform several of the abovementioned functions by taking a number of spectral and video images with the same image sensor. Design details of the developed prototypes and results of clinical tests illustrating their functionality are presented and discussed.

Keywords: multispectral skin imaging; skin autofluorescence and photobleaching; photoplethysmography imaging

---

1. Introduction

Biomedical imaging has become a powerful tool for diagnostics and monitoring of human health condition. Apart from routine clinical imaging modalities (e.g., x-ray, ultrasound, endoscopy, computed tomography, magnetic resonance imaging), a number of advanced "open air" optical imaging methods and technologies have been introduced recently. Their main advantages are remote operation (avoids infection) and non-invasiveness (does not change the structure of tissues). Besides, digital imaging ensures quantitative documentation on the skin condition and its changes.

There are several commercially available skin diagnostic imaging devices for dermatologists (e.g., *SIAscope* [1], *MelaFind* [2], confocal microscopes [3], multi-photon tomographs [4]), but most of them are bulky, cable-connected to computers and also too expensive for GPs or small clinics. With a perspective on personalized medicine, new more compact and less expensive self-sustaining designs for skin imaging are preferable. The recently commercialized pocket-size digital dermatoscopes [5], video-microscopes [6] and smartphone-based solutions [7] have shown promising potential for primary skin diagnostics. Further developments of portable skin imaging technologies would facilitate their wider and more efficient implementation in hospitals and clinics. They may also prove useful for home monitoring of skin condition, follow-up after skin therapies and for some forensic applications, e.g., for age estimation of bruises [8].

This review paper (which follows a previous review [9]) presents the operational principles, designs and clinical test results of ten portable in-vivo skin imaging prototypes developed over the last five years at the Biophotonics Laboratory of the University of Latvia. Four groups of imaging devices are presented. Multi-spectral imagers offer possibilities for distant mapping of specific skin parameters (e.g., distribution of skin chromophore concentrations) so facilitating better diagnostics of skin malformations. Autofluorescence photobleaching rate imagers show a promising potential for skin tumor identification and margin delineation. Photoplethysmography video-imagers ensure remote detection of cutaneous blood pulsations and can provide real-time information on cardiovascular parameters and anesthesia efficiency. Finally, multimodal skin imagers perform several of the abovementioned functions by taking a number of spectral and video images with the same image sensor. All devices are portable and most of them wireless; original software solutions (not discussed here) provide fast data processing for obtaining clinically significant tissue parameters.

2. Materials and Methods

2.1. Prototype Devices for Multispectral Skin Imaging

Multispectral imaging is a method based on acquisition of a limited number (typically three to 10) of images within relatively narrow non-overlapping spectral bands—so-called spectral images [10]. The captured spectral images of skin can be further converted into parametric images, e.g., 2-D maps that specify distribution of skin chromophore concentrations [11,12]. In the visible spectral range, a relatively simple 3-chromophore skin model can be applied for obtaining chromophore distribution maps over the imaged area [13]. The hardware implementing this approach should ensure easy capture of three narrowband spectral images of skin as fast as possible. One option for that is subsequent narrowband illumination by means of different color LEDs and capturing one spectral image under each illumination mode [11]. This approach was examined earlier by a compact research grade RGB camera-LED illumination ring system [14]. As the next steps, three prototype devices comprising commercial consumer cameras and spectrally specific illuminators were developed.

2.1.1. RGB-LED Add-On Illumination System for Smartphones

Thanks to the rapid development of communication technologies, a number of smartphone camera-based health assessment software applications are available, both in ambient light and under white LED illumination from the same phone [15,16]. Such applications may provide, for instance, information about the potential malignancy of skin lesions [7]. To extend the smartphone applications for skin evaluation, we developed a technique for mapping the main skin chromophores using a RGB light source specially designed as add-on for various smartphone models.

The system design scheme is presented at Figure 1. The smartphone is fixed on a flat sticky surface with a window for its rear camera [17], which is surrounded from bottom by a ring of LEDs mounted within cylindrical screening spacers (6 cm between the skin and camera). The ring includes four types of LEDs, with four diodes of each type: white—to find and adjust location of the skin malformation, and colored—with emission in blue (maximum at 460 nm), green (maximum at 535 nm), and red (maximum at 663 nm) spectral bands (Figure 1b) which are suitable for mapping of three skin chromophores. LEDs are operated in continuous mode and switched on and off manually or automatically by a special software using a Bluetooth connection between the smartphone and the illumination system. Illumination and image detection are performed normally to the skin surface. Two orthogonally oriented polarizers are used in front of the LEDs and smartphone camera, respectively, to reduce detection of skin specular reflection. Five AA 2800 mAh rechargeable battery blocks provide the system power supply.

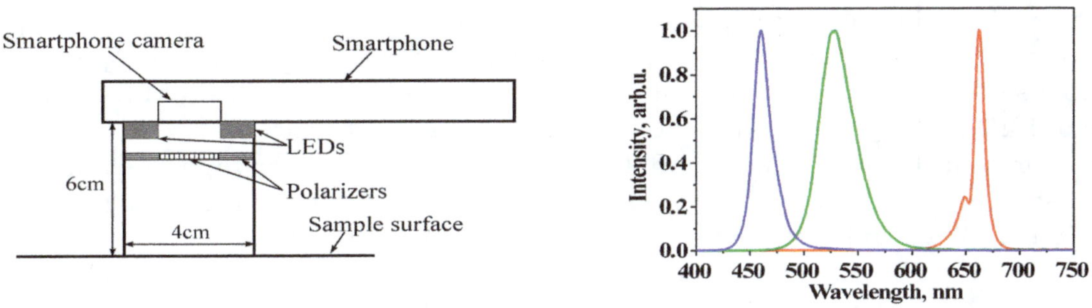

(a) (b)

Figure 1. Design scheme of smartphone RGB illuminator (**a**) and normalized emission spectra of the used color LEDs (**b**) [18].

Figure 2a provides more design details of the prototype. A driver placed in the compartment 10 ensures Bluetooth wireless connection between the smartphone and illumination unit and enables automatic sequential on-off switching of the color LEDs within less than 1 s (one image for each illumination band) by command from the smartphone touchscreen. Specially developed software transmits the obtained spectral images via mobile network to a remote server that converts them into distribution maps of the three main skin chromophores (melanin, oxy- and deoxy-hemoglobin) and then transmits the maps back for displaying on the smartphone touchscreen. More details on the RGB-LED smartphone add-on prototype and its tests are provided in [17,18].

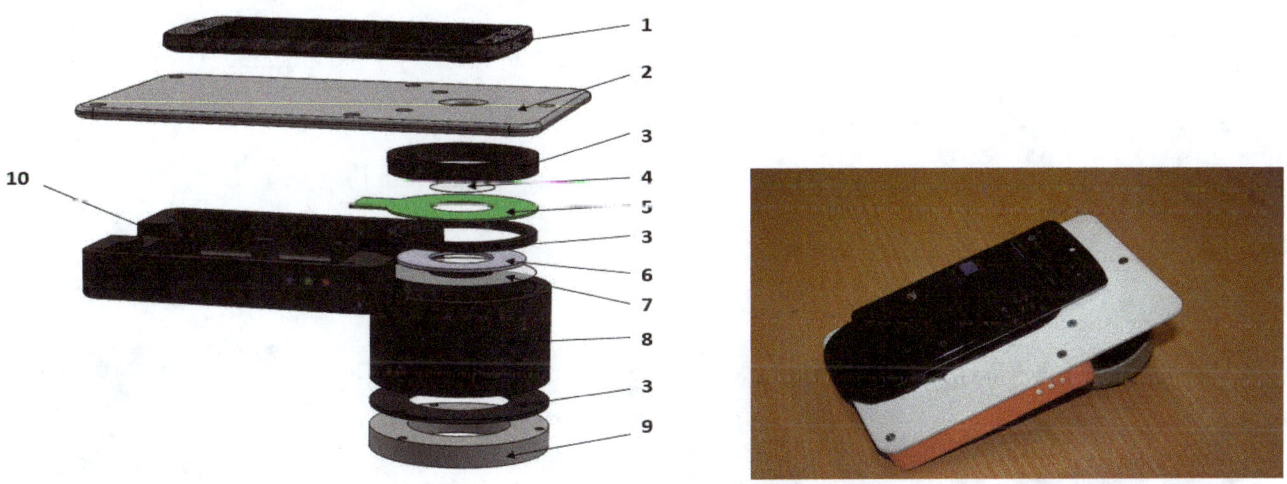

(**a**) (**b**)

Figure 2. Design details of the smartphone-LED prototype device (**a**) and its outlook with a smartphone on it (**b**): 1—smartphone, 2—sticky fixing platform with a camera window, 3—holding ring, 4—polarizer of the detected light, 5—LED ring comprising four sets of LEDs, 6—light diffuser, 7—illumination polarizer (oriented orthogonally to the polarizer 4), 8—screening spacer, 9—silicone skin contact ring, 10—compartment for batteries and electronic components [17].

2.1.2. Modified Multispectral Video-Microscope

A number of digital microscopes nowadays are small handheld devices connected to a PC via a USB cable; they can be applied also for visual skin assessment [19]. A typical digital microscope consists of a webcam with a high-powered macro-lens and a built-in LED light source. Advantages of such microscopes are their compactness, low power consumption and relatively low price, typically a few hundreds of USD. Most of the digital microscopes have white illumination source(s) and some of them–also ultraviolet illuminators [20]. These devices, however, cannot be used for detailed spectral analysis of skin. To overcome this drawback, we adapted a standard digital microscope (model *DinoLite* AD413, series AM-4013) for multispectral imaging by replacing the built-in LEDs with specifically selected color LEDs and by developing the LED management software.

Figure 3 presents the block diagram of the custom-modified microscope. A standard white/UV LED illuminator ring has been removed and replaced by a lab-designed illuminator ring comprising sixteen LEDs combined in four groups: (1) four infrared 940 nm LEDs; (2) four red 660 nm LEDs; (3) four green 545 nm LEDs; and (4) four blue 450 nm LEDs. To each group of LEDs a current of 80 mA is fed by LED drivers that are controlled by a FTDI USB controller. The two-port USB hub provides control over the LEDs and the original CMOS image sensor of the microscope. The power support, LED switching and CMOS control are executed through the USB interface.

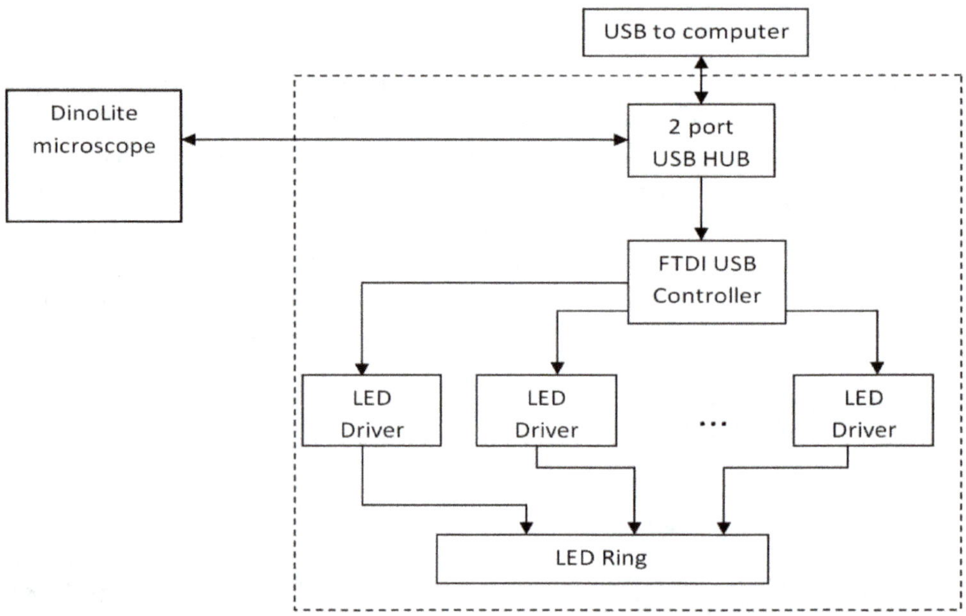

Figure 3. Block diagram of the modified video-microscope [21].

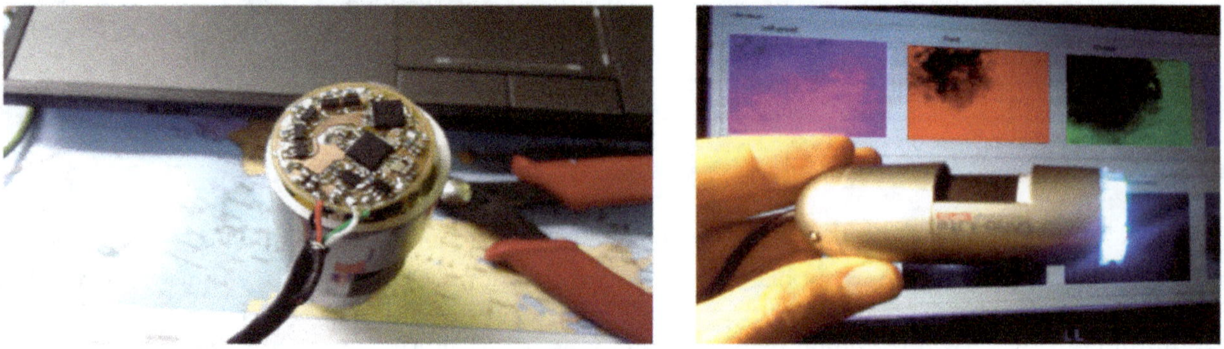

a b

Figure 4. The developed LED control unit (**a**) and the modified video-microscope with replaced illumination unit (**b**) [21].

The custom-designed control unit module is installed on the rear side of microscope as shown on Figure 4a. The lab-made 16-LED ring is mounted on the front side (Figure 4b); it is even more compact than the original 8-LED *DinoLite* ring. For better homogeneity of skin illumination, a diffuser film is attached to the new LED-ring. To avoid detection of the directly reflected radiation from the skin surface (thus distinguishing the diffusely reflected radiation from the upper layers of skin), a pair of orthogonally-oriented polarizing filters are added: one of them directly after the diffuser, and the other-in front of the camera sensor matrix. The microscope is computer-controlled. The custom-developed program written in MatLab with a standard FTDI USB driver and a custom LED driver (written in C programming language) performs the control over LEDs and the acquisition of images. The software provides two image processing modes: (1) the preview mode, for focusing the microscope to the skin object, and (2) the video acquisition/processing mode, where the software performs sequential switching of LEDs and triggering of the video sensor. Each single measurement includes capturing of four frames (taken within the four wavelength bands). After recording, the images are stored in a 4-image matrix and saved as a data file for further processing. The image processing software allowed mapping of three above-mentioned skin chromophores, erythema index and the melanoma/nevus differentiation parameter [22]. More details on the modified video-microscope and its tests are available in [21,23,24].

2.1.3. Prototypes for Smartphone Monochromatic Spectral Imaging of Skin at Multi-Laser Illumination

If skin is evenly illuminated by several laser sources, monochromatic spectral images can be extracted from a single RGB image file [25], thus making it possible to map several chromophores in a single snapshot. Such an approach speeds-up the image processing and excludes image artefacts caused by the tissue movements. First demonstration of skin hemoglobin snapshot RGB mapping under double-wavelength laser illumination was reported at [26]. Later mapping of three main skin chromophores under triple-wavelength laser illumination was demonstrated with laboratory [27] and smartphone-based [28] setups.

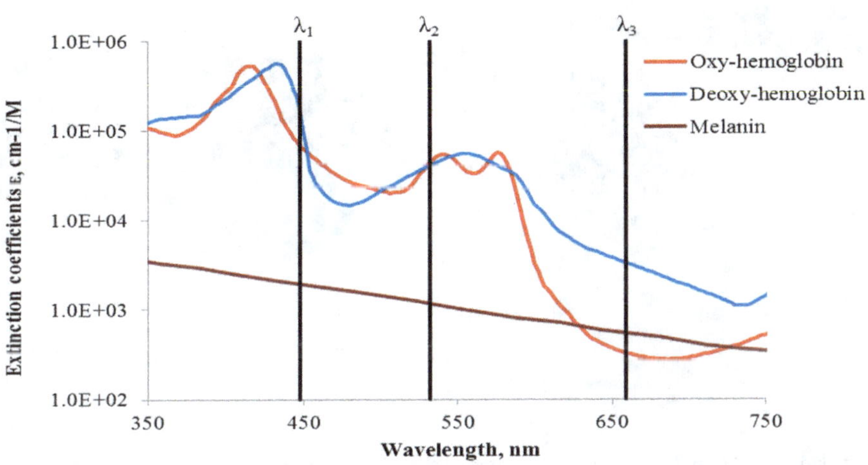

Figure 5. Absorption of three main skin chromophores [29,30] at three fixed wavelengths [28].

The general concept of snapshot skin chromophore mapping at fixed wavelengths is illustrated at Figure 5. Let us suppose that an RGB color image of skin is captured under illumination that comprises only three equal intensity spectral lines at wavelengths λ_1, λ_2 and λ_3 (the vertical lines in Figure 5). With respect to the spectral sensitivity of RGB image sensor and the cross-talk between its detection bands at the fixed wavelengths, three monochromatic spectral images can be extracted from the color image data set by the technique described in [25,31]. If the skin surface reflection is suppressed (e.g., by means of two crossed polarizers), variations in chromophore composition induce changes of the diffusely reflected light intensities at each of the fixed wavelengths. Such variations in the pathology region relatively to the healthy skin can be estimated by measuring reflected light intensities from equally sized regions of interest in the pathology (I_j) and the adjacent healthy skin (I_{oj}). The ratios I_j/I_{jo} at each pixel or pixel's group of three monochromatic spectral images contain information on the concentration increase or decrease of all three regarded chromophores, which can be further mapped over the whole image area [28].

A compact smartphone-compatible three wavelength illuminator has been designed, assembled and tested in the laboratory and clinics. Figure 6 shows the design details (left) and outlook of operating prototype with smartphone on it (right). Flat ring-shaped laser diffuser [17] ensures uniform three wavelength illumination of the round target area with diameter 40 mm. The illumination wavelengths 448 nm, 532 nm and 659 nm are emitted by three pairs of compact 20 mW power laser modules (models *PGL-DF-450nm-20mW-15011564, PGL-VI-1-532nm-20mW-15030443* and *PGL-DF-655nm-20mW-150302232* from Changchun New Industries Optoelectronics Tech. Co., Ltd., Changchun, China). Laser modules (1, Figure 6a—showing three out of six) of each equal-wavelength pair are mounted at opposite sides on the internal wall of a hollow 3D-printed plastic shielding cylinder 2; the round bottom opening of this cylinder is in contact with skin and forms the field of view for the smartphone camera, situated 80 mm apart. All six coaxial laser beams are pointed to the 45-degree conical reflecting edge of a Plexiglass transparent disc 3 (beam collector); after reflections they are turned radial towards the internal ring-shaped flat milky-Plexiglas diffuser 4. In result, the flat diffuser 4 evenly illuminates the 65 mm distant skin target area simultaneously by the three laser wavelengths.

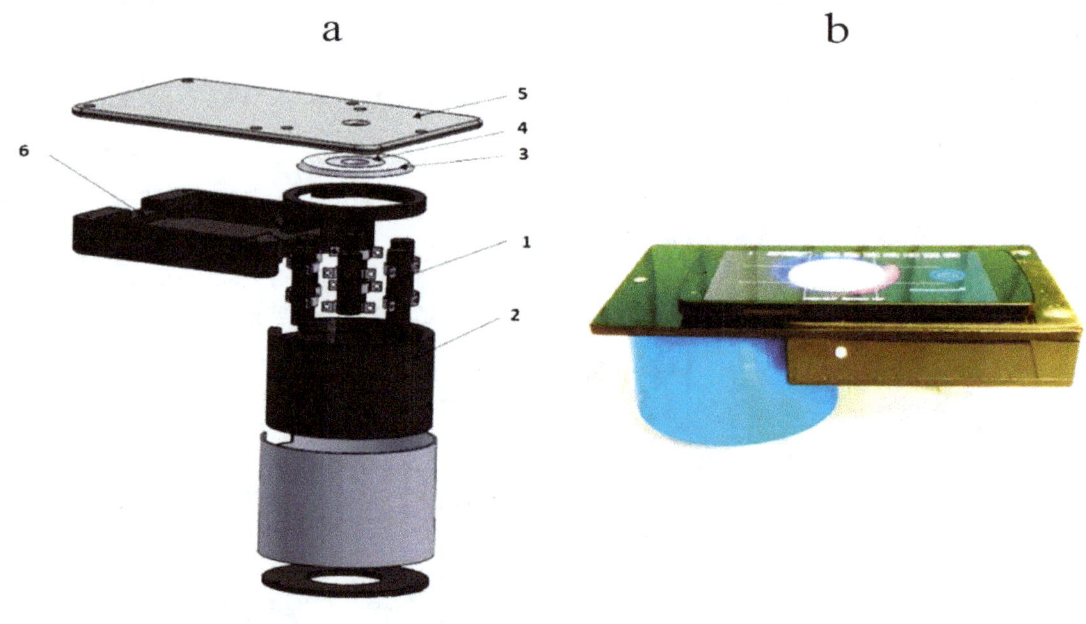

Figure 6. Design scheme of the 3-wavelength laser add-on illuminator (**a**) and the mobile prototype with smartphone on it (**b**): 1—laser modules (3 pairs, 448-532-659nm), 2—shielding cylinder, 3—collector of laser beams, 4—flat ring-shaped diffuser of laser light, 5—sticky platform for the smartphone, 6—electronics compartment [28].

The smartphone is placed on flat sticky platform 5 (Figure 6a) with a round window for the smartphone rear camera, co-aligned with the internal opening of the diffuser 4. The round camera window is covered by a film polarizer; another film with orthogonal direction of polarization covers the diffuser 4 from bottom, so avoiding detection of skin surface-reflected light by the smartphone camera. We used a model *Google Nexus5* smartphone comprising an 8Mpx *SONY IMX179* image sensor with known RGB-sensitivities; spatial resolution of the imaging system was better than 0.1 mm.

The single-snapshot RGB technique is not applicable for express-mapping of more than three skin chromophores. The double-snapshot approach [32] for obtaining four monochromatic images has been implemented in a model device comprising switchable four laser illuminator and a smartphone. Figure 7 shows the design scheme and outlook of a smartphone add-on illuminator intended for mapping of four skin chromophores, e.g., melanin, oxy-hemoglobin, deoxy-hemoglobin and bilirubin. Two of the laser modules can be manually switched on and off, so providing two sets of 3-wavelengths illumination (405, 532, 650 nm and 450, 532, 650 nm). Four rechargeable AA-type batteries are used for power supply. Relatively uniform illumination of round skin spot (dia. 18 mm) is provided by an advanced optical design which also reduces laser speckle artefacts [33]. More details on the multi-laser smartphone add-on prototypes and their test results can be found in [17,28,34].

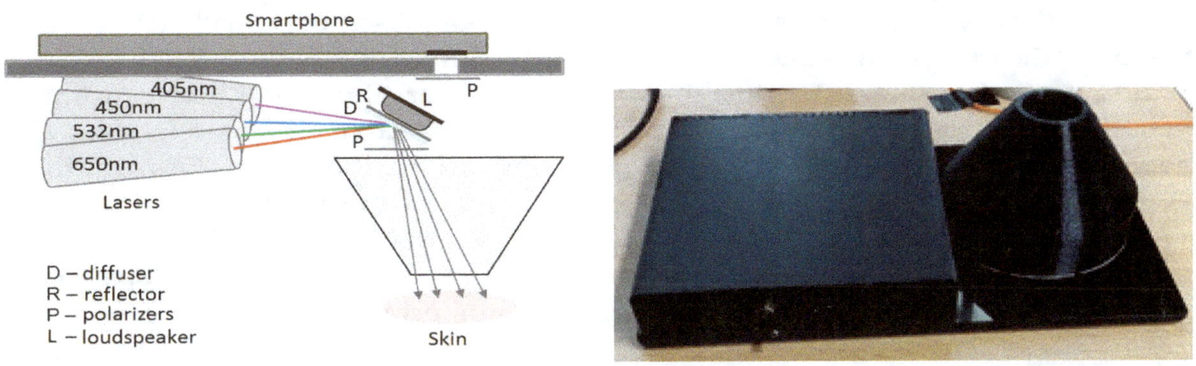

(a) (b)

Figure 7. Design scheme (**a**) and outlook (**b**) of the prototype device for switchable 4-wavelengths skin illumination [33,34].

2.2. *Prototype Device for Skin Fluorescence Imaging With a Smartphone*

If the light is absorbed in skin, it can be further re-emitted at longer wavelengths as autofluorescence (AF), i.e., self-fluorescence without any specific additives on or inside the skin. There is a number of fluorescing compounds called fluorophores in the upper skin, each with its specific emission spectrum. Even if excited by a narrow laser line, several emission spectra overlap and skin autofluorescence spectrum usually is bell-shaped, without a pronounced structure. Besides, a phenomenon called autofluorescence photobleaching (AFPB) normally takes place: the in-vivo skin emitted intensity decreases during continuous optical excitation and does not fully recover after interruptions of the excitation (Figure 8). AFPB causes some interesting effects like low power radiation induced "fingerprints" on in-vivo skin [35].

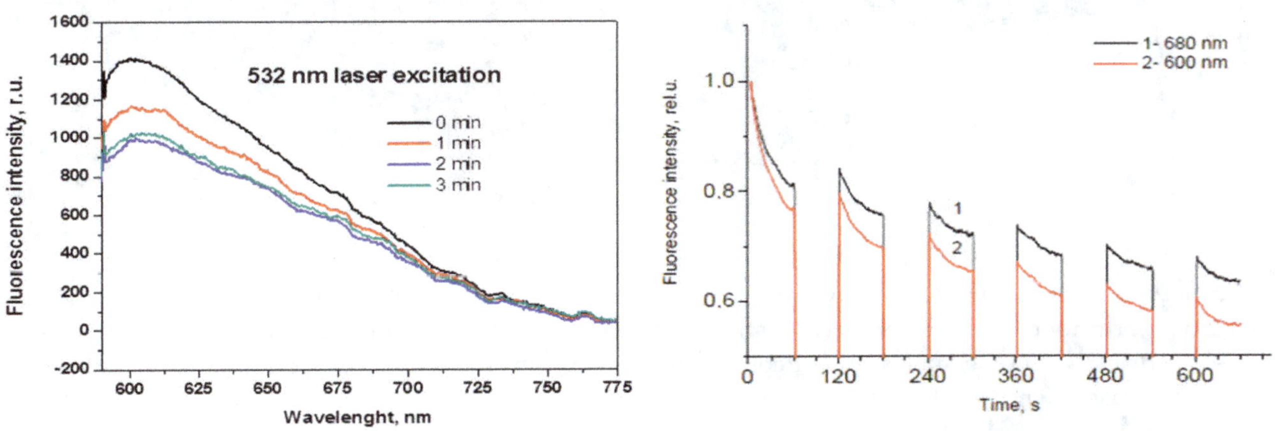

(a) (b)

Figure 8. Skin autofluorescence photobleaching at continuous 532nm laser irradiation (~85 mW/cm^2): (**a**)—temporal changes of the emission spectrum [36]; (**b**)—partial recovery of the autofluorescence intensity at two wavelengths after interrupted excitation [37].

The decrease of skin autofluorescence intensity during the laser exposure in most cases can be approximated by a double-exponential expression:

$$I(t) = a\exp(-t/\tau_1) + b\exp(-t/\tau_2) + A \quad (1)$$

where I—autofluorescence intensity at a fixed wavelength band, t—time, a and b—weighting coefficients, A—the "bottomline" constant, and τ_1, τ_2—the "fast" and "slow" AFPB rate coefficients, respectively. The "fast" AFPB (when sharp intensity decrease is observed) usually takes place during the first 5–15 s of the irradiation, while the "slow" AFPB continues up to several min.

Our first set-up for skin AFPB imaging comprised laser illuminator and consumer photo camera equipped with a band-pass filter in front of the objective; it was operating at a slow video-mode (~2 frames/s) [38]. After the image processing, distribution of τ-values over the imaged skin area was mapped and analyzed. This study showed that the τ-values are sensitive to skin structural changes—e.g., AFPB rates detected from melanin-pigmented nevi were always slower than those detected from healthy skin. Thus, the AFPB rate measurements and spatial mapping may have a potential for skin diagnostics and recovery monitoring, as well as for better skin tumor margin delineation.

As the next step, a smartphone-compatible technique for acquisition and analysis of violet LED excited skin fluorescence intensity and AFPB rate distribution images has been developed and clinically tested [39]. Design of the prototype device is illustrated on Figure 9. For parametric mapping of skin AF intensity decrease rates, a sequence of AF images under continuous 405 nm LED (model LED Engin LZ1-00UA00-U8, spectral band half-width 30 nm) excitation at a power density of ~20 mW/cm^2 with framerate 0.5 fr/s is recorded for 20 s. Four battery-powered violet LEDs placed within a cylindrical light-shielding wall (which also ensures a fixed 60 mm distance between the smartphone camera and skin) evenly irradiate a 40 mm round spot of the examined skin tissue. A long pass filter (>515 nm) is placed in front of the smartphone camera to prevent detection of the exciting LED emission. The battery/electronics compartment comprises a set of rechargeable batteries and a Bluetooth Low Energy (BLE) module with a driver for communications between the smartphone and illumination unit.

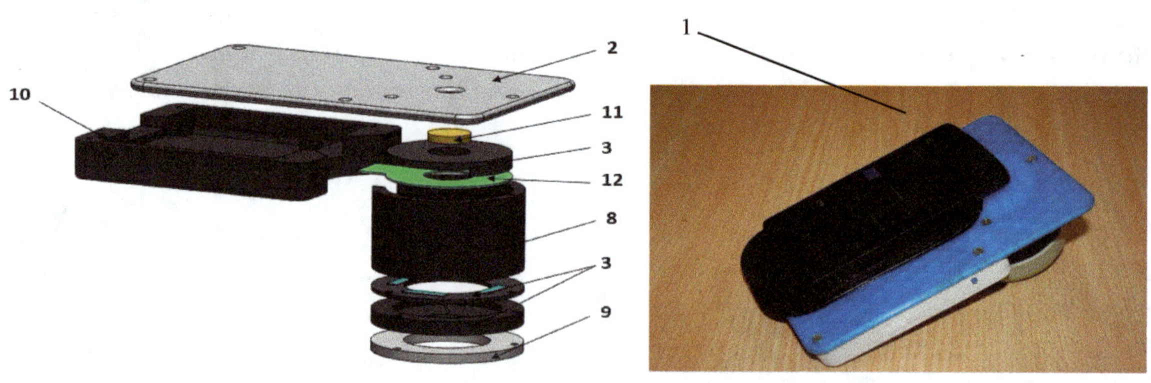

(a) (b)

Figure 9. Design scheme (**a**) and outlook (**b**) of the prototype device for skin fluorescence imaging with a smartphone: 1—smartphone, 2—sticky fixing plate with camera window, 3—mounting rings, 8—cylindrical screening spacer, 9—silicone skin-contact ring, 10—battery/electronics compartment, 11—long-pass filter, 12—LED ring [17].

The recorded RGB fluorescence images were further separated to exploit the R- and G-images for imaging of skin autofluorescence in the red and green spectral bands, respectively. Due to spectral cut-off by the 515 nm long pass filter, the B band images served only for reference. A *Samsung Galaxy Note 3* smartphone comprising integrated CMOS RGB image sensor with resolution of 13 MP was used for image acquisition. All images were taken at the following settings: ISO-100, white balance—daylight, focus—manual, exposure time—fixed 200 ms. More details on the skin fluorescence imager design and its test results are provided in [17,39].

2.3. Photoplethysmography Video-Imaging Prototypes

The incident cw light can be reflected from the skin surface and also may enter its epidermal and dermal layers where light can be absorbed and/or scattered. A part of back-scattered photons have been travelled via the skin dermal layer where arterial blood volume periodically changes with each heartbeat. As a consequence, also total blood absorption changes with each heartbeat and the back-scattered light intensity is modulated—the detected so-called remission photo-plethysmography (PPG) signal comprises a relatively stable DC component, determined by absorption of the "static" skin structures, and a pulsatile AC component caused by the periodically changing blood absorption [40]. The pulsatile remission PPG signals can be detected not only by specially designed skin contact probes [41], but also distantly, e.g., by video-imaging of skin with subsequent signal processing [42]. This technique is called PPG-imaging (PPGI) or remote PPG (rPPG). The captured video-signals consist of a number of image frames taken at a definite frame rate, e.g., 20 frames per second. Consequently, during one heart activity cycle (~1 s) 20 skin images are obtained, each at different phase of the sub-cutaneous pulse wave. If consecutive frames are compared, the skin-remitted light intensity detected from a fixed area increases and decreases with time, forming the periodic PPGI signal. Specific software [43] allows extracting the arterial pulsations from the video-signal over the whole imaged skin area. The amplitude of PPG peaks may differ between the image pixels due to different blood perfusion of the skin tissues—especially if there is a burn or other dermal skin damage. After the image processing, parametric maps of the PPG signal amplitude distribution (or blood perfusion maps) can be constructed [44].

2.3.1. PPGI Prototype for Palm Anesthesia Monitoring

Figure 10 illustrates the recently designed PPGI prototype device for distant monitoring of anesthesia efficiency during the palm surgeries. The system was intended for recording signals from the curved surface of the hand (dorsal or ventral aspect). The illuminator comprised four bispectral light sources, each consisting of two high-power LED emitters (Roithner LaserTechnik GmbH, Vienna, Austria; green: λ = 530 nm, 3 W and infrared: λ = 810 nm, 1 W). To achieve uniform illumination of skin surface, adjustable LED intensity control was introduced via PC based custom developed software. The two wavelengths of illumination were chosen in order to control blood pulsations at two different vascular depths in real time [45].

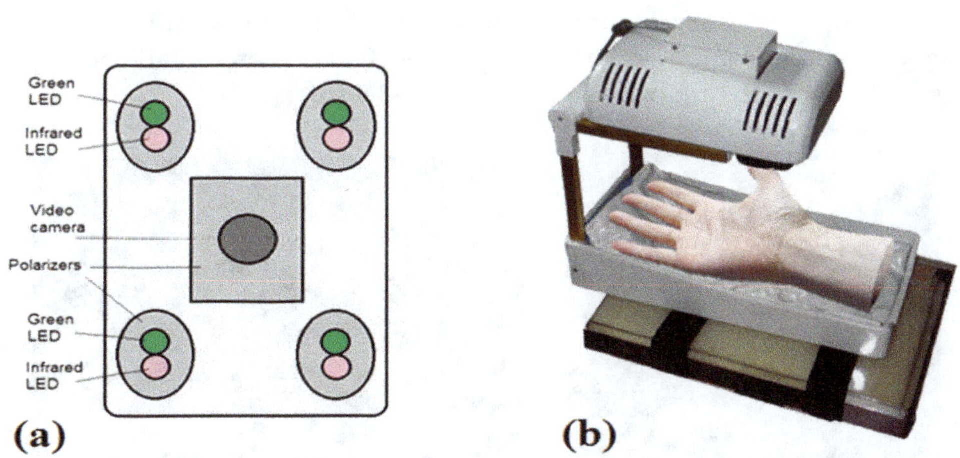

Figure 10. Dual wavelength photoplethysmography imaging device: bottom view of the imaging system-camera and light sources (**a**) and the whole device with vacuum pillow supporting the palm (**b**) [46].

The microcontroller board (Arduino Nano, Arduino, New York, NY, USA) provided sequential switching of green and IR LEDs and triggering of the captured video frames. The camera control was performed by *uEye* software using manual trigger mode, fixed exposure time, 2 × 2 pixels binning and triggered at 60 frames/s. The monochromatic camera (8 bit CMOS *IDS-uEye UI-1221LE*) was equipped with an *S-mount* 1/2 inch F = 4 mm low distortion, wide-field lens (Lensagon, Lensation GmbH, Karlsruhe, Germany). The camera lens was placed at 15 cm distance from the skin surface so ensuring full view of adult palm (20 cm × 15 cm field of view). In order to reduce skin specular reflectance, orthogonally oriented polarizers were placed behind the camera and all four light sources, respectively. The plastic parts were produced by a 3D printer (*Prusa i3*, custom made, Latvia). The device comprised a plastic enclosure filled with an adjustable vacuum pillow (40 × 20 AB Germa, Kristianstad, Sweden) as the palm support.

2.3.2. Universal Compact PPPGI Prototypes

Another, much smaller PPGI prototype device (Figure 11) for more universal applications related to skin microcirculation control has been developed, as well. It involves near-infrared LED illuminator and a video camera, both placed in custom designed 3D-printed case (4 cm × 4 cm × 4 cm). The illuminator comprises a ring of twelve circularly oriented near-infrared LEDs (peak wavelength 760 nm, current 20 mA each), connected in parallel; stabilized illumination is provided by LED driver (cat4104). Video acquisition is performed by a board-level CMOS video camera (*IDS uEye UI-1221LE*), resolution 752 × 480 pixels, maximum framerate 87 fps., 8-bit monochrome). The camera is equipped with low-distortion S-mount 4 mm lens (Lensagon). In order to reduce skin specular reflectance, cross-oriented polarizers are placed behind the light sources and in front of the camera, respectively. The infrared cut-off filter KC-15 (>700 nm) also is placed in the front of the camera, in order to minimize the influence of ambient illumination. USB-2 cable connection to PC ensures both video-signal processing and the power supply.

For real clinical applications, it is a good choice to use surgical lamp as a light source. A simple and convenient PPGI system for contactless monitoring of anesthesia effectiveness before and during surgical procedures has been developed (Figure 12). The system involves compact lightweight camera (CMOSIS, ADC-8/10/12-bits, resolution 640 × 480 pixels, 502 frames/s, Ximea-xiQ, Cubert GmbH, Ulm, Germany) with a low-distortion lens (3.5 mm f/2.4, Edmund Optics, Barrington, NJ, USA) and green band-pass filter (half-bandwidth 520–580 nm). Both are placed in a custom designed 3D-printed case, adapted for handle attachment to the warm-white-light surgical lamp (Prismalix PRX800, ALM, Soma Technology Inc., Bloomfield, CT, USA), see Figure 12b. The camera is connected via USB-3 cable to a laptop computer which also serves as the power supply of camera. Video acquisition frame rate is 100 Hz (equal to the lamp blinking frequency), so temporal variations of the lamp intensity do not affect the PPGI signal, filtered in the frequency range 0.7–3.0 Hz. More details on the developed PPGI prototype devices and their software can be found in [42–44,46,47].

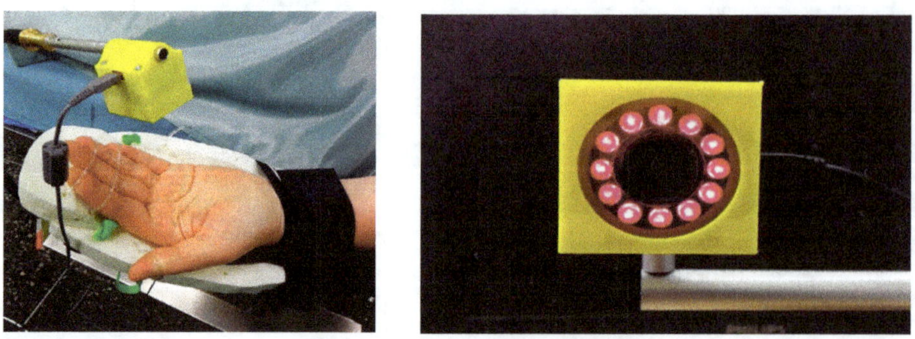

Figure 11. The compact PPGI prototype device in operation (**left**) and the front view of the device (**right**).

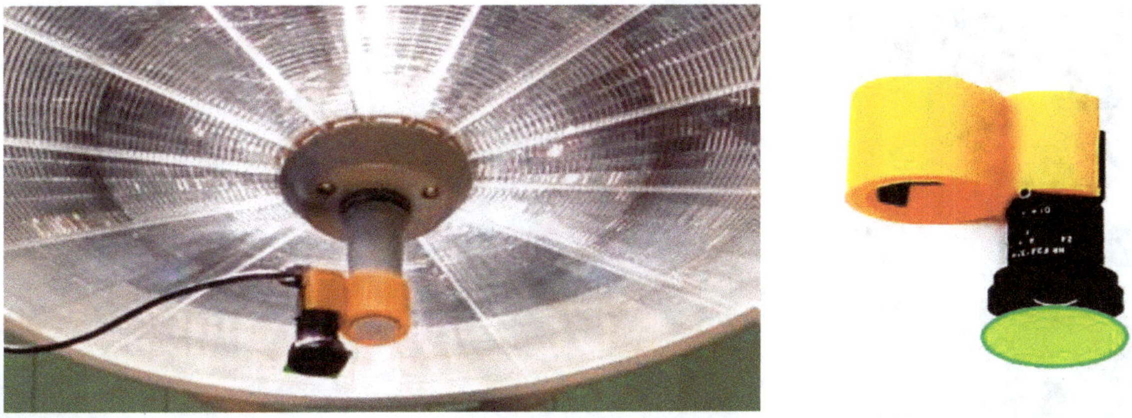

(a) (b)

Figure 12. The PPGI device attached to a surgical lamp (**a**) and the design of its holder (**b**) [47].

2.4. Multimodal Skin Imagers

2.4.1. SkImager—A Concept Device for Multimodal Skin Imaging

A proof-of-concept prototype device based on inexpensive components and smart software was developed for compact and handy wireless skin diagnostics and monitoring. The multimodal imaging includes capturing by a single camera a number of spectral and video-images from the skin pathology area, with subsequent extraction of clinically significant information. The device captures four consecutive imaging series: (i) RGB image of skin at white polarized LED illumination, helping to reveal hidden subcutaneous structures; (ii) four spectral images at narrowband LED illumination for mapping of the main skin chromophores; (iii) video-images under green LED illumination for mapping of skin blood perfusion; (iv) autofluorescence video-images under UV LED irradiation for mapping of the skin fluorophores. Polarized LED light is used for illumination, and round skin spot of diameter 34 mm is imaged by a CMOS sensor via cross-oriented polarizing filter. To improve the reliability of diagnostics, manipulation with maps of different parameters (i.e., extraction, summing, and division of images) is proposed, as well. Our first prototype version was described earlier [48].

A more advanced prototype device with the preliminary brand-name *SkImager* [49] has been developed (Figure 13). It is a battery-powered fully self-contained wireless device. Its main building blocks are CMOS image sensor, LED illumination system, on-chip microcomputer, touchscreen, memory card and rechargeable battery. The functional diagram of the device is presented at Figure 13c. A *Tegra 2 T20* (Nvidia, Santa Clara, CA, USA) system on chip (SoC) module with a dual-core *Cortex-A9* processor (clock frequency 1 GHz, ARM Inc., San Jose, CA, USA) is used as a central processing unit. It provides smooth operation of all components of the device. A 3 Mpix RGB CMOS matrix with 3.2 micron pixel size (MT9T031) serves as the image sensor; it is connected to the central processor via 10-bit parallel line. Removable SD memory card stores the image information that can be transferred to external processor, e.g., PC. It can be done also via Mini-USB connector which also ensures software installations and updates from outside. On-board and off-board calculations can be performed to extract parametric maps of the examined skin area. The main information input-output device is the built-in 4.3 inch/480 × 272 pixels touchscreen. It displays the operation mode and state of the device (battery charge level, clock, state of the memory card). Power switch button is placed on the side above the slot of memory card (Figure 13b). The device has its holder with integrated contacts for battery charging (Figure 13a). The Li-ion battery (3.6 V, 4.6 Ah) ensures up to 15 h of operation, providing about 100 full measurement cycles. The power consumption under the maximum load (display switched-on, spectral and video image recording and processing) is 3 Watts, or 1 Watt in the waiting mode. Dimensions of the device are 121 mm × 205 mm × 101 mm, weight about 440 g.

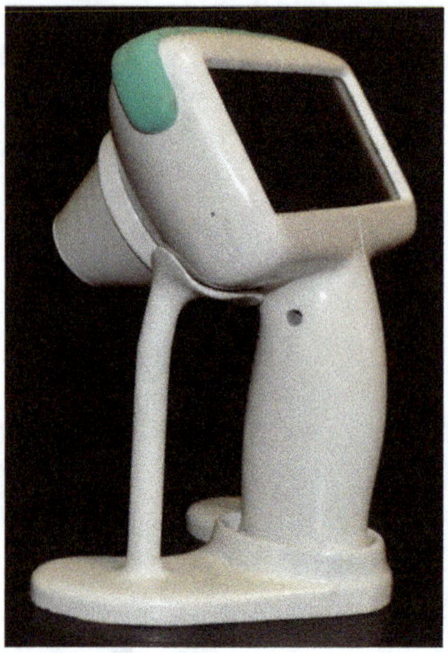

(a)

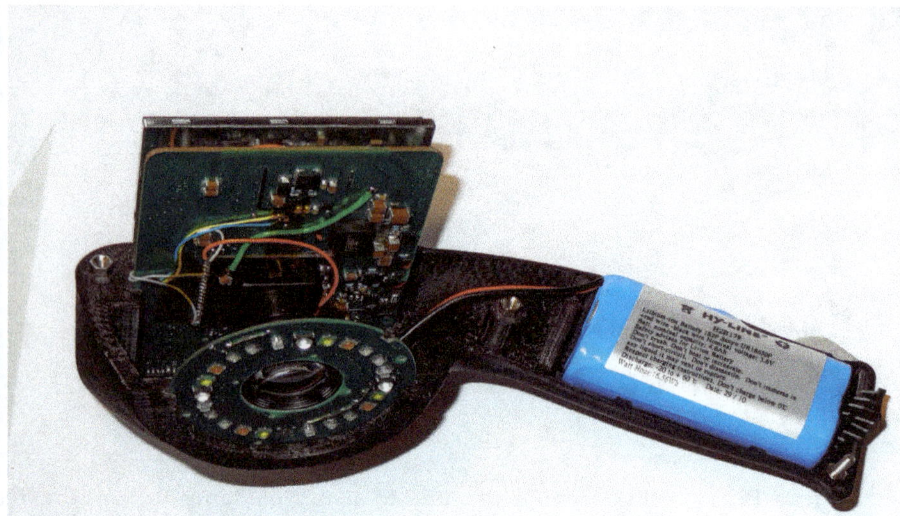

(b)

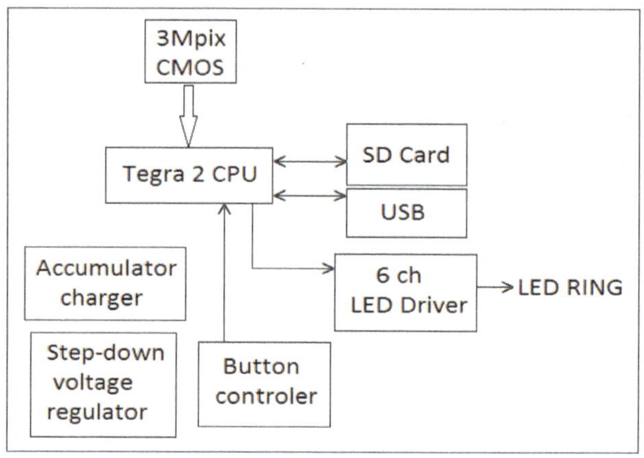

(c)

Figure 13. The *SkImager* prototype device in its battery-charging holder (**a**); internal design details (**b**) and functional scheme (**c**) [49].

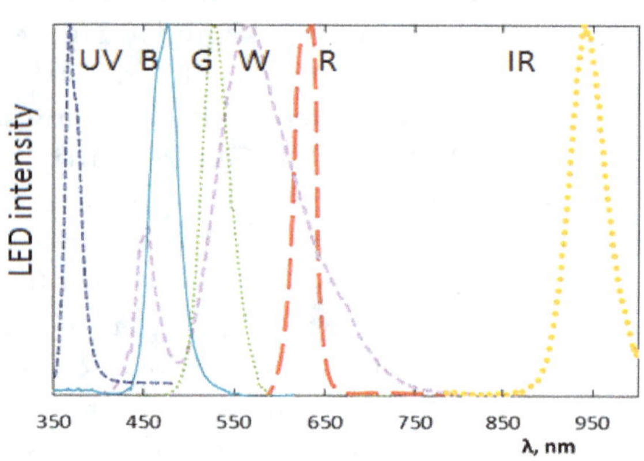

(a)

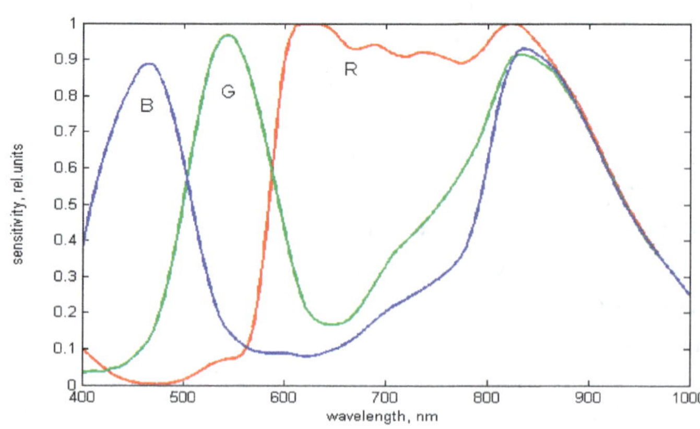

(b)

Figure 14. The measured emission bands of the exploited LEDs (**a**) and spectral sensitivity bands of the CMOS image sensor (**b**) exploited in the *SkImager* prototype [49].

The spectrally-specific skin illumination is performed by a ring of LEDs, surrounding the objective of image sensor—Figure 13b. In total 24 LEDs are operated—six sets of four diodes, emitting at six various wavelength bands (peaks at 365 nm, 450 nm, 540 nm, 660 nm, 940 nm and white—Figure 14a). Each set of equal LEDs is powered separately by the 6-channel LED driver (Figure 13c), in order to provide the same illumination intensity and constant signal output by the visible and NIR emitting diodes. In order to minimize detection of the surface-reflected light, crossed film polarizers cover the LED ring and camera objective (S-Mount M12 × 0.5), respectively. To keep fixed 55 mm distance to the skin, two easily changeable conical tips are used, with the target field diameters 34 mm and 11 mm, respectively. The latter is intended for more curved skin locations, e.g., on nose. Internal surfaces of the tips are black coated and multiple-step shaped, in order to suppress any side-reflected light. The RGB CMOS (Aptina Imaging, Nampa, ID, USA) image sensor with resolution of 2048 × 1536 pixels and maximal framerate 25 frames/s is used. Spectral sensitivity bands of the CMOS sensor (with removed NIR filter) are shown in Figure 14b. More details on the *SkImager* prototype and its test results are provided in [49,50].

2.4.2. The Modular Multimodal Skin Imager

Another prototype for multimodal skin imaging has been designed as a 3D-printed modular device that comprises three main modules (Figure 15):

1. Processing, wireless transmission and power block,
2. Camera and lens block,
3. Illumination block.

The first (processing and communication) module uses embedded computer—Raspberry Pi [51] as the main processing unit. Wireless connections are realized by WiPi USB dongles, and rechargeable battery is used as the power source. Charging is performed by connecting USB cable, similar as for mobile phones. All elements use standard interfaces and can be replaced just by plugging cable to the new device. The second (imaging) module holds an IDS uEye UI-3581LE-C-HQ camera [52] and the Lensagon BVM8020014 lens. Camera uses USB interface and allows upgrading to a new camera without any changes in hardware and software. IDS camera manufacturer was preferred since it has wide range of cameras and all of them share the same physical and software design. By using two lens mounts—"C type" and "S type"—lenses can be interchanged easily, as well.

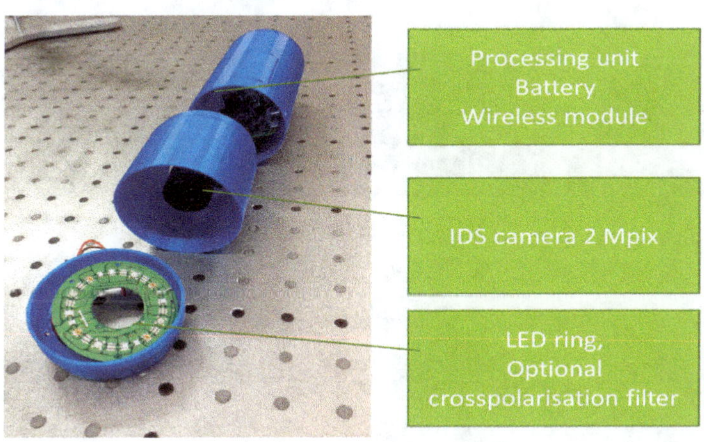

Figure 15. Photo of the 3D-printed modular multimodal imaging prototype [53].

The third (illumination) module ensures three imaging modes: multispectral imaging of diffuse reflectance (spectral bands with maxima at 435 nm, 535 nm, 660 nm, 740 nm and 940 nm), fluorescence spectral imaging (excitation at 405 nm) and 635 nm laser speckle imaging. Custom printed board was created for managing skin illumination by narrowband LEDs. It uses standard interface for selecting current illumination band, therefore light source change requires less effort than in fully customized existing designs.

By using her/his own smartphone or laptop, the user connects to the device's WiFi network and controls imaging process through the Internet browser. During the first step, the operating system's procedure for connecting to the WiFi network (with a password-controlled access) is performed. On the step two users selects whether he/she requires a new image capture or wishes to view the previous results. During the third step user targets the skin region to be captured by viewing live video stream from the camera. Image is captured by pressing a physical button located on the device. The capturing process can be repeated a number of times. After all skin images are acquired, user can switch to the last—results viewing step. Typical time delay between finishing the image capture procedure and obtaining the results is less than 10 s. More details on this device and its tests are presented in [53].

3. Results

The developed skin imaging prototypes were initially tested in laboratory and then in real clinical environments. All clinical studies were performed with written consent of the involved volunteers under official approval by the local ethics committee. Some results of the clinical measurements, aimed at checking functionality and appropriateness of the prototypes, are briefly presented below.

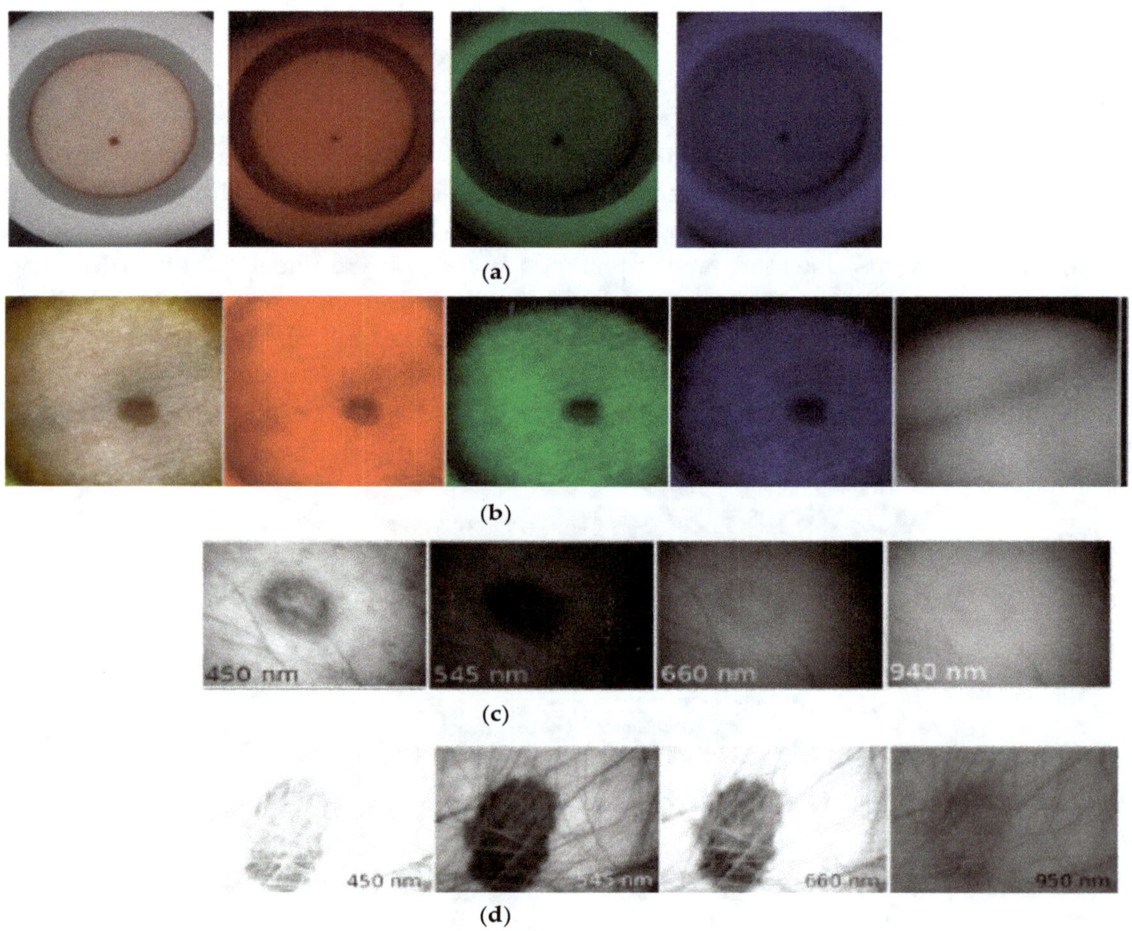

Figure 16. Spectral images of skin malformations taken by different prototypes: (**a**) nevus taken by smartphone—RGB LED prototype at white, red, green and blue illumination [18]; (**b**) nevus taken by SkImager at white, red, green, blue and NIR illumination [49]; (**c**) papilloma taken by modified video-microscope at blue, green, red and NIR illumination [23]; (**d**) melanoma taken by modified video-microscope at blue, green, red and NIR illumination [23].

3.1. Clinical Spectral Images and Chromophore Maps of Skin

Figure 16a illustrates spectral images of a skin nevus taken under white, red, green, and blue illumination of the RGB-LED system by *NEXUS5* smartphone camera, in comparison with spectral images of another nevus, taken under similar illumination by the *SkImager* prototype (Figure 16b). Qualitative agreement of nevi spectral images in the visible range can be observed. *SkImager* and the modified video-microscope provide also NIR spectral images at peak wavelength 940–950 nm which penetrates in skin deeper than the visible light [54]. If the NIR images of skin nevus, papilloma and melanoma are compared (Figure 16b–d), notable differences are seen. Nevus and papilloma images in NIR practically disappear while the melanoma NIR-image still has sufficient contrast, indicating to pathology in deeper skin layers accordingly to the clinical expectations [55].

Nine vascular and pigmented skin lesions were examined by the mobile laser illuminator system [28]. Aim of this study was to check ability of the prototype to provide physiologically feasible skin pigmentation information on already diagnosed skin malformations. After processing the clinical images, skin chromophore maps were constructed and changes of malformation's chromophore content with respect to the adjacent healthy skin evaluated. As initially expected, we observed notable melanin content increase in all cases of both pigmented malformations—nevi and seborrheic keratosis, without essential changes in the hemoglobin content. Increase of oxy-hemoglobin content and decrease of deoxy-hemoglobin (if compared to the surrounding healthy skin) was observed in all examined vascular malformations—hemangiomas, without notable changes in skin melanin content (Figure 17). This result is a good illustration of increased arterial blood supply in skin hemangiomas and confirms functionality of the multi-laser prototype.

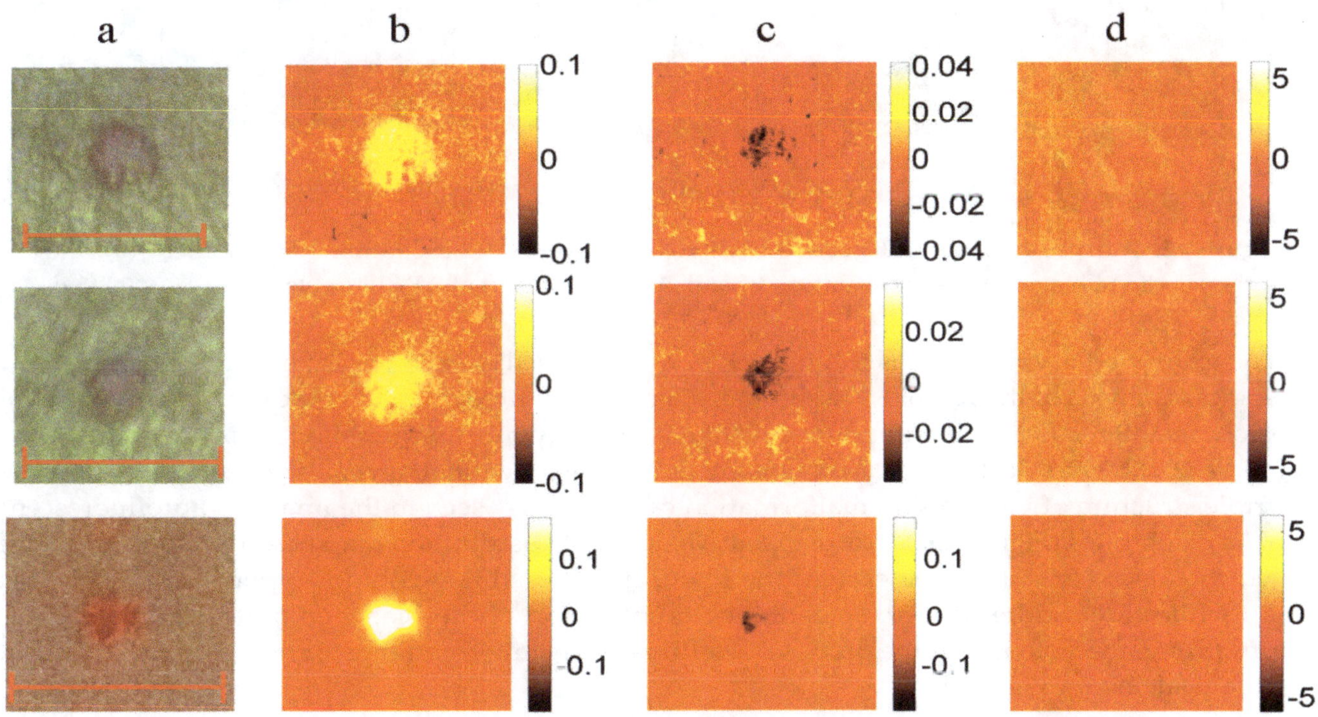

Figure 17. RGB image ((**a**) scale bar 5 mm) and the corresponding maps of chromophore concentration changes for three cases of a vascular hemangioma: (**b**)—oxy-hemoglobin; (**c**)—deoxy-hemoglobin; (**d**)—melanin. Units of the color scale-milimoles [28].

3.2. Fluorescent and Photo-Bleaching Rate Images of Skin Tumors

Overall 50 patients with 150 different skin neoplasms were inspected with the smartphone based fluorescence imager. For more detailed image analysis 13 basal cell carcinomas (BCC) and 1 atypical nevus were selected [39]. In order to visualize the skin AF intensity decrease rates during the photo-bleaching, the following image processing expression was applied:

$$N(C) = (I_{t0}[C] - I_t[C])/I_{t0}[C] \tag{2}$$

where N(C) represents normalized AF intensity decrease map for each pixel (or pixel group) during the excitation period, $I_{t0}[C]$—AF image at the excitation start moment, $I_t[C]$—AF image after 20 s of continuous excitation and C—color component of the RGB image—red (R), green (G) and blue (B), respectively. The values of RGB components were defined from the image data by a special program developed in MATLAB®.

In all BCC cases (confirmed by cytological examination) the fluorescent images showed lowered AF intensity in malignant tissue as compared with the healthy surrounding skin, which may be attributed to lower concentration of fluorophores and increased blood perfusion caused by the malignant process. A case of solid BCC is illustrated in Figure 18. The G-band AF intensity image (Figure 18b) shows relatively low intensity within the tumor area, with clear margins between tumor and surrounding healthy skin. The tumor area also shows higher AF intensity photobleaching rate (Figure 18c) in comparison with the surrounding healthy skin. Both AF intensity and photobleaching images appear to be useful for non-contact delineation of skin tumor margins.

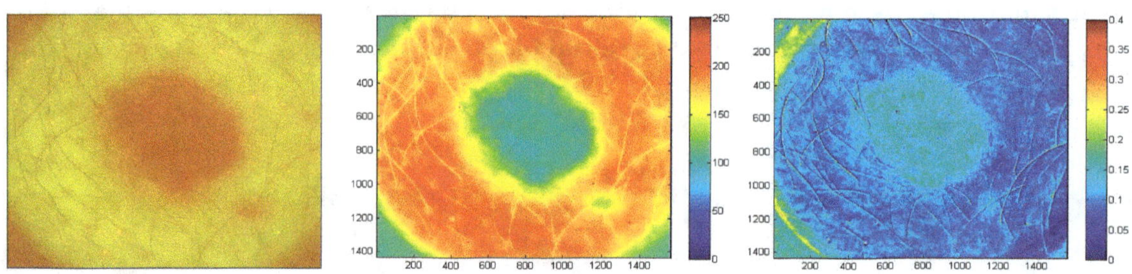

(a) (b) (c)

Figure 18. Images of solid BCC: filtered AF color image at the excitation start moment (**a**), the corresponding G-band fluorescence image (**b**) and normalized map of AF photo-bleaching rates (**c**) [39].

The examined atypical nevus (Figure 19) before surgical excision was suspected as melanoma. Histological analysis of the removed tissue sample revealed three different types of tissue cells within the lesion area. Specifically, the upper part of the pathology mostly prevailed by intradermal nevus, the middle part by dysplastic nevus, and the lower part by junctional nevus. Not visible by naked eye, such triple structure of in-vivo skin malformation can be clearly seen in the image of autofluorescence photobleaching rates (Figure 19c). Normalized AF decrease distribution map before surgery/histology showed the fastest intensity decrease in the lower (junctional nevus) and upper side (intradermal nevus), while the middle part (dysplastic nevus) of lesion photo-bleached slower. This example confirms promising potential of the proposed AFPB rate imaging technique for non-contact diagnostics of oncological changes in skin.

3.3. Skin Blood Perfusion Measurements With the PPGI Prototypes

In order to evaluate ability of the double-wavelength PPGI prototype (Figure 10) to discriminate between cutaneous superficial and deep plexus perfusion, hyperemia of superficial plexus was induced by vasodilatory liniment (Transvasin, Seton, UK) [46]. PPGI signal amplitudes at both spectral bands of illumination (peak wavelengths 530 nm and 810 nm) were recorded; Laser Doppler imaging (LDI) signals were captured in parallel by a certified commercial device. Ten healthy volunteers (five males and five females, skin type II) were recruited to participate.

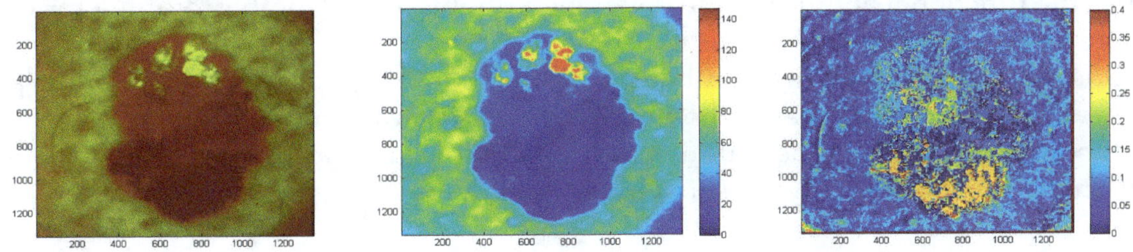

(a) (b) (c)

Figure 19. Color filtered AF image of skin atypical nevus at the excitation start moment (**a**), the corresponding G-band fluorescence image (**b**) and normalized AF photo-bleaching rates (**c**) [39].

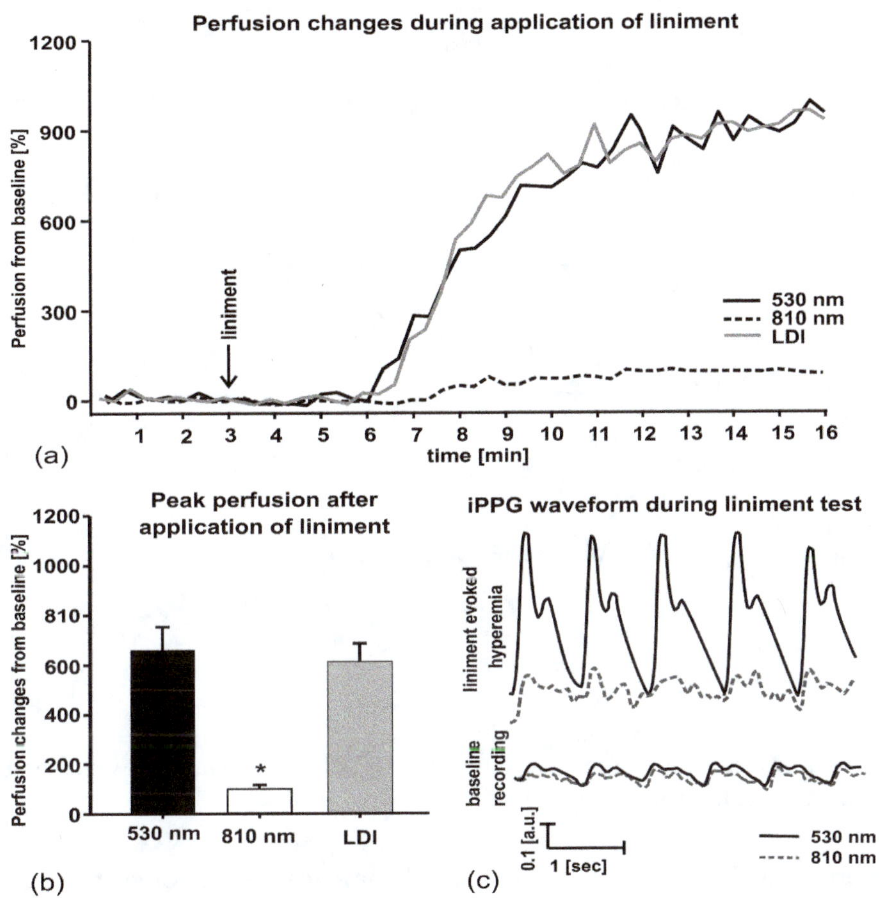

Figure 20. Liniment-induced skin perfusion changes as registered with the double-wavelength PPGI prototype and commercial LDI device (**a**), peak perfusion increase from the baseline (**b**) and the PPGI signal waveforms before and after provocation (**c**) [46].

The subjects were seated on a comfortable reclined chair with the right hand at the dorsal aspect, fixed on the vacuum pillow support (Figure 10b) and kept at heart level, with fingers tightly fitted to avoid movements. The protocol involved 3-min recording of the baseline followed by topical application of liniment and signal recording for 12 min. Within three to four min after application of liniment the reddening of skin appeared, indicating to hyperemia. Green PPGI measurements showed essential (about six times) increase of superficial skin perfusion, well correlated to that measured by the LDI device, while the NIR PPGI signal amplitude (reflecting arterial blood perfusion in deeper dermal layers) only slightly increased—see Figure 20. This result convincingly demonstrates the functional abilities of the developed double-wavelength prototype for non-contact skin microcirculation monitoring.

Local anesthesia affects the sympathetic vascular tone, resulting in vasodilation and raised skin blood perfusion. This increases the amplitude of fast-varying signal detected by the PPGI prototypes—see Figure 21 for illustration. Such physiological response makes possible to detect remotely, if and when anesthesia works just by following the changes in amplitude of the detected PPG signals.

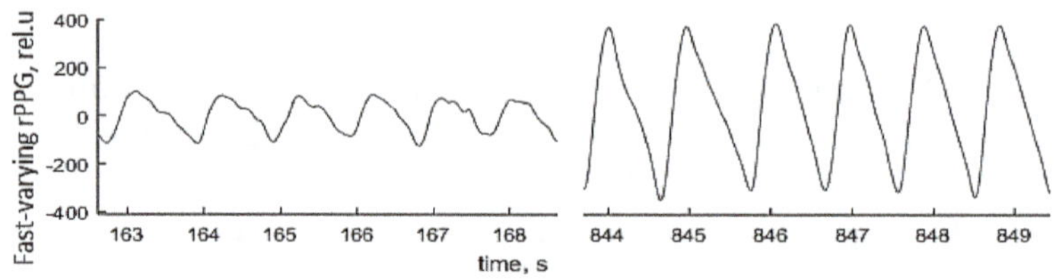

Figure 21. The palm PPGI signal waveforms before (**left**) and after (**right**) administration of local anesthetic [47].

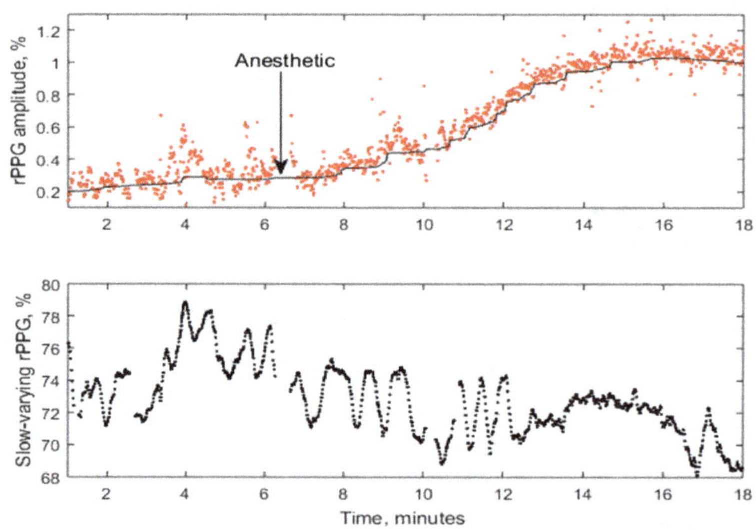

Figure 22. The averaged amplitude of fast-varying PPG signal (**above**) and slow-varying signal (**below**) during the regional anestesia procedure [47].

Figure 22 presents the PPG signal amplitude dynamics in response to regional anesthesia of patient's palm before surgery, as detected by the PPGI prototype attached to the surgical lamp (Figure 12). The graph above shows the beat-to-beat amplitude dynamics while the graph below represents temporal variation of the slow-varying PPGI component. Gradual increase of perfusion with subsequent rise of the PPGI signal amplitude (the upper graph) was observed few min after the administration of local anesthetics. The plateau phase—stable increased skin perfusion induced by the anesthetic—was reached approximately 10 min later and indicated the possible surgery starting time.

Figure 23 shows several screenshots of palm video fused with PPG-amplitude (PPGA) maps during anesthetic action before the surgery. As the local anesthetic affected four different nerves, subsequent microcirculation changes at four different palm skin zones (dermatomes) were observed. The PPGA maps showed increased microcirculation in dermatomes immediately after the local anesthetic was administered (stages 2–6). To conclude, the obtained results confirm clinical efficiency of the developed PPGI prototypes for remote patient anesthesia monitoring before and during surgeries.

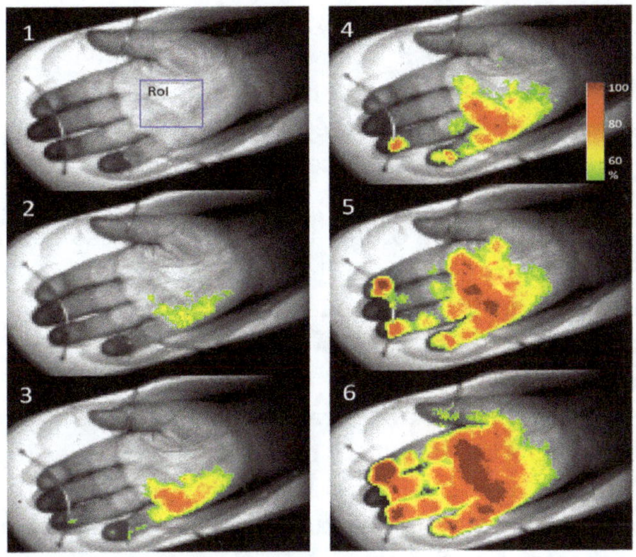

Figure 23. PPGA maps before (1) and after the administration of local anesthetic: 2—1 min, 3—3 min, 4—5 min, 5—6 min, 6—7 min later [47].

4. Discussion

The principles of operation and design features of ten recently developed prototype devices for diagnostic skin imaging have been presented, along with some clinical test results confirming their practical applicability. The laboratory-made prototypes were mainly intended as proof-of-principle devices, able to examine suitability of the developed design concepts and software solutions for further implementation in real clinical environments. Diagnostic sensitivity/specificity, influence of skin color, epidermal thickness and/or optical clearing have not been considered at this stage, as they can be evaluated only after statistically representative clinical trials.

Tests of the multispectral skin imaging prototypes led to conclusions on critical conditions to be met for successful extraction of skin parametric maps (e.g., chromophore distribution maps) from the captured spectral images. The most important ones are uniformity of skin illumination at all used spectral bands, long-term repeatability of all spectral illumination parameters, possibly narrow spectral bandwidths (monochromatic spectral images preferred) and short image acquisition time (single snapshot mode preferred). The developed designs are intended for imaging of relatively flat skin areas; the curved ones (e.g., nose, fingers) still remain an issue due to uneven illumination and varying focal distance. Speckle free multi-laser illumination [33] seems to be a good challenge for multi-spectral skin diagnostic imaging in future. If smartphones or consumer cameras are used for skin image capturing, all automatic settings must be switched off to avoid unexpected artifacts. Besides hardware, also the spectral image processing software has a lot of space for improvements, in order to speed up the image conversion processes and to use more adequate algorithms for calculation of clinically significant parameters.

Fluorescent skin imaging is relatively less complicated non-contact diagnostics technique. It was shown that even a simple and inexpensive smartphone-illuminator system (Figure 9) can provide clinically interesting data for skin tumor identification and margin delineation. Imaging of skin autofluorescence photo-bleaching rates certainly has a good potential for such clinical applications. A technical challenge to be solved is ensuring motionless conditions during the recording of fluorescent images for at least 15 s from any location of the body. The camera-skin motions can be easily avoided if the skin surface is relatively flat (e.g., on the back), while obtaining high quality fluorescent video-files from curved body locations (e.g., face, arms) would require further developments of special holders and skin spacers. Like in the case of multi-spectral imaging, software development for fast and accurate fluorescent image processing is still an issue, as well.

The developed photoplethysmography imaging prototypes and software have revealed new challenges for distant non-contact monitoring of skin blood perfusion changes at different vascular depths and under anesthesia. The latter application seems to be most successful if the camera is attached to the surgical lamp or originally integrated there. Stabilized DC power supply to the lamp is preferred, but the AC supply also does not influence the results much if the video frame rate is selected equal to the light pulsation frequency. Fusion of PPGA images with real body images (Figure 22) seems to be efficient for future on-line monitoring of the anesthesia process details.

Tests of the developed multimodal imaging prototypes have confirmed their proposed functionality. However, from the point of clinical users the number of offered options seems to be too high and more specialized devices based on the tested concepts eventually might be more successful in the medical device market.

Implementation of new design ideas and practical tests of the prototypes will promote better understanding of the challenges and drawbacks of in-vivo skin imaging technologies. Their clear advantages are remote and nearly real-time operation, as well as ability of quantitative pathology documentation. On the other hand, image-based clinical criteria for skin pathology diagnostics either do not exist or are in very early stage of development. Routine healthcare needs "golden standards" for fair assessment of patient's condition and for setting up the recovery strategy, and from this point optical imaging techniques still have to be checked at numerous clinical measurements before becoming a standard of care. Even if some of the above-described skin imaging prototypes would appear clinically acceptable, lots of efforts will be needed in future to establish and validate specific image parameters related to clinically significant threshold levels of particular skin pathologies.

Acknowledgments: Preparation of this review was mainly supported by the Latvian national research program SOPHIS under the grant agreement #10-4/VPP-4/11. The prototypes were developed also in frame of projects funded by the European Regional Development Fund. Author is deeply grateful to all collaborators (co-authors of the below-listed papers and patent applications) for their significant contributions. Fruitful discussions of the results in frame of the EC COST action BM1205 are highly appreciated.

References

1. MoleMate Siascope Handheld Melanoma Screening System. Available online: http://www.wms.co.uk/Dermatology/Dermatoscopes,Lights_and_Magnifiers/MoleMate_Siascope_Handheld_Melanoma_Screening_System (accessed on 9 April 2017).
2. MelaFind. Available online: http://www.melafind.com/melafind/ (accessed on 9 April 2017).
3. Que, S.K.T.; Grant-Kels, J.M.; Rabinovitz, H.S.; Oliveiro, M.; Scope, A. Application of handheld confocal microscopy for skin cancer diagnosis. *Dermatol. Clin.* **2016**, *34*, 469–475. [CrossRef] [PubMed]
4. DermaInspect. Available online: http://www.jenlab.de/DermaInspect.29.0.html?&L=en%3E%22 (accessed on 9 April 2017).
5. Dermlight. Available online: https://dermlite.com/ (accessed on 9 April 2017).
6. Dlite Microscope. Available online: http://skinandhairscope.com/Products/Dlite/Dlite.php (accessed on 9 April 2017).
7. Skinvision. Available online: https://www.skinvision.com/technology-skin-cancer-melanoma-mobile-app (accessed on 12 March 2017).
8. Vidovič, L.; Milanič, M.; Randeberg, L.L.; Majaron, B. Quantitative characterization of traumatic bruises by combined pulsed photothermal radiometry and diffuse reflectance spectroscopy. *Proc. SPIE* **2015**, *9303*, 930307. [CrossRef]
9. Spigulis, J. Biophotonic technologies for noninvasive assessment of skin condition and blood microcirculation. *Latv. J. Phys. Techn. Sci.* **2012**, *49*, 63–80.
10. Multispectral Imaging. Available online: http://www.imaging.org/site/PDFS/Reporter/Articles/REP27_4_CIC20_TOMINAGA_p177.pdf (accessed on 12 March 2017).
11. Jakovels, D.; Spigulis, J.; Rogule, L. RGB mapping of hemoglobin distribution in skin. *Proc. SPIE* **2011**, *8087*, 80872B.

12. Jakovels, D.; Kuzmina, I.; Berzina, A.; Valeine, L.; Spigulis, J. Noncontact monitoring of vascular lesion phototherapy efficiency by RGB multispectral imaging. *J. Biomed. Opt.* **2013**, *18*, 126019. [CrossRef] [PubMed]
13. Jakovels, D.; Spigulis, J. 2-D mapping of skin chromophores in the spectral range 500–700 nm. *J. Biophoton.* **2010**, *3*, 125–129. [CrossRef] [PubMed]
14. Jakovels, D.; Spigulis, J. RGB imaging device for mapping and monitoring of hemoglobin distribution in skin. *Lith. J. Phys.* **2012**, *52*, 50–54. [CrossRef]
15. Philips Vital Signs Camera. Available online: http://www.vitalsignscamera.com/ (accessed on 12 March 2017).
16. The Best Heart Disease iPhone & Android Apps of the Year. Available online: http://www.healthline.com/health-slideshow/top-heart-disease-iphone-android-apps#5 (accessed on 12 March 2017).
17. Spigulis, J.; Lacis, M.; Kuzmina, I.; Lihacovs, A.; Upmalis, V.; Rupenheits, Z. Method and Device for Smartphone Mapping of Tissue Compounds. Lv. Patent WO 2017012675 A1, 26 January 2017.
18. Kuzmina, I.; Lacis, M.; Spigulis, J.; Berzina, A.; Valaine, L. Study of smartphone suitability for mapping of skin chromophores. *J. Biomed. Opt.* **2015**, *20*, 090503. [CrossRef] [PubMed]
19. Dino-Lite for Healthcare. Available online: http://www.dino-lite.com/applications_list.php?index_id=8 (accessed on 12 March 2017).
20. Dino-Lite AM4115-FUT. Available online: http://www.dino-lite.com/products_detail.php?index_m1_id=0&index_m2_id=0&index_id=61 (accessed on 12 March 2017).
21. Rubins, U.; Zaharans, J.; Lihacova, I.; Spigulis, J. Multispectral video-microscope modified for skin diagnostics. *Latv. J. Phys. Techn. Sci.* **2014**, *51*, 65–70. [CrossRef]
22. Diebele, I.; Kuzmina, I.; Lihachev, A.; Spigulis, J.; Kapostinsh, J.; Derjabo, A.; Valaine, L. Clinical evaluation of melanomas and common nevi by spectral imaging. *Biomed. Opt. Express* **2012**, *3*, 467–472. [CrossRef] [PubMed]
23. Bekina, A.; Diebele, I.; Rubins, U.; Zaharans, J.; Derjabo, A.; Spigulis, J. Multispectral assessment of skin malformations by modified video-microscope. *Latv. J. Phys. Techn. Sci.* **2012**, *49*, 4–8.
24. Bekina, A.; Rubins, U.; Lihachova, I.; Zaharans, J.; Spigulis, J. Skin chromophore mapping by means of a modified video-microscope for skin malformation diagnosis. *Proc. SPIE* **2013**, *8856*, 88562G.
25. Spigulis, J.; Elste, L. Method and Device for Imaging of Spectral Reflectance at Several Wavelength Bands. Lv. Patent WO2013135311 A1, 19 September 2013.
26. Spigulis, J.; Jakovels, D.; Rubins, U. Multi-spectral skin imaging by a consumer photo-camera. *Proc. SPIE* **2010**, *7557*, 75570M.
27. Spigulis, J.; Oshina, I. Snapshot RGB mapping of skin melanin and hemoglobin. *J. Biomed. Opt.* **2015**, *20*, 050503. [CrossRef] [PubMed]
28. Spigulis, J.; Oshina, I.; Berzina, A.; Bykov, A. Smartphone snapshot mapping of skin chromophores under triple-wavelength laser illumination. *J. Biomed. Opt.* **2017**, *22*, 091508. [CrossRef] [PubMed]
29. Prahl, S. Tabulated Molar Extinction Coefficient for Hemoglobin in Water. Available online: http://omlc.ogi.edu/spectra/hemoglobin/summary.html (accessed on 30 November 2016).
30. Sarna, T.; Swartz, H.M. The Physical Properties of Melanin. Available online: http://omlc.ogi.edu/spectra/melanin/eumelanin.html (accessed on 30 November 2016).
31. Spigulis, J.; Elste, L. Single-snapshot RGB multispectral imaging at fixed wavelengths: proof of concept. *Proc. SPIE* **2014**, *8937*, 89370L.
32. Spigulis, J.; Oshina, I. Method and Device for Chromophore Mapping under Illumination by Several Spectral Lines. Lv. Patent 15106 B, 20 March 2016.
33. Rubins, U.; Kviesis-Kipge, E.; Spigulis, J. Device for Obtaining Speckle-Free Images at Illumination by Scattered Laser Beams. Lv. Patent P-17-17, 10 May 2017.
34. Oshina, I.; Spigulis, J.; Rubins, U.; Kviesis-Kipge, E.; Lauberts, K. Express RGB mapping of three to five skin chromophores. *OSA Tech. Dig.* **2017**, in press.
35. Lihachev, A.; Lesins, J.; Jakovels, D.; Spigulis, J. Low power cw-laser signatures on human skin. *Quant. Electron.* **2010**, *40*, 1077–1080. [CrossRef]
36. Lihachev, A. Kinetics of Laser-Excited In-Vivo Skin Autofluorescence and Remission. Ph.D. Thesis, University of Latvia, Riga, Latvia, 2010.
37. Lesinsh, J.; Lihachev, A.; Rudys, R.; Bagdonas, S.; Spigulis, J. Skin autofluorescence photobleaching and photo-memory. *Proc. SPIE* **2011**, *8092*, 80920N.

38. Spigulis, J.; Lihachev, A.; Erts, R. Imaging of laser-excited tissue autofluorescence bleaching rates. *Appl. Opt.* **2009**, *48*, D163–D168. [CrossRef] [PubMed]
39. Lihachev, A.; Derjabo, A.; Ferulova, I.; Lange, M.; Lihacova, I.; Spigulis, J. Autofluorescence imaging of Basal Cell Carcinoma by smartphone RGB camera. *J. Biomed. Opt.* **2015**, *20*, 120502. [CrossRef] [PubMed]
40. Allen, J. Photoplethysmography and its application in clinical physiological measurement. *Physiol. Meas.* **2007**, *28*, R1. [CrossRef] [PubMed]
41. Spigulis, J. Optical non-invasive monitoring of skin blood pulsations. *Appl. Opt.* **2005**, *44*, 1850–1857. [CrossRef] [PubMed]
42. Rubins, U.; Upmalis, V.; Rubenis, O.; Jakovels, D.; Spigulis, J. Real-time photoplethysmography imaging system. *Proc. IFMBE* **2011**, *34*, 183–186.
43. Rubins, U.; Spigulis, J.; Miscuks, A. Photoplethysmography imaging algorithm for continuous monitoring of regional anesthesia. In Proceedings of the 2016 ACM/IEEE 14th Symposium on Embedded Systems for Real-Time Multimedia, Pittsburgh, PA, USA, 6–7 October 2016. [CrossRef]
44. Rubins, U.; Spigulis, J.; Miscuks, A. Application of color magnification technique for revealing skin microcircuration changes under regional anaesthetic input. *Proc. SPIE* **2013**, *9032*, 903203.
45. Spigulis, J.; Gailite, L.; Lihachev, A.; Erts, R. Simultaneous recording of skin blood pulsations at different vascular depths by multi-wavelength photoplethysmography. *Appl. Opt.* **2007**, *46*, 1754–1759. [CrossRef] [PubMed]
46. Marcinkevics, Z.; Rubins, U.; Zaharans, J.; Miscuks, A.; Urtane, E.; Ozolina-Moll, L. Imaging photoplethysmography for clinical assessment of cutaneous microcirculation at two different depths. *J. Biomed. Opt.* **2016**, *21*, 35005. [CrossRef] [PubMed]
47. Rubins, U.; Miscuks, A.; Lange, M. Simple and convenient remote photoplethysmography system for monitoring regional anesthesia effectiveness. In Proceedings of the EMBEC-NBC2017, Tampere, Finland, 12–15 June 2017, in press.
48. Spigulis, J.; Garancis, V.; Rubins, U.; Zaharans, E.; Zaharans, J.; Elste, L. A device for multimodal imaging of skin. *Proc. SPIE* **2013**, *8574*, 85740J.
49. Spigulis, J.; Rubins, U.; Kviesis-Kipge, E.; Rubenis, O. SkImager: A concept device for in-vivo skin assessment by multimodal imaging. *Proc. Est. Acad. Sci.* **2014**, *63*, 213–220. [CrossRef]
50. Spigulis, J.; Rubins, U.; Kviesis-Kipge, E. Multimodal Imaging Device for Non-Contact Skin Diagnostics. Lv. Patent 14749 B, 20 November 2013.
51. Embedded Linux on Board Computer Description. Available online: https://www.raspberrypi.org/ (accessed on 12 March 2017).
52. Industrial USB Cameras Description. Available online: https://en.ids-imaging.com/ (accessed on 12 March 2017).
53. Bliznuks, D.; Jakovels, D.; Saknite, I.; Spigulis, J. Mobile platform for online processing of multimodal skin optical images: Using online Matlab server for processing remission, fluorescence and laser speckle images, obtained by using novel handheld device. In Proceedings of the 2015 International Conference on BioPhotonics (BioPhotonics), Florence, Italy, 20–22 May 2015. [CrossRef]
54. Anderson, R.R.; Parrish, J.A. The optics of human skin. *J. Invest. Dermatol.* **1981**, *77*, 13–19. [CrossRef] [PubMed]
55. Rigel, S.D.; Robinson, K.J.; Ross, I.M.; Friedman, R. *Cancer of the Skin: Expert Consult*, 2nd ed.; Elsevier Health Sciences: Amsterdam, The Netherlands, 2011; pp. 99–123.

Design of Liver Functional Reserve Estimation Technique Based on Optical Densitometry

Ekaterina Savchenko [1,*], Ilya Kolokolnikov [1], Elena Velichko [1], Victor Osovskikh [2], Lyubov Kiseleva [2] and Zhyldyz Musakulova [3]

1 Institute of Physics, Nanotechnology and Telecommunications, Peter the Great St. Petersburg Polytechnic University, 195251 St. Petersburg, Russia; kin_kolin@mail.ru (I.K.); velichko-spbstu@yandex.ru (E.V.)
2 Department of Anesthesiology and Resuscitation Russian Research Center for Radiology and Surgical Technologies, 197758 St. Petersburg, Russia; osoff@mail.ru (V.O.); luba_kiseleva@mail.ru (L.K.)
3 Computer Information Systems, International University of Kyrgyzstan, Bishkek 720007, Kyrgyzstan; mjyldyz@rambler.ru
* Correspondence: savchenko-spbstu@mail.ru

Abstract: This work is aimed at creating a modified invasive technique for assessing the liver's functional reserves. A study of the degree of hepatodepression is carried out by measuring the plasma elimination of indocyanine green using the method of optical densitometry. This paper presents test results for an aqueous solution and an albumin solution, as well as the results of measurements of plasma elimination of indocyanine green for patients with liver disease. Perfecting the proposed method will make an important scientific contribution to modern diagnostic medicine. Diagnosing the stages in the progression of the disease and its developing complications can make it possible to rapidly correct the patient's treatment algorithm, achieving positive outcomes in medical practice.

Keywords: optical densitometry; liver diagnosis; indocyanine green; liver functional reserve; optical density; plasma disappearance rate

1. Introduction

One of the pressing issues in modern hepatology is assessing the degree of hepatic depression [1–5]. As of 2019, 325 million people worldwide have been infected with viral hepatitis B or C, and 1.4 million people die from it every year, while the need for resection occurs in 80% of cases in patients with hepatitis C and B [2].

Liver disease can be divided into diffuse and focal. The underlying pathophysiological mechanisms of the progression of diffuse liver disease are inflammation, vascular insufficiency, or abnormal accumulation of substances. Chronic liver failure is most frequently caused by viral hepatitis and fatty degeneration of hepatocytes of alimentary origin. Fulminant liver failure is mainly caused by hepatitis viruses and xenobiotics (including drugs). Diffuse liver disease is traditionally treated by hepatologists. The progression of chronic liver failure naturally raises the question about a radical method of treatment that is liver transplantation. Unfortunately, the existing clinical criteria for prediction are not perfect, which means that patients are not placed on the waiting list for transplantation in a timely manner. In the case of focal lesions (primary tumor, metastases, parasitic cyst, and abscess), the surgical strategy consists of removing pathological lesions while ensuring sufficient function of remaining organ volume. Experimental data indicate that the mass of liver tissue sufficient to meet the needs of the body is about 1% of body weight. However, this refers to fully functional tissue. In case of combined focal and diffuse lesions, such estimates will be low. Another branch of medicine where functional assessment of the liver plays a crucial role is treatment of organ failure in patients in critical condition. It is known that the hepatic component is the most difficult to control.

The study of the functional status of the liver currently includes the parameters of synthesis (prothrombin, cholesterol, and albumin), cellular integrity (transaminase), detoxification (ammonia) excretion, and cholestasis (bilirubin, alkaline phosphatase, and gamma-glutamyl transpeptidase) in combination with various imaging techniques. These "static" tests of hepatic function have limitations, especially when it comes to prognosis of survival or liver function tests in patients in critical condition [6]. Currently, only dynamic tests based on studies of the clearance of exogenously introduced substances can give a global picture of organ function [7]. Some tests can be used repeatedly within a limited time frame, for example, allowing to determine the limit of resection more thoroughly in conditions of temporary vascular isolation of the organ.

Dozens of substances were proposed as dynamic markers (both natural participants of metabolic reactions, and xenobiotics), along with methods for their detection. Only a few have reached widespread clinical use. One of the markers that has become firmly rooted in the practice of hepatology is indocyanine green (ICG) [8]. It is a water-soluble non-toxic fluorescent dye used for diagnostics of the cardiovascular system since 1956 [9]. After indocyanine green is administered intravenously, it is distributed only to the intravascularly space, binding to plasma proteins, and is removed from the blood only by hepatocytes. ICG refers to exogenous markers with rapid hepatic elimination, respectively, the rate of excretion depends on the function of hepatocytes and the hepatic blood flow rate.

The gold standard for determining the rate of ICG elimination is the method of sequential samples. Blood samples taken at regular intervals after the introduction of ICG are centrifuged, and the plasma is subjected to photometry (spectrophotometry) at a wavelength of 805 nm [10,11]. The disadvantages of sequential sampling are the long times it takes, and the additional personnel required. Thanks to the unique physical characteristics of indocyanine green, determination of ICG elimination rate by pulse densitometry was first introduced in the late 1990s. While a large number of publications confirm a high correlation of invasive and non-invasive techniques, there are certain problems related to pulse densitometry [10–14]. In particular, impaired capillary blood flow [15,16], obesity, and tremor of the extremities prevent obtaining reliable data [14]. This problem is especially important) in patients in critical condition. If non-invasive measurements fail, not only are expensive drugs lost, but new measurements are inevitably delayed to ensure that the previous dose of the indicator has been eliminated. Unfortunately, the technique for non-invasive determination of absolute ICG concentration and the related opportunities for calculating the circulating blood volume have also not been developed any further.

To solve this problem, we propose to use a combination of invasive and non-invasive methods for determining the rate of dye elimination on a single platform, with the possibility of post-processing the data obtained by pulse densitometry. The goal of this work is to develop the first stage, namely, an invasive method for measuring the plasma elimination of indocyanine green for diagnosing hepatic function.

2. Experimental Setup of Optical Densitometry

An experimental setup that we developed (Figure 1) was used to conduct measurements of plasma elimination of indocyanine green for diagnostics of hepatic function.

Light emitted from diode (**1**) passes though the test solution. Part of the radiation is absorbed, and part of the radiation is backscattered [17,18]. The emitting diode has an emission spectrum narrower than the peak absorption spectrum of the dye in the near infrared region; therefore, a monochromatic filter in the circuit is not required. The prepared solution of known concentration of indocyanine green is placed in cuvette (**2**). Photodetector (**3**) is used to detect the transmitted radiation. The distance between the emitting diode and the photodetector is 100 mm. Measured at this distance, the intensity of light passing through the cuvette with water without dye is 100 μW. The cuvette with the solution is placed 50 mm from the emitting diode. Measurements are made every 0.4 s.

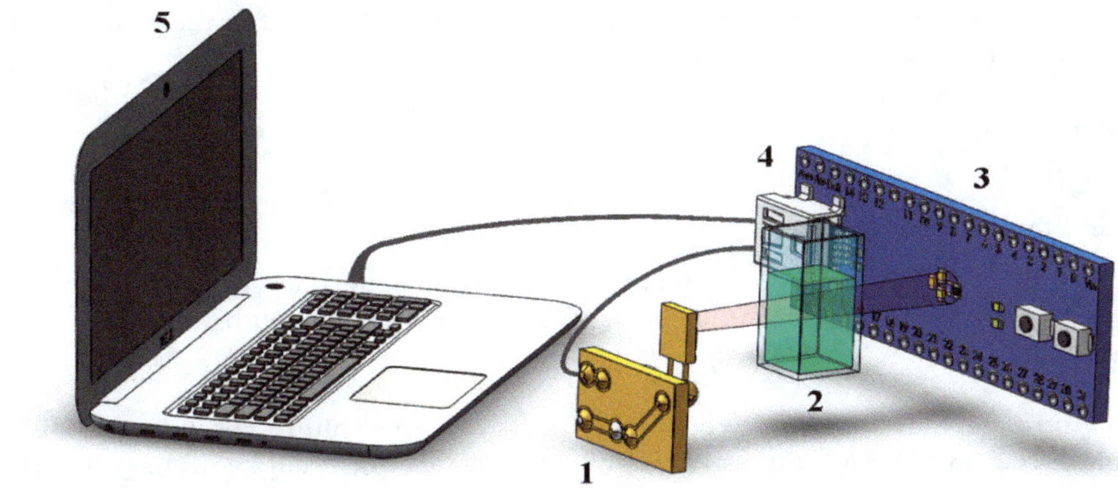

Figure 1. Experimental setup: (**1**) emitting diode, (**2**) sample cell, (**3**) photodetector, (**4**) microcontroller, and (**5**) computer.

Microcontroller (**4**) controls the collection of data by the Serial Peripheral Interface bus. The emitting diode is powered by the MCU pins and has only two modes: on and off. Communication with the photodetector is performed through the I2C interface. Data from the microcontroller for further processing are displayed on user device (**5**), which is a personal computer or an android device via USB.

The signal fluctuations of the medium optical density occur during the measurements. Their deviation from the average value, as a rule, does not reach 0.5% [19,20]. Fluctuations in optical density can be conditioned by fluctuations of dye concentration, intensity measurement error is mostly determined by photodetector quantization error. Figure 2 presents an example of the received signal.

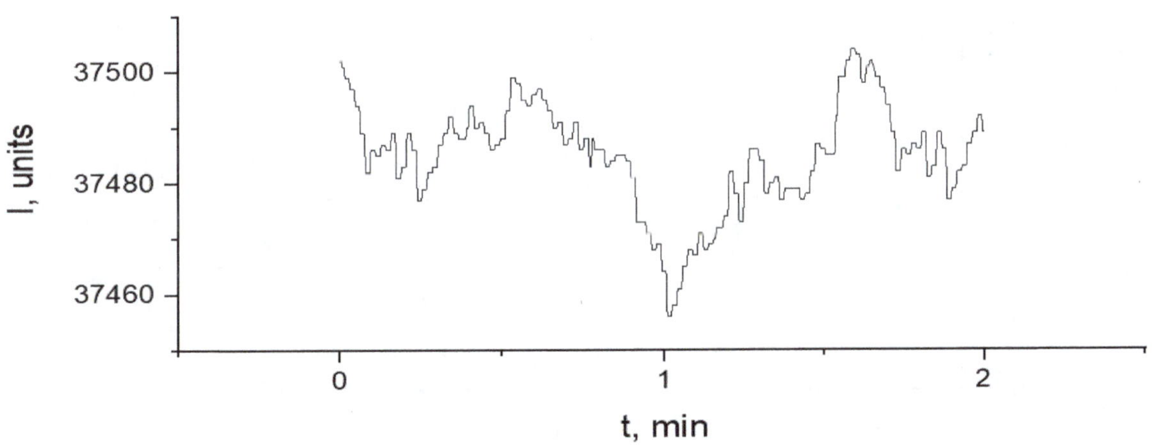

Figure 2. Example of time dependence of intensity of the light transmitted by 20% albumin solution without dye: I–the intensity of the light transmitted, t–recording time of the signal.

The developed experimental setup has several advantages compared with other photometric methods.

- Small dimension: The size of the experimental setup is 15 × 7 × 5 cm. The number of elements in this installation is minimized.
- Noise immunity: To improve the noise immunity, the Butterworth low pass filter and median filter were used.
- Cost-effectiveness: Optimized device design allows using cheaper optical elements. Emitting diode with 810 nm was used as a light source. (Which is cheaper than deuterium and tungsten sources)

- Simplicity of use: This experimental setup does not require additional training of users for carrying out experimental studies.
- Quick real-time presentation of the results: Processing of experimental studies takes up to several minutes.

3. Results and Discussion

This paper presents test measurements of the developed experimental setup and the proposed software. Solutions of the indocyanine green dye with water and with albumin were used as test samples.

At the first stage, measurements were made for an aqueous solution of indocyanine green at a low dye concentration. These samples were prepared by adding small portions of the dye with a known concentration in distilled water. Figure 3 shows a graph of the obtained experimental results for measuring the concentration of an aqueous solution of green indocyanine at a low dye concentration and their approximation by the exponent. The measurement result is calculated by averaging the signal values. The error bars marked on the graph reflect the value of the random experimental error calculated by estimation of the mean value (10 measurements), and confidence interval with a confidence level of 95%.

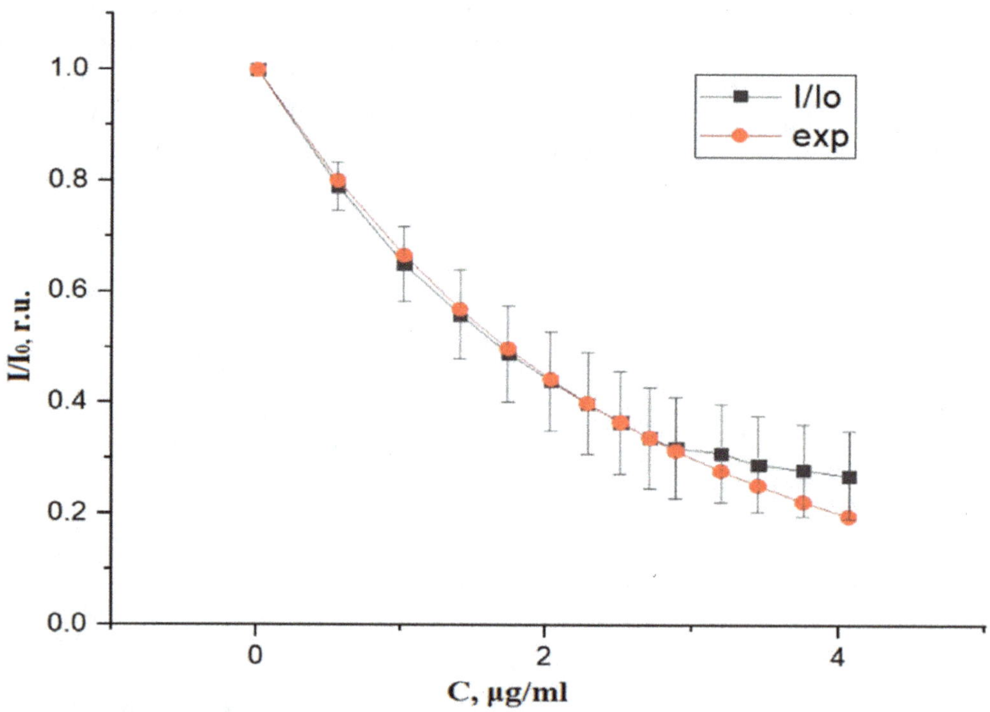

Figure 3. Ratio of intensity (I) of the light transmitted by aqueous solution of green indocyanine at low dye concentration (C) to intensity (I_0) of the light transmitted by water, and its approximation by an exponential function (exp).

Measurements at a low dye concentration are approximated by an exponent with a selected coefficient.

To test the operability of the developed experimental setup, we also performed experiments for a 20% albumin solution, gradually adding the dye to the test medium. The experimental results of measurements with low concentrations of indocyanine green in a 20% albumin solution and their exponential approximation are presented in Figure 4.

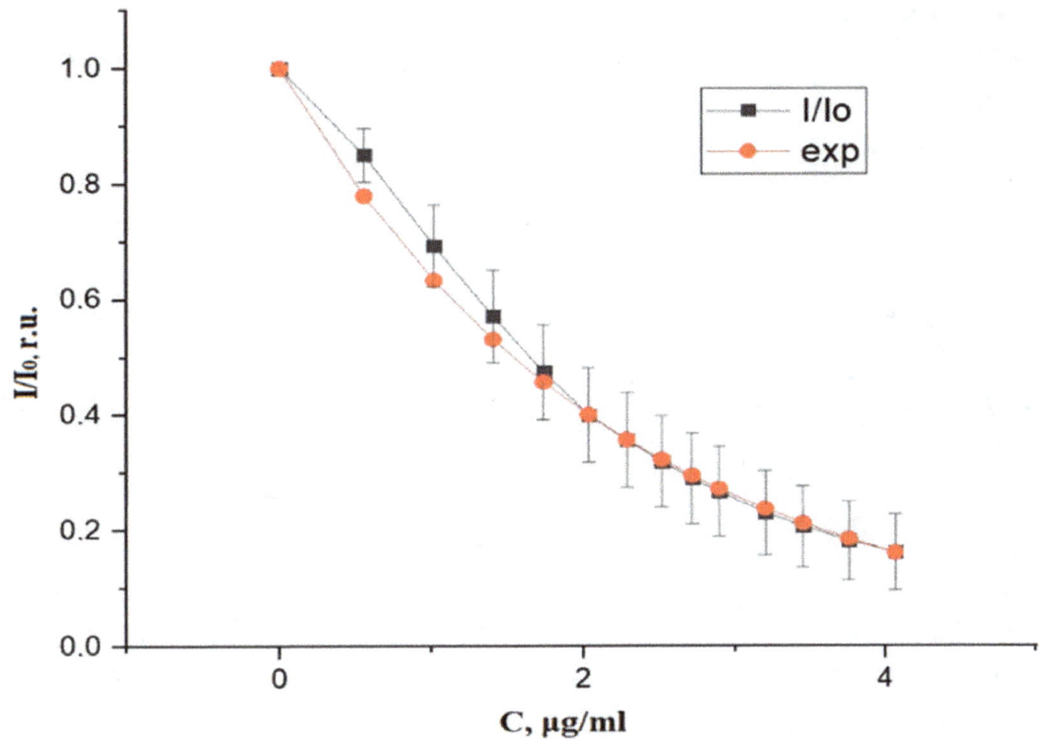

Figure 4. Ratio of the intensity of the light transmitted by dye albumin solution to intensity of light transmitted by solution of albumin and its approximation by an exponential function.

An experiment with a 20% albumin solution in the dye concentration range showed agreement with the theoretical data. However, in contrast to the experiment with water, it was not possible to choose an exponent that could approximate the beginning of the graph at a concentration near zero.

At the second stage of the measurements, we studied blood plasma samples from patients with liver pathology. Plasma samples were taken from 23 patients with liver pathology as part of routine ICG serial blood testing at the department of anesthesiology and intensive care of Russian Research Center of Radiology and Surgical Technologies. Plasma samples form a series each consisting of a set of measurements during the study of one patient. We have studied the samples taken before administering the dye, which are used to determine the optical density of the blood plasma itself. The intensity I_0 of the light passing through the plasma without dye allows to calculate the relative concentration of the dye in subsequent samples:

$$C_{rel} = -\ln\left(\frac{I}{I_0}\right). \tag{1}$$

In addition, plasma samples taken 2, 7, 12, and 17 min after dye administration were investigated. Figure 5 shows the results for a plasma sample from one of the patients with liver pathology.

Experiments with plasma allowed us to estimate the rate of dye elimination in the blood of patients. By calculating the relative concentration of the dye in these samples and comparing them, we can estimate the PDR (plasma disappearance rate) parameter by approximating a series of concentrations with an exponent with a selected coefficient for the argument. Measurements of the concentration ratio in the samples taken after 2 and 17 min determine the value of the PDR parameter, defined as the percentage by which the dye concentration decreases in 15 min. Figure 6 presents the results of experiments with plasma aimed at assessing the rate of elimination of the dye in the blood of patients.

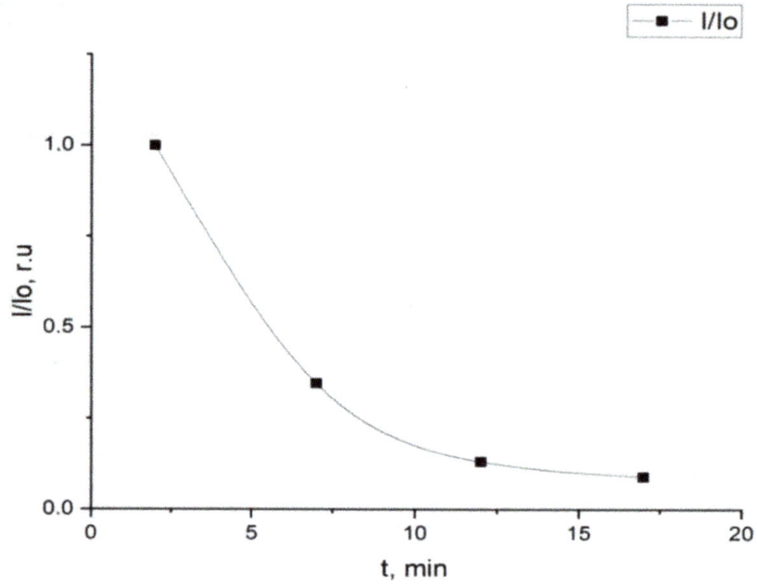

Figure 5. Ratio of intensity of the light transmitted by the dye blood plasma solution to the intensity of light transmitted by blood plasma solution from the time the plasma was taken from the patient.

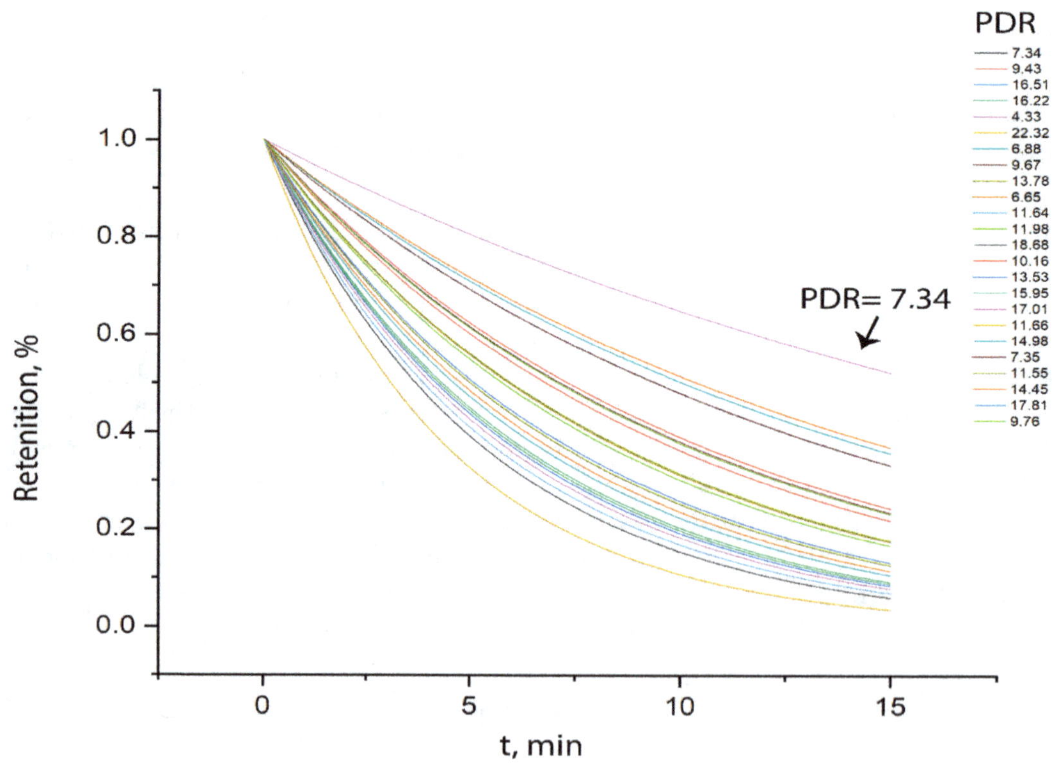

Figure 6. Plasma dye elimination curves corresponding to individual series.

The metabolic function of the liver of patients can be assessed based on these results. The faster the liver removes the dye from the circulatory system, the lower the ratio of the concentration in the subsequent sample to the concentration in the previous one after the same period. The liver of those patients whose curves are located lower purifies the blood better than the liver of those whose curves are higher.

To compare the results obtained by evaluating the concentration of the dye in the plasma, parallel studies were carried out by the method of sequential sampling on a commercial DU® 800 UV/Visible

Spectrophotometer. Figure 7 shows the relationship between the optical densities of the samples measured using a spectrophotometer (D_2) and the optical densities of the samples measured using our experimental setup (D_1).

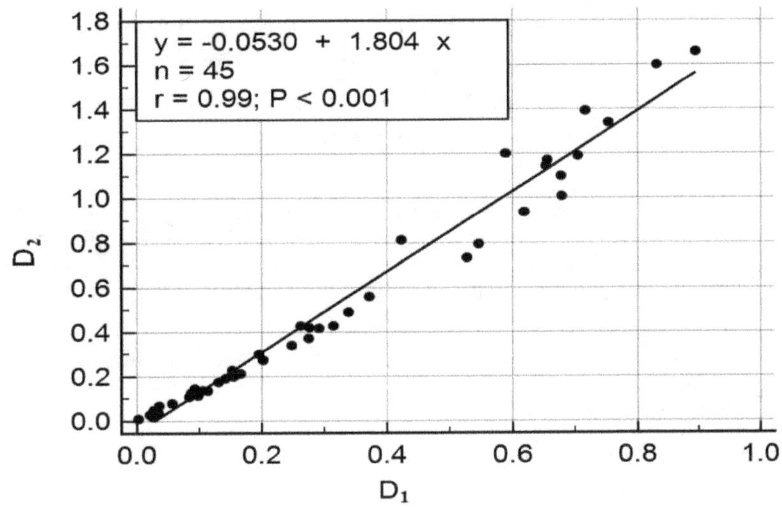

Figure 7. Comparison of the optical densities, D, obtained by two methods: D_2–the optical densities of the samples measured using a spectrophotometer and D_1–the optical densities of the samples measured using our experimental setup.

PDR values were also calculated by two methods. The comparison of the results is shown in Figure 8.

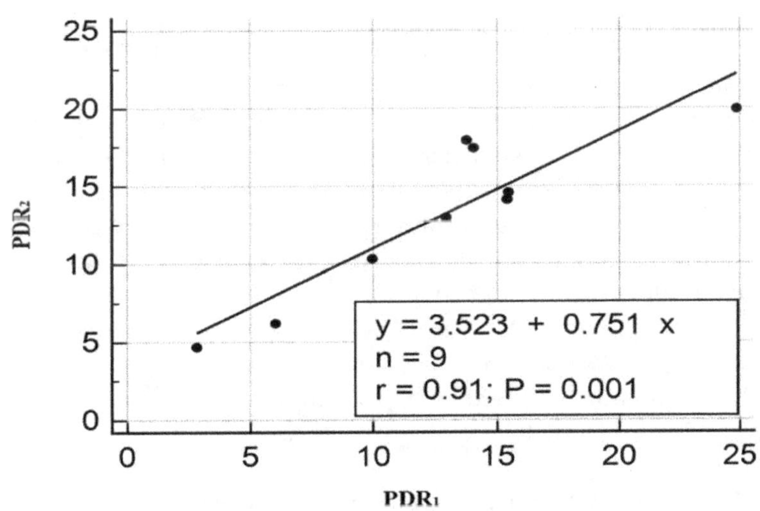

Figure 8. Comparison of plasma disappearance rate (PDR) parameters calculated from the measurements obtained with DU® 800 UV/Visible Spectrophotometer at the Department of Anesthesiology and Intensive Care of Russian Research Center for Radiology and Surgical Technologies (PDR_2), and with our experimental setup (PDR_1).

Figures 7 and 8 show that there is a correlation between the two measurement methods. The preliminary results obtained for assessing the concentration of indocyanine green in various liquids can be the basis for further studies [21]. This development can be included in the smart medical autonomous distributed system for diagnostics based on machine learning technology [22].

4. Conclusions

In this study, we developed an experimental setup, a program for collecting and displaying data, and an experimental technique for assessing the concentration of green indocyanine in various solutions. The experimental studies involved measurements with an aqueous dye, an albumin solution, and blood plasma correlated with the data from a commercial DU® 800 UV/Visible spectrophotometer. The main (advantages) of a device are cost-effectiveness, simplicity of use and quick real-time presentation of the results. The developed system will make it possible to diagnose liver function and predict its recovery with higher accuracy compared with existing approaches.

Author Contributions: Funding acquisition, supervision, E.V.; methodology, formal analysis, V.O.; investigation, I.K.; experiment in Russian Research Center for Radiology and Surgical Technologies, L.K.; writing—original draft preparation, E.S. and I.K.; and machine learning consultation and data evaluation, Z.M. All authors have read and agreed to the published version of the manuscript.

Acknowledgments: We express our gratitude to the Russian Research Center for Radiology and Surgical Technologies for providing biological samples, to S.V. Ermak for comprehensive assistance and valuable scientific advice, and to E.K. Nepomnyashchaya for illustration design.

References

1. Rosen, H.R. Chronic hepatitis C infection. *N. Engl. J. Med.* **2011**, *364*, 2429–2438. [CrossRef] [PubMed]
2. World Health Organization. Available online: https://www.who.int/campaigns/world-hepatitis-day/2019 (accessed on 3 July 2020).
3. Williamson, R.M.; Price, J.F.; Glancy, S.; Perry, E.; Nee, L.D.; Hayes, P.C. Prevalence of and risk factors for hepatic steatosis and nonalcoholic fatty liver disease in people with type 2 diabetes: The Edinburgh Type 2 Diabetes Study. *Diabetes Care* **2011**, *34*, 1139–1144. [CrossRef] [PubMed]
4. Aijaz, A.; Perumpail, R.B.; Harrison, S.A. High prevalence of hepatic fibrosis in the setting of coexisting diabetes and hepatic steatosis: A case for selective screening in the general population? *Hepatology* **2016**, *63*, 20–22.
5. Mueller, A.R.; Platz, K.P.; Kremer, B. Early postoperative complications following liver transplantation. *Best Pract. Res. Clin. Gastroenterol.* **2004**, *18*, 881–900. [CrossRef]
6. Bonfrate, L.; Grattagliano, I.; Palasciano, G.; Portincasa, P. Dynamic carbon 13 breath tests for the study of liver function and gastric emptying. *Gastroenterol. Rep.* **2014**, *3*, 12–21. [CrossRef] [PubMed]
7. Sakka, S.G. Assessing liver function. *Curr. Opin. Crit. Care* **2007**, *13*, 207–214. [CrossRef] [PubMed]
8. Kunikowska, A.J.; Wildgruber, M.; Schulte-Frohlinde, E.; Lahmer, T.; Schmid, R.M.; Huber, W. Liver function assessment using indocyanine green plasma disappearance rate in a young male with icteric leptospirosis: A case report. *BMC Infect. Dis.* **2019**, *19*, 473. [CrossRef] [PubMed]
9. Slakter, J.S.; Yannuzzi, L.A.; Guyer, D.R.; Sorenson, J.A.; Orlock, D.A. Indocyanine-green angiography. *Curr. Opin. Ophthalmol.* **1995**, *6*, 25–32. [CrossRef] [PubMed]
10. Haruna, M.; Kumon, K.; Yahagi, N.; Watanabe, Y.; Ishida, Y.; Kobayashi, T.; Aoyagi, T. Blood Volume Measurement at the Bedside Using ICG Pulse Spectrophometry. *Anesthesiology* **1998**, *89*, 1322–1328. [CrossRef] [PubMed]
11. Osamu, O.; Tetsuya, K.; Hiroyuki, S.; Soichiro, I.; Shin, T.; Akimasa, N. ICG Pulse Spectrophotometry for Perioperative Liver Function in Hepatectomy. *J. Surg. Res.* **2002**, *103*, 109–113.
12. Kovac, N.; Peric, M. Liver function assessment by indocyanine green plasma disappearance rate in patients with intra-abdominal hypertension after "non-hepatic" abdominal surgery. *Curr. Med. Res. Opin.* **2018**, *34*, 1741–1746. [CrossRef] [PubMed]
13. Mayr, U.; Fahrenkrog-Petersen, L.; Batres-Baires, G.; Herner, A.; Rasch, S.; Schmid, R.M.; Lahmer, T. Largevolume paracentesis effects plasma disappearance rate of indocyanine green in critically ill patients with decompensated liver cirrhosis and intraabdominal hypertension. *Ann. Intensive Care* **2018**, *8*, 1–10.
14. Pantanali, C.A.; Gonzalez, D.E.; D'Albuquerque, L.A.; Andraus, W.; Barzallo, P.; Asperti, A.M. Lessons Learned with the LiMON Method of Indocyanine Green Elimination. *EC Gastroenterol. Dig. Syst.* **2018**, *5*, 297–304.

15. Li, H.-m. Microcirculation of liver cancer, microenvironment of liver regeneration, and the strategy of Chinese medicine. *Chin. J. Integr. Med.* **2016**, *22*, 163–167. [CrossRef] [PubMed]
16. Tian, H.; Qi, W. Quantitative analysis of microcirculation blood perfusion in patients with hepatocellular carcinoma before and after transcatheter arterial chemoembolisation using contrast-enhanced ultrasound. *Eur. J. Cancer* **2016**, *68*, 82–89. [CrossRef] [PubMed]
17. Davydov, R.V.; Antonov, V.I.; Yushkova, V.V.; Grebenikova, N.M.; Dudkin, V.I. A new algorithm for processing the absorption and scattering signals of laser radiation on a blood vessel and human tissues. *J. Phys. Conf. Ser.* **2019**, *1236*, 012079. [CrossRef]
18. Bisyarin, M.A.; Kotov, O.I.; Hartog, A.H.; Liokumovich, L.B.; Ushakov, N.A. Influence of a variable Rayleigh scattering-loss coefficient on the light backscattering in multimode optical fibers. *Appl. Opt.* **2017**, *56*, 4629. [CrossRef] [PubMed]
19. Kotov, O.; Chapalo, I. Signal-to-noise ratio for mode-mode fiber interferometer. In *Optical Measurement Systems for Industrial Inspection X*; SPIE Optical Metrology: Munich, Germany, 2017.
20. Liokumovich, L.B.; Kostromitin, A.O.; Ushakov, N.A.; Kudryashov, A.V. Method for Measuring Laser Frequency Noise. *J. Appl. Spectrosc.* **2020**, *86*, 1106–1112. [CrossRef]
21. Privalov, V.E.; Rybalko, A.V.; Charty, P.V.; Shemanin, V.G. Effect of noise and vibration on the performance of a particle concentration laser meter and optimization of its parameters. *Tech. Phys.* **2007**, *52*, 352–355. [CrossRef]
22. Velichko, E.; Nepomnyashchaya, E.; Baranov, M.; Galeeva, M.A.; Pavlov, V.A.; Zavjalov, S.V.; Savchenko, E.; Pervunina, T.M.; Govorov, I.; Komlichenko, E. A Concept of Smart Medical Autonomous Distributed System for Diagnostics Based on Machine Learning Technology. In *Internet of Things, Smart Spaces, and Next Generation Networks and Systems*; Springer: Cham, Switzerland, 2019; pp. 515–524.

10

Excimer Laser Surgery: Biometrical Iris Eye Recognition with Cyclorotational Control Eye Tracker System

Bojan Pajic [1,2,3,4], Zeljka Cvejic [2], Zoran Mijatovic [2,*], Dragan Indjin [5] and Joerg Mueller [1]

1 Swiss Eye Research Foundation, Eye Clinic ORASIS, 5734 Reinach AG, Switzerland; bpajic@datacomm.ch (B.P.); joerg.mueller@nova-optik.ch (J.M.)
2 Faculty of Sciences, Department of Physics, University of Novi Sad, Trg Dositeja Obradovica 4, Novi Sad 21000, Serbia; zeljkac@uns.ac.rs
3 Medical Faculty, Military Medical Academy, University of Defans Belgrade, Belgrade 11000, Serbia
4 Division of Ophthalmology, Department of Clinical Neurosciences, Geneva University Hospitals, Genève 1205, Switzerland
5 School of Electronic and Electrical Engineering, University of Leeds, Leeds LS2 9JT, UK; d.indjin@leeds.ac.uk
* Correspondence: mijat@uns.ac.rs

Academic Editor: Vittorio M. N. Passaro

Abstract: A prospective comparative study assessing the importance of the intra-operative dynamic rotational tracking—especially in the treatment of astigmatisms in corneal refractive Excimer laser correction—concerning clinical outcomes is presented. The cyclotorsion from upright to supine position was measured using iris image comparison. The Group 1 of patients was additionally treated with cyclorotational control and Group 2 only with X-Y control. Significant differences were observed between the groups regarding the mean postoperative cylinder refraction ($p < 0.05$). The mean cyclotorsion can be calculated to 3.75° with a standard deviation of 3.1°. The total range of torsion was from −14.9° to +12.6°. Re-treatment rate was 2.2% in Group 1 and 8.2% in Group 2, which is highly significant ($p < 0.01$). The investigation confirms that the dynamic rotational tracking system used for LASIK results in highly predictable refraction quality with significantly less postoperative re-treatments.

Keywords: cyclorotation control eye tracker system; Excimer laser; refractive surgery

1. Introduction

In recent years, several improvements in the diagnostic aspects of refractive corneal surgery have been introduced which have contributed to improved precision and the availability of new clinical information such as wavefront aberration maps and three-dimensional corneal maps with high precision elevation data [1,2].

From the indication and algorithm points of view, parallel developments have been started by expanding the treatment ranges for high levels of astigmatism, aspheric ablation profiles, and the correction of high order aberrations [3–6].

These developments have resulted in the therapeutic components of a refractive platform that needs to be equipped with new technologies in order to provide a laser system capable of delivering superior precision and to utilize a new level of available information. It is well known that the eye can rotate several degrees when a person moves from a sitting position to a prone position. Having in mind that wavefront and topographic data are collected in the sitting position and that refractive surgery is performed in supine position, there is a great chance for potential error. Therefore, if the laser is tracking the center of the pupil, it would be most impossible to detect a rotational change because the center of the pupil may not be affected.

One of the essential components required to achieve this goal is a sophisticated eye tracking technology. The automated system that utilizes an eye tracking feature is a part of today's novel refractive laser systems.

Technolas 217z100P eye tracking system is a video-based system that uses infrared (IR) radiation to illuminate and capture the image by combining the advantages of being independent of the surrounding iris color conditions and the illumination level of the surgical field.

The relevance of cyclotorsion and its impact on the effectiveness of the ablation process are well known and several other systems have begun to include compensating technologies into their platforms [7]. As the observed rotational misalignment during the ablation cannot be neglected, the eye tracking system could improve surface ablation results when treating high astigmatism or when being wavefront guided.

2. Materials and Methods

We measured and adjusted the eye tracker system of Technolas 217z100P™ (Technolas, Munich, Germany) in LASIK (LASer-assisted In situ Keratomileusis) treatments on a total of 88 eyes in this study, 44 eyes with rotational tracker in Group 1 and 44 eyes with only X/Y tracker system in Group 2. For patients where bilateral treatment was performed, only data from the right eyes were used. The cyclotorsion from upright to supine position was measured using iris image comparison and it was not necessary to mark the cornea. All flaps created with the LDV high frequency femtosecond laser and energy range in nJ, were designed to deliver equivalent geometric dimensions 110 μm flap thickness, 9.5 mm flap diameter with superior hinge angle. The mean age of patients was: 36 ± 7.9 years (range: 23–61 years) in Group 1 and 36 ± 8.2 years (range: 21–62 years) in Group 2. The preoperative mean refractive spherical equivalent in Group 1 was −3.43 ± 2.61 D (range −10.5 to −0.75 D) and −3.69 ± 2.55 D in Group 2 (range −8.75 to −1.00 D) (the left part of the Figures 1 and 2 marked as before surgery).

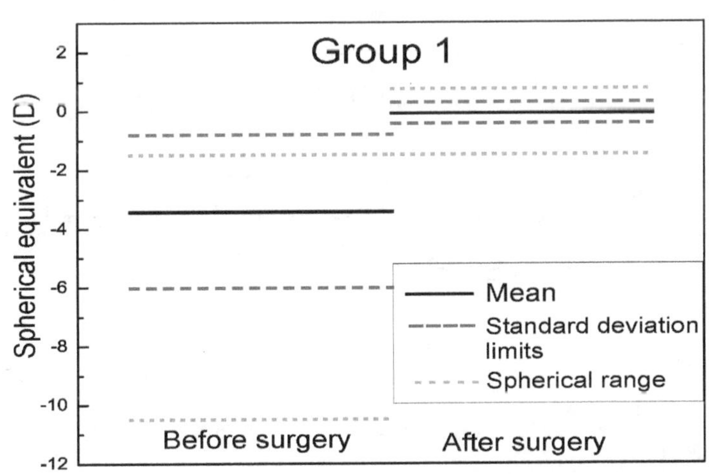

Figure 1. Refractive spherical equivalent pre- and postoperative Group 1.

The mean cylinder was −1.14 ± 1.00 D (range −5.75 to 0.00 D) in Group 1 and −1.12 ± −1.0 D (range −6.00 to −0.00 D) in Group 2 (the left part of the Figures 3 and 4 marked as – before surgery).

There was no significant difference between the groups regarding the mean preoperative spherical equivalent and cylinder refraction ($p > 0.05$).

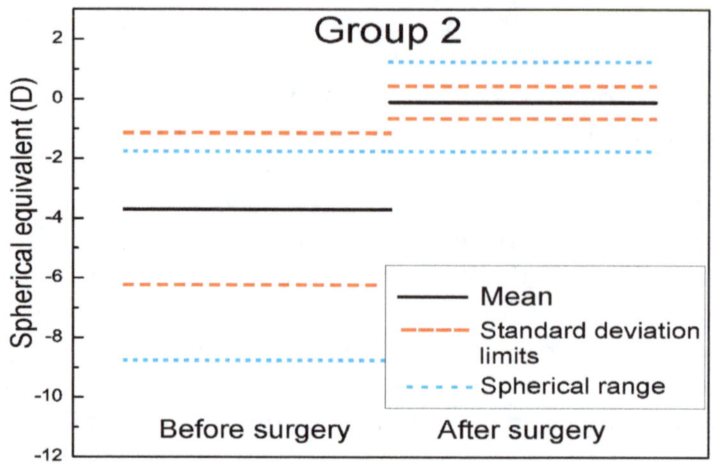

Figure 2. Refractive spherical equivalent pre- and postoperative Group 2.

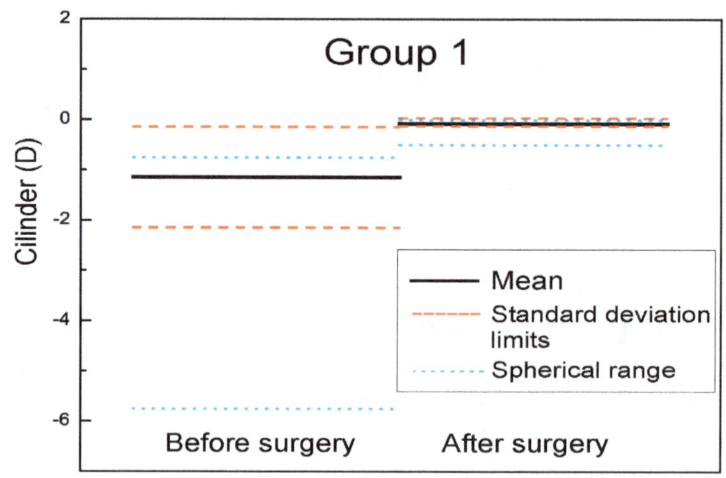

Figure 3. Mean cylinder pre- and postoperative Group 1.

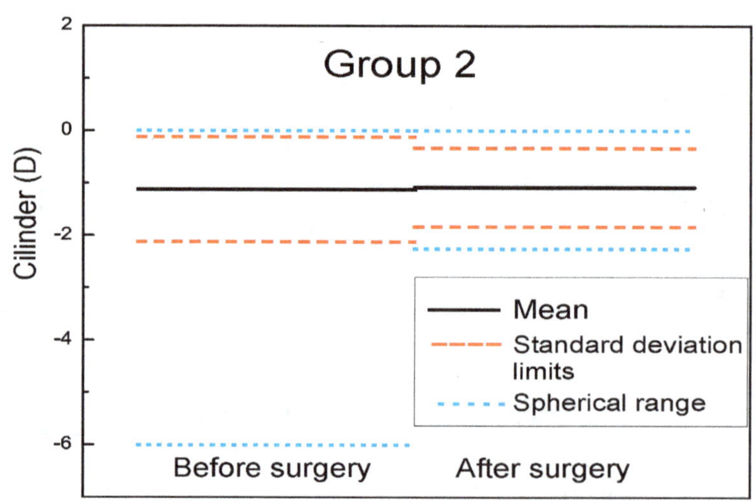

Figure 4. Mean cylinder pre- and postoperative Group 2.

By introducing the rotational eye tracker in the Technolas 217z100P™ the already approved X/Y tracker, which compensates actively for transversal movements of the eye, will be upgraded to compensate for misalignments in rotation. While it uses the acquired iris images only, additional objectively acquired information is needed to provide a rotational tracking capability. The 217z100P rotational tracker module is based on iris pattern recognition technology. It is well known that iris patterns are similar to finger prints with unique biometric properties of the individual. By using the appropriate technology, not only the individual eye can be recognized but also specific match parameters—such as rotational misalignment between two images of the same iris—can be obtained. The basic data used to analyze iris patterns are acquired infrared images of the iris. With special image processing and normalization technologies, the iris images are processed to account for differences in illumination conditions (large and small pupils) or even from different systems (such as Zywave wavefront sensor and laser system). The Zywave wavefront sensor is a diagnostic system which utilizes the same wavelength to acquire an Infrared (IR) image forms, the eye, and the corresponding iris [8]. Finally, the process described above results in a digital code which is created as follows: determine automatically pupil boundary and limbus boundary of the reference image (Figure 5).

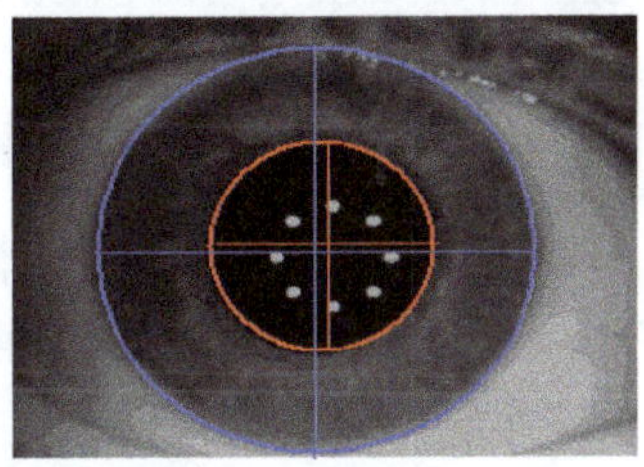

Figure 5. Pupil and limbus boundary recognition of the reference image.

Certain sanity checks are applied to ensure that the automatically identified pupil and limbus geometries are within reasonable measures. The visible iris pattern defined as the structures between the pupil boundary and the limbus edge are used to create a normalized band (Figure 6).

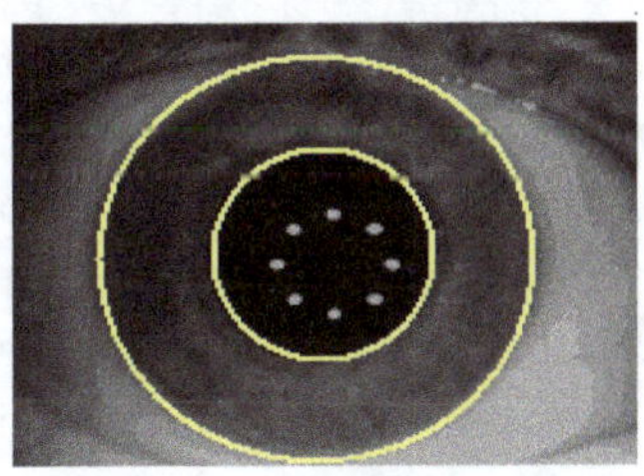

Figure 6. Visible iris pattern definition.

All operations which lead to the final digital iris code are performed within this normalized band (Figure 7).

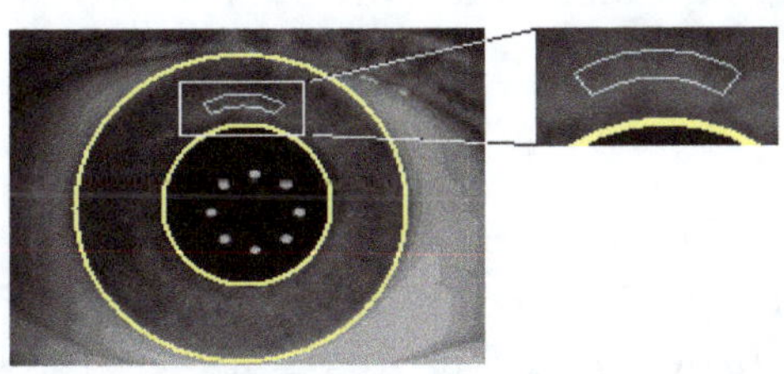

Figure 7. Digital iris code performance.

Within this band of iris image data, a unique digital code is generated. The basic data stream of this digital code consists of information obtained at 980 different iris locations. This iris code is, therefore, a unique code for this specific iris pattern and is used to detect potential torsional deviations between two different images from the same iris. The output parameters of the rotational eye tracker system—such as pupil radius/center and limbus radius/center—are given in resolution less than 30 μm. The rotation angle between images is within ±14.8° and with the resolution of 0.7° (=360°/512). Response time is 40 ms (i.e., 25 Hz).

During the static cyclotorsion compensation, the first step is a diagnostic phase which consists of obtaining IR iris image and deriving digital iris code from this reference iris image. This is followed with a planning phase where obtained data are transferred to the laser system. The next phase is a cyclotorsion compensation phase in which the patient's head is aligned in the supine position. After that, the second IR iris image is acquired for comparison between the reference and actual iris code.

During to intra-operative rotational compensation phase (dynamic cyclotorsion compensation), the referenced image is used as the first image for providing the iris code. Afterwards, a new iris image and code are required, while laser system is treating the patient's eye. The next step is determining rotational angle to achieve maximum overlap of iris code and transferring this info to the laser software. The correct treatment pattern is determined according to the rotational angle.

To observe and track the eye movements of a patient during surgery, the laser is equipped with two different cameras for the eye tracking system. One camera detects eye movements in the x/y direction. It is optimized for the area around the pupil and operational frequency is 240 Hz. The other eye-tracker camera detects the rotational movements of the eye and has a wider display window, so that the iris and limbal region can be observed. Operational frequency of this camera is 25 Hz. The slower frequency of the rotational eye tracker camera is justified with the slow speed of cyclotoric movements of eyes, while the x/y tracker must handle very fast saccadic movements in the x/y direction.

Due to the different observation angles of the two camera systems, it is also possible to detect movements in the height of an eye (also called Z-tracking) by the observation of the pupil centers obtained from the both cameras. The Z-tracking is opposite to the lateral and torsional tracking of a passive tracking system which simply deactivates the laser application if the eye moves outside of a given range of ±0.5 mm of the nominal Z-position. It should also be mentioned that the lateral eye tracker system works independently from the other two systems (rotational and Z-tracking). All mentioned eye tracking modules can block a laser pulse if the position is not accurate. The surgeon is able to deactivate the rotational eye-tracker system (including Z-tracking) at any time of surgery, while the x/y tracker can remain activated. If it is needed, the user can manually deactivate the x/y tracker too.

The system delivers the cyclorotational angle from a supine to horizontal position and additionally the dynamic eye tracker systems records the angle differences during the surgery. This results in an overall angle from the beginning until the end of surgery. This value is taken for the mean calculation of all eyes where the surgeries were undertaken with the cyclorotational eye tracker system, referred to as Group 1.

3. Results

The six-month postoperative mean refractive spherical equivalent was −0.08 ± 0.36 D in Group 1 (range −1.5 to +0.75 D) and −0.11 ± 0.55 D in Group 2 (range −1.75 to +1.25 D) (the right part of the Figures 1 and 2 marked as after surgery). In Figures 1 and 2, it is very well revealed the refractive clinical outcome: preoperative vs. six months postoperative.

The mean cylinder was −0.08 ± 0.05 D (range −0.5 to 0.0 D) in Group 1 and −1.08 ± 0.75 D (range −2.25 to 0.0 D) in Group 2 (the right part of the Figures 3 and 4 marked as after surgery). In Figure 8, the double angle scatter plot of the cylinder value and angle is shown for the Group 1. Only a small range of astigmatism power and angle can be seen in contrast to the Group 2 where results for a double angle scatter plot analysis are shown in Figure 9.

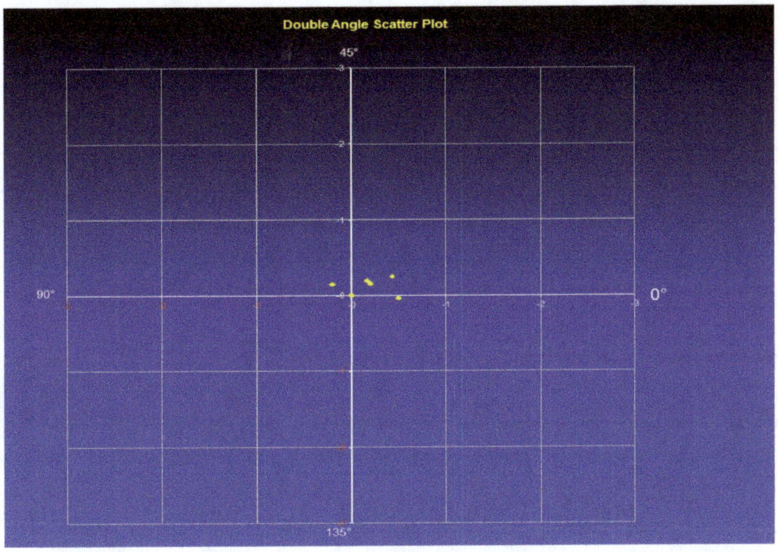

Figure 8. Double angle scatter plot for group 1.

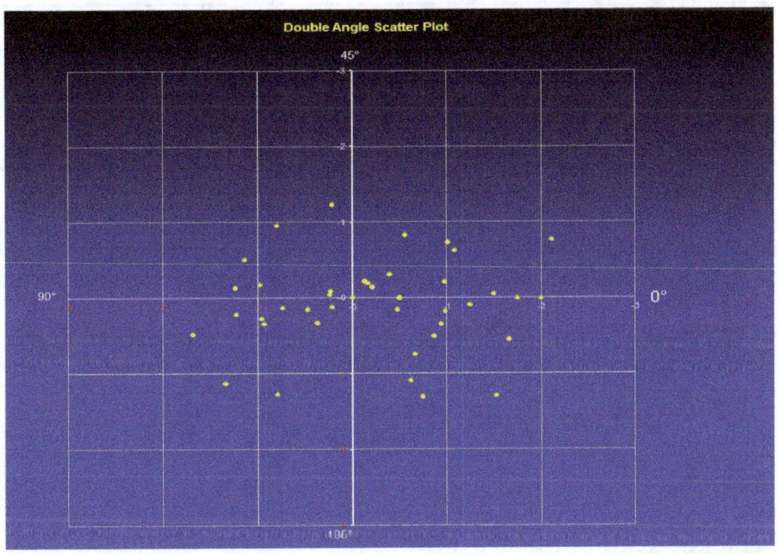

Figure 9. Double angle scatter plot for group 2.

There is no much difference between the groups related to the mean postoperative spherical equivalent ($p > 0.05$) but significant difference in outcomes was observed related to the mean cylinder ($p = 0.0043$). The cylinder range of 2.25 D in Group 2 is remarkably high compared with the results obtained for Group 1, where only a range of 0.5 was measured. From supine to horizontal patient position there was an average static cyclotorsion deviation of $-1.45°$ in Group 1. During the surgery the average cyclotorsion was calculated to be 3.75° with a standard deviation of 3.1°. Torsion was ranged from $-14.9°$ to $+12.6°$.

In the Group 1, the safety of BSCVA (Best Spectacle-Corrected Visual Acuity) remained unchanged in 5 cases, 25 cases gained 1 line, 10 cases gained 2 lines, and 4 cases gained more than 2 lines of visual acuity (Figure 10).

In the Group 2, the safety of BSCVA remained unchanged in 17 cases, 1 case lost 2 lines, 1 case lost 1 line, 22 cases gained 1 line, and 3 cases gained 2 lines of visual acuity (Figure 11).

Re-treatment rate is 2.2% in the Group 1 compared to 8.2% in Group 2. The difference is highly significant ($p < 0.01$).

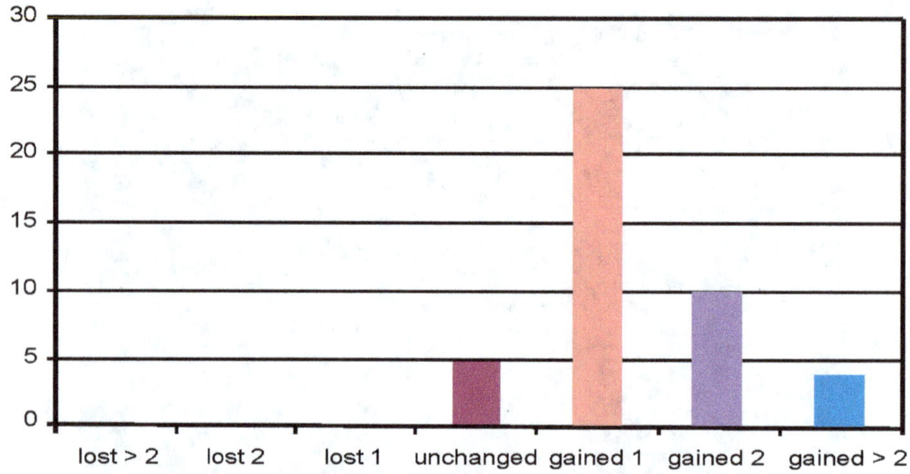

Figure 10. Treatment safety of Group 1.

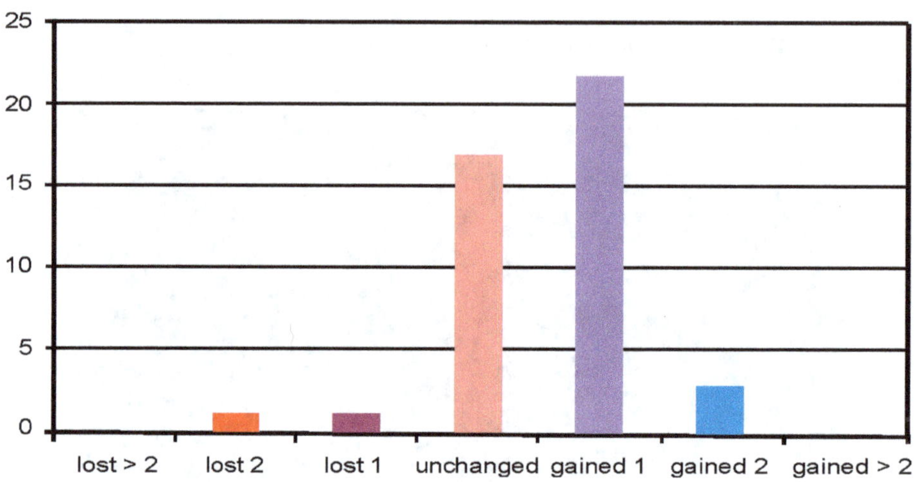

Figure 11. Treatment safety of Group 2.

4. Discussion

The rotational eye-tracker system has the ability not only to correct the rotation of an eye due to a change of the body position but also the ability to correct cyclotoric movements intra-operatively. This intra-operative cyclotorsion can occur, for example, due to a loss of fixation of the patient, excitement, or small head rotations. To ensure accurate pulse position during treatment the recognition process is continuously active during laser ablation. These images are continuously compared to the reference image, which is the last image of the initial recognition process. For each image, the quality factor and rotation angle is calculated and the remaining pulse list is rotated to the actual valid rotation angle. Therefore, even if intra-operative cyclotorsions occur, the dynamic application of the iris recognition process and the following correction ensure accurate pulse positioning during the treatment. During laser treatment, the images of the eye can lose contrast, for example due to dehydrating of the corneal surface, consequently, the difference between the reference image and the actual real time image is increased. In this case, the software is capable of recording a new reference image with the last valid rotation angle and continues to track the rotation angle using the new reference image. In our study, a highly significant difference was observed between the postoperative cylindric correction with and without a cyclotorsion control. The mean cyclotorsion was 3.75° with a standard deviation of 3.1°. The total range of torsion was from −14.9° to +12.6°. If a cylindric refraction of 4 D should be corrected with a cyclorotation of 10° without a cyclotorsion control and a correction error of 1D will be expected calculated mathematically with vector analysis. It has been shown in other studies that 50%—and in some case up to 65%—of the population has a cyclotorsion difference between standing and horizontal positions of more than 2° [7,9,10]. The cyclorotation can increase in individuals even up to 17° [7,11]. This confirms that the cyclotorsion control is a very important tool regarding the clinical outcome. In Group 2 we detected one eye which lost one line and another eye that lost two lines of visual acuity. In our opinion, the higher grade of astigmatism error in Group 2 leads to higher aberrations and, consecutively, to a decrease of the best-corrected visual acuity in these specific cases. Our results show good agreement with other published literature [7,12–14]. Different studies investigated the amount of cyclotorsion of eyes during LASIK treatments. Swami et al. [9] marked 240 eyes preoperatively while the patients were seated. Immediately before beginning the treatment, they measured the rotational misalignment of the eyes on the supine patients and found a mean cyclotorsion of 4.1° (±3.7°) while 8% of the eyes showed a deviation greater than 10°. Ciccio et al. [7] repeated the measurements, marking the horizontal axis of 1019 eyes prior to wavefront measurements, and detected the mark on the supine patient under the laser. The angle of misalignment was measured and analyzed whereby a mean rotational angle of the eyes from seated to supine patient of 4.05° (±2.9°) was observed. Moreover, they found a difference between left eyes and right eyes in the predominant trend of the rotation with 46% of the patients showing bilateral excyclotorsion and only 1.7% displaying bilateral incyclotorsion.

As already mentioned, it is well known that iris patterns are unique properties of an individual (such as finger prints) and the probability of finding two objects with the same iris pattern is extremely low. The challenge is to utilize this fact in a way that the realization provides an accurate determination of the special alignment of the unique pattern when compared to a reference image of the same eye. The strategy to fulfil these criteria is developed by means of using a sophisticated approach to analyze the complex iris structures and to transform this information into a digital code of the iris. This code should be sufficiently unique but still compact enough to provide a realistic processing time according to the desired application.

A central iris recognition and comparison module is used in all the applications mentioned. This module is the main tool in the process of identification of the iris patterns as well as in the determination of the rotational misalignment between two specific images. The initial point for an iris recognition process is always the availability of two iris images that can be compared to each other. Depending on whether or not they belong to the same eye, the key question is whether there is a measurable rotational angle between the two images.

The study was approved by the local institutional review board (Kantonalethikkommission Nr 2006/11, Aargau) and adhered to the tenets of the Declaration of Helsinki.

5. Conclusions

In this study, we present the results of 88 treatment sessions, 44 with and 44 without a cyclorotational eye tracker system. There was no significant difference of clinical outcome regarding the spherical equivalent, however there was a highly significant difference regarding the cylinder treatment. The advantage of iris recognition ensures a much better laser spot position during the surgery while it is not always the case in an only X/Y eyetracker control procedure. The dynamic cyclorotational eye tracker system leads to a high level of cylinder control during corneal refractive surgery with the Excimer laser. Therefore, the proposed system used for LASIK results in highly predictable refraction quality with significantly less postoperative re-treatments.

Acknowledgments: This work was supported by European Cooperation in Science and Technology (COST) Action BM1205.

Author Contributions: Bojan Pajic and Zeljka Cvejic conceived and designed the experiments; Bojan Pajic and Jörg Müller performed the experiments; Zoran Mijatovic and Jörg Müller analyzed the data; Dragan Indjin contributed analysis tools; all authors wrote the paper.

References

1. Taravella, M.J.; Davidson, R.S. Corneal Topography and Wavefront Imaging—IV Chapter. In *Ophthalmology*, 4th ed.; Yanoff, M., Duker, J.S., Eds.; Elsevier Saunders: Philadelphia, PA, USA, 2014; pp. 168–173.
2. Zhon, C.; Chair, X.; Yuan, L.; He, Y.; Ren, Q. Corneal higher-order aberrations after customized aspheric ablation and conventional ablation for myopic correction. *Curr. Eye Res.* **2007**, *32*, 431–438. [CrossRef]
3. Mrochen, M.; Kaemmerer, M.; Seiler, T. Wavefront-guided laser in situ keratomileusis: Early results in three eyes. *J. Refract. Surg.* **2000**, *16*, 116–121. [PubMed]
4. McDonald, M.B. Summit Autonomous custom cornea LASIK outcomes. *J. Refract. Surg.* **2000**, *16*, 617–618.
5. Smolek, K.M. Method for Expressing Clinical and Statistical Signicance of Ocular and Corneal Wavefront Error Aberrations. *Cornea* **2012**, *31*, 212–221. [CrossRef] [PubMed]
6. Seiler, T.; Kaemmerer, M.; Mierdel, P.; Krinke, H.E. Ocular optical aberrations after photorefractive kerarectomy for myopia and myopic astigmatism. *Arch. Ophthalmol.* **2000**, *118*, 17–21. [CrossRef] [PubMed]
7. Ciccio, A.E.; Durrie, D.S.; Stahl, J.E. Ocular cyclotorsion during customized laser ablation. *J. Refract. Surg.* **2005**, *21*, S772–S774. [PubMed]
8. Holladay, J.T.; Dudeja, D.R.; Chang, J. Functional vision and corneal changes after laser in situ keratomileusis determined by contrast sensitivity, glare testing and corneal topography. *J. Cataract. Refract. Surg.* **1999**, *25*, 663–669. [CrossRef]
9. Chernyak, D.A. Cyclotorsion eye motion occurring between wavefront measurement and refractive surgery. *J. Cataract. Refract. Surg.* **2004**, *30*, 633–638. [CrossRef] [PubMed]
10. Tjon-Fo-Sang, M.J.; De Faber, J.T.H.N.; Kingma, C.; Beckhuis, W.H. Cyclotorsion: A possible cause of residual astigmatism in refractive surgery. *J. Cataract. Refract. Surg.* **2002**, *28*, 599–602. [CrossRef]
11. Fea, A.M.; Sciandra, L.; Annetta, F.; Musso, M.; Dal Vecchio, M.; Grignolo, F.M. Cyclotorsional eye movements during a simulated PRK procedure. *Eye* **2006**, *20*, 764–768. [CrossRef] [PubMed]
12. Swami, A.U.; Steinert, R.F.; Osborne, W.E. Rotational malposition during laser in situ keratomileusis. *Am. J. Ophthalmol.* **2002**, *133*, 561–562. [CrossRef]
13. Neuhann, I.M.; Lege, B.A.; Hassel, J.M. Static and Dynamic rotational eye tracking during LASIK treatment of myopic astigmatism with Zyoptix laser platform and Advanced Control Eye Tracker. *J. Refract. Surg.* **2010**, *26*, 17–27. [CrossRef] [PubMed]
14. Prakash, G.; Agarwal, A.; Kumar, D.A. Surface ablation with iris recognition and dynamic rotational eye tracking-based tissue saving treatment with the Technolas 217z excimer laser. *J. Refract. Surg.* **2011**, *27*, 323–331. [CrossRef] [PubMed]

11

Performance Characterization of a Switchable Acoustic Resolution and Optical Resolution Photoacoustic Microscopy System

Mohesh Moothanchery and Manojit Pramanik *

School of Chemical and Biomedical Engineering, Nanyang Technological University, 62 Nanyang Drive, Singapore 637459, Singapore; mmohesh@ntu.edu.sg

* Correspondence: manojit@ntu.edu.sg

Academic Editors: Dragan Indjin, Željka Cvejić and Małgorzata Jędrzejewska-Szczerska

Abstract: Photoacoustic microscopy (PAM) is a scalable bioimaging modality; one can choose low acoustic resolution with deep penetration depth or high optical resolution with shallow imaging depth. High spatial resolution and deep penetration depth is rather difficult to achieve using a single system. Here we report a switchable acoustic resolution and optical resolution photoacoustic microscopy (AR-OR-PAM) system in a single imaging system capable of both high resolution and low resolution on the same sample. Lateral resolution of 4.2 μm (with ~1.4 mm imaging depth) and lateral resolution of 45 μm (with ~7.6 mm imaging depth) was successfully demonstrated using a switchable system. In vivo blood vasculature imaging was also performed for its biological application.

Keywords: photoacoustic imaging; AR-PAM; OR-PAM; microscopy; deep tissue imaging

1. Introduction

Photoacoustic microscopy (PAM) is an emerging hybrid in vivo imaging modality, combining optics and ultrasound, which can provide penetration beyond the optical diffusion limit with high resolution. This approach can provide deeper imaging than other optical modalities and has been successfully applied to in vivo structural, functional, molecular, and cell imaging [1–9]. PAM overcomes the limitations of other existing optical modalities combining optical contrast with ultrasound resolution. In PAM, the contrast is related to the optical properties of the tissue, but the resolution is not limited by optical diffusion due to multiple photon scattering. Unlike optical coherence tomography (OCT), PAM does not rely on ballistic or backscattered light. Any light, including both singly and multiply scattered photons, contributes to the imaging signal. As a result, the imaging depth in PAM is relatively large. The key advantages of PAM include (1) combination of high optical contrast and high ultrasonic resolution; (2) good imaging depth; (3) no speckle artifacts; (4) scalable resolution and imaging depth with the ultrasonic frequency; (5) use of non-ionizing radiation (both laser and ultrasound pose no known hazards to humans); and (6) relatively inexpensive.

In PAM, a short laser pulse irradiates the tissue/sample. Due to absorption of light by the tissue chromophores (such as melanin, hemoglobin, and water), there is a temperature rise, which in turn produces pressure waves emitted in the form of acoustics waves. A wideband ultrasonic transducer receives the acoustic signal (known as photoacoustic (PA) waves) outside the tissue/sample boundary. In acoustic resolution photoacoustic microscopy (AR-PAM) deep tissue imaging can be achieved with weak optical and tight acoustic focusing [10–12]. Since AR-PAM lateral resolution is dependent on the ultrasound focus, one can achieve high lateral resolution (~45 μm with 50 MHz focused ultrasound transducer with numerical aperture (NA) 0.44) with an imaging depth of up to 3 mm, as the PA signal in AR-PAM does not depend on the ballistic photons. Resolving single capillaries acoustically need ultrasonic transducers greater than 400 MHz central frequency; however, at this frequency the penetration depth will be less than 100 μm. In optical resolution photoacoustic microscopy (OR-PAM), the lateral resolution can be improved by a tight optical focus; one can achieve a lateral resolution of up to 0.5 μm in the reflection mode and up to 0.2 μm lateral resolution in the transmission mode [13–20]. There were other techniques employed to attain super resolution imaging capability including nonlinear enhancement [17,21], use of double excitation process [22], and use of a photonic nanojet [23,24]. OR-PAM can clearly resolve single capillaries or even a single cell [25]. However, the penetration depth is rather limited due to light focusing and it can image up to ~1.2 mm inside the biological tissue [19]. Therefore, in summary AR-PAM can image deeper, but with lower resolution and OR-PAM can image with very high resolution but limited imaging depth. The imaging speed of the AR- and OR-PAM system mainly depends on the pulse repetition rate of the laser source [26].

Not many efforts have been put to integrate both these systems together. Mostly, two different imaging scanners are used for imaging. However, hybrid imaging with both optical and acoustic resolution PAM enables imaging with scalable resolution and depth. In one approach, the optical and ultrasound focus have been shifted for doing both AR- and OR-PAM. However, since the light focus and ultrasound focus are not aligned, the image quality and resolution was not optimal [27]. In another approach, an optical fiber bundle was used to deliver light for OR- and AR-PAM [28]. In this approach, they have used two separate lasers (high energy laser at 532 nm for the AR and a low energy high repetition rate laser at 570 nm for the OR), making the system inconvenient, expensive, and not suitable for applications including oxygen saturation measurements [29]. In any of these techniques, AR-PAM was not having dark field illumination and hence there were strong photoacoustic signals from the tissue surface. The use of dark field illumination can reduce the generation of strong photoacoustic signals from the skin surface hence deep tissue imaging can be performed using ring-shaped illumination as the detection sensitivity of deep photoacoustic signals will be higher compared to brightfield illumination [12]. Here, we report a switchable AR- and OR-PAM (AR-OR-PAM) imaging system capable of both high-resolution imaging as well as low resolution deep tissue imaging on the same sample utilizing dark field illumination. We use the same laser for both systems. The AR-OR-PAM system was characterized in terms of spatial resolution and imaging depth using phantom experiments. In vivo blood vasculature imaging was performed on mouse ear for demonstrating its biological application.

2. System Description

2.1. The Switchable Acoustic Resolution-Optical Resolution-Photoacoustic Microscopy (AR-OR-PAM) System

The schematic of the AR-OR-PAM system is shown in Figure 1a. Figure 1b shows the photograph of the switchable AR-OR-PAM scanning head. This AR-OR-PAM system employs a nanosecond tunable laser system, consisting of a diode-pumped solid-state Nd-YAG laser (INNOSLAB, Edgewave, Wurselen, Germany) and a dye laser (Credo-DYE-N, Sirah dye laser, Spectra Physics, Santa Clara, CA, USA). The laser system was tunable between 559–576 nm using Rhodamine 6G dye. The wavelength range can be changed depending on the dye used. For example, using DCM dye, the wavelength range can be changed to 602–660 nm. For AR-PAM scanning, the laser beam was diverted using a right angle prism, RAP1 (PS915H-A, Thorlabs, Newton, NJ, USA), placed on a computer controlled motorized stage (CR1/M-Z7, Thorlabs). The diverted beam passed through another right angle prism, RAP2 (PS915H-A, Tholabs), and a variable neutral density filter, NDF2 (NDC-50C-4M, Thorlabs), and coupled on to a multimode fiber, MMF (M29L01, Thorlabs) using a combination of objective (M-10X, Newport, Irvine, CA, USA) and XY translator (CXY1, Thorlabs), which acts as the fiber coupler (FC). The fiber out was fixed on the stage using a translator (TS) (CXY1, Thorlabs). The beam out from the fiber passed through a collimating lens, L1 (LA1951, Thorlabs), and then passed through a conical lens (Con.L), having an apex angle of 130° (1-APX-2-B254, Altechna, Vilnius, Lithuania) to provide a ring-shaped beam. The conical lens was placed on a translating mount, TM1 (CT1, Thorlabs). The ring shaped beam was allowed to focus weakly onto the subject with the focal region coaxially overlapping the ultrasonic focus inside the tissue using a homemade optical condenser (OC) (cone angles: 70°, 110°), having a 50 MHz ultrasonic transducer (UST) (V214-BB-RM, Olympus-NDT, Waltham, MA, USA) in the center. An acoustic lens (AL) (LC4573, Thorlabs) having a radius of curvature of 4.6 mm and a 6 mm diameter was attached using a UV curing optical adhesive (NOA61, Thorlabs) to the bottom of the transducer, which provided an acoustic focal diameter of ~46 μm. In an optically clear medium, the optical focus was around 2 mm in diameter, which was wider than the ultrasonic focus. This type of dark field illumination is beneficial for deep tissue imaging where there are no strong signals from the tissue surface. The laser repetition rate (LRR) was set to be 1 kHz, and the laser energy at focus can be varied up to 30 μJ per pulse. The optical illumination on the object surface was donut shaped with a dark center so that no strong photoacoustic signals were produced from the surface on the object within the ultrasonic field of view. In our setup, all components were integrated and assembled in an optical cage setup. For AR, both 30 mm and 60 mm optical cages (OC connected in 60 mm cage) were used. The use of the cage system made the AR setup compact and easier to assemble and align.

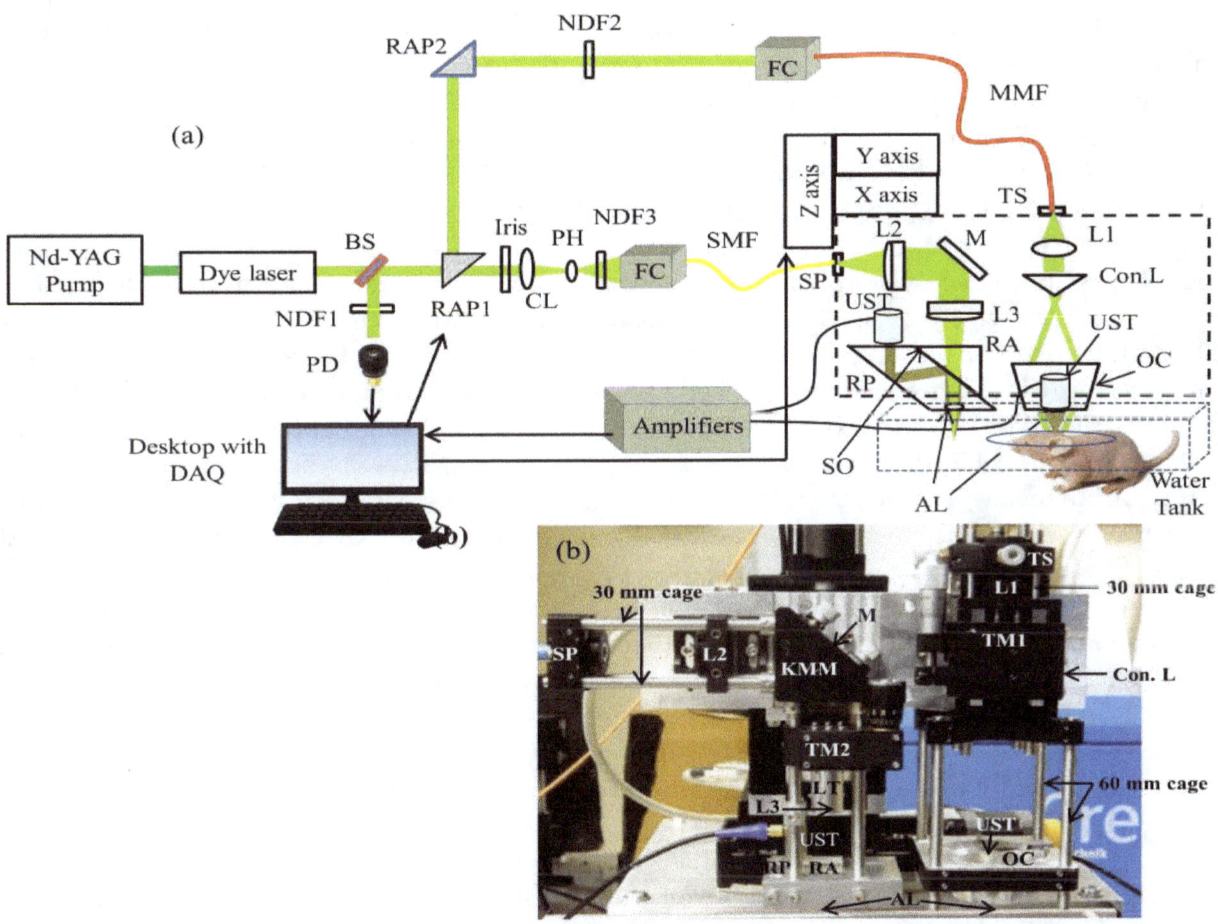

Figure 1. (**a**) Schematic of the Acoustic Resolution—Optical Resolution—Photoacoustic Microscopy (AR-OR-PAM) imaging system. BS: beam sampler; NDF: neutral density filter; RAP: right angle prism; PD: photodiode; CL: condenser lens; PH: pinhole; FC: fiber coupler; UST: ultrasound transducer; MMF: multimode fiber; SMF: single mode fiber; DAQ: data acquisition card; TS: translation stage; Con.L: conical lens; L1: convex lens; L2 & L3: achromatic lens; RA: right angle prism; RP: rhomboid prism; OC: optical condenser; M: mirror; SP: slip plate; LT: lens tube; TM: translation mount; KMM: kinematic mirror mount; AL: acoustic lens; (**b**) Photograph of the prototype AR-OR-PAM system.

For the OR-PAM setup, the rotational stage (holding the RAP1) would rotate at 90° so that the laser beam went straight and was reshaped by an iris (ID12/M, Thorlabs) and then focused by a condenser lens, CL (LA4327, Thorlabs), and passed through a 50 μm pinhole, PH (P50S, Thorlabs), for spatial filtering. The filtered beam was attenuated by a variable neutral density filter, NDF3 (NDC-50C-4M, Thorlabs), and launched on to a single-mode fiber, SMF (P1-460B-FC-1, Thorlabs), using a single mode fiber coupler, FC (F-91-C1, Newport). The output port of the single-mode fiber was placed on a slip plate positioner, SP (SPT1, Thorlabs). The output beam from the SMF was then collimated by an achromatic lens, L2 (32-317, Edmund Optics, Barrington, New Jersey, United States) was reflected by a stationary elliptical mirror, M (PFE10-P01, Thorlabs), was fixed on a Kinematic mirror mount, KMM (KCB1, Thorlabs), and filled the back aperture of another identical achromatic lens, L3, placed on a translation mount, TM2 (SM1Z, Thorlabs). The achromatic lens was placed on the translation mount with the help of a lens tube, LT (SM05L10, Thorlabs). The effective clear aperture of the achromatic lens through the tube was 10.9 mm, which makes the effective numerical aperture (NA) of the achromatic lens as 0.11. The beam then passed through an optoacoustic beam combiner consisting of a right angled prism, RA (PS615, Thorlabs) and a rhomboid prism, RP (47-214, Edmund optics) with a layer of silicon oil, SO (DMPS1M, Sigma Aldrich, St. Louis, MI, USA) in between. The silicon oil layer acts as optically transparent and acoustically reflective film. An acoustic lens, AL (LC4573, Thorlabs) provided acoustic focusing (a focal diameter of ~46 μm), was attached at the bottom of the rhomboid prism. The ultrasonic transducer, a 50 MHz center frequency (V214-BB-RM, Olympus-NDT), was placed on top of the rhomboid with an epoxy layer from a single part of a two part epoxy (G14250, Thorlabs) for effective coupling. To maximize the detection sensitivity, the optical and acoustic foci were aligned confocally. The laser repetition rate for the OR-PAM was set to 5 kHz and the laser energy at focus could be varied up to 200 nJ per pulse. Like AR, the OR systems components were also integrated and assembled in a 30 mm optical cage system.

The AR-OR combined system was attached to a homemade plate that helps in switching between AR and OR scanhead easily by sliding the scanhead on top of the imaging area. At present, the y-axis translation stage used has a range of 5 cm; therefore, the switching between the AR and OR systems was done by manual sliding. However, if one uses the y-axis translation stage with a 10 cm range, manual transition can be avoided. The AR-OR combined scanner head was attached to a 3-axis motorized stage (PLS 85 for X and Y axis, VT 80 for Z axis, PI—Physik Instrumente, Karlsruhe, Germany). All three stages were controlled by a 3-axis controller (SMC corvus eco, PI micos) connected to the computer. For photoacoustic imaging, the bottom of the AR-OR-PAM scanner head was submerged in a water-filled tank (13 cm × 30 cm) for acoustic coupling. An imaging window of 7 cm × 7 cm was opened at the bottom of the tank and sealed with a polyethylene membrane for optical and acoustic transmission. The PA signal acquired by the UST was amplified by two amplifiers (ZFL-500LN, Mini Circuits, Brooklyn, NY, USA) each having a 24 dB gain, and was recorded using a data acquisition (DAQ) card, (M4i.4420, Spectrum, Grosshansdorf, Germany) in a desktop computer (Intel xeon E5-1630 3.7 GHz processor, 16 GB RAM, 64 bit windows 10 operating system). The DAQ card had a 16 bit analog-to-digital converter (ADC), a 250 Ms/s sampling rate, 2 channels, and a 4 GB on-board memory. The same desktop computer was used for both AR and OR-PAM systems. The scanning and data acquisition was controlled using Labview software (National Instrument). Two-dimensional continuous raster scanning of the imaging head was used during image acquisition. The time-resolved PA signals were multiplied by the speed of sound, 1540 m/s in soft tissue [30] to obtain an A-line. Multiple A-lines were captured during the continuous motion of the Y stage to produce a two-dimensional B-scan. Multiple B-scans of the imaging area were captured and stored in the computer. MATLAB (MathWorks, Natick, MA, USA) was used to process and obtain the maximum amplitude projection (MAP) photoacoustic images.

The synchronization of the data acquisition and the stage motion was controlled by the signal from a photodiode (PD) (SM05PD1A, Thorlabs). A beamsampler, BS (BF10-A, Thorlabs), was placed in front of the laser beam diverted a small portion of the beam (5%) to the PD. A neutral density filter,

NDF 1 (NDC-50C-4M, Thorlabs), was placed in front of the PD to control the energy falling on the PD. The PD signal can also used for compensating pulse-to-pulse laser energy variations during data acquisition. All experiments were done at a laser wavelength of 570 nm in this work.

2.2. Laser Safety

For in vivo imaging, the maximum permissible pulse energy is governed by American National Standards Institute (ANSI) laser safety standards [31]. The safety limit varies with illumination wavelength, pulse duration, exposure duration, and exposure area. The maximum pulse energy by a single laser pulse (MPE_{SP}) on the skin surface should not exceed $MPE_{SP} = 2C_A 10^{-2}$ J/cm^2, where C_A the wavelength correction factor, is unity for visible wavelength range (400–700 nm). The irradiance should not exceed 200 mW/cm^2 if a point on skin is exposed to more than 10 s. In the case of raster scanning, a point on the skin will not be exposed for 10 s; hence, the maximum permissible exposure (MPE_{AVE}) is limited by 1.1 $C_A t^{0.25}$ mJ/cm^2, where t denotes the exposure duration in seconds.

For AR-PAM, the diameter of the optical focus at the ultrasound focus was 2 mm. Having a minimum pixel separation of 15 μm, an average of 133 (N) adjacent laser pulses overlap at the ultrasound focus. At 1 kHz LRR, the exposure time was 133 ms, so the maximum pulse energy for the pulse train (MPE_{TRAIN}) was 664 mJ/cm^2 (1.1 $C_A t^{0.25}$). The MPE_{SP} for the pulse train was $MPE_{AVG} = MPE_{TRAIN}/N = 664/133 = 5$ mJ/cm^2. The current AR-PAM system can deliver per pulse energy of 0.32 mJ/cm^2 (30 μJ/pulse, 2 mm diameter focus), which is well below the MPE_{SP} safety limit. For AR-PAM experiments, we used a pulse energy of 30 μJ/pulse for imaging depth and 6 μJ/pulse for the resolution test and in vivo ear blood vasculature imaging.

For OR-PAM, we believe the effect of optical aberrations at the prism surface and acoustic lens might have reduced the objective NA from 0.11 to 0.075, which will give a spot size diameter of 3.9 μm (which agrees with our lateral resolution). Assuming the optical focus is 150 micron below the skin surface for in vivo imaging, the surface spot size was 22.5 μm in diameter. Having a minimum pixel separation of 2 μm, an average of 11 (N) adjacent laser pulses overlaps on the skin surface. At 5 kHz LRR, the exposure time was 2.4 ms. Therefore, the MPE_{TRAIN} was 238 mJ/cm^2. The MPE_{SP} for the pulse train was $MPE_{AVG} = MPE_{TRAIN}/N = 238/11 = 21.6$ mJ/cm^2. The current OR-PAM system can deliver an MPE_{SP} of 20.4 mJ/cm^2 (90 nJ/pulse, 0.075 NA) at the skin surface (close to the safety limit). For OR-PAM experiments, we used a pulse energy of 20 nJ/pulse for the resolution test and 90 nJ/pulse for imaging depth and in vivo ear blood vasculature imaging.

3. Experimental Methods

In order to evaluate the system performance of the switchable AR-OR-PAM system, a series of experiments were conducted to determine the spatial resolution and the maximum imaging depths for both AR- and OR-PAM. In vivo imaging was also done using the switchable system to show the biological imaging capability of the system.

3.1. Spatial Resolution Quantification

The lateral resolution of the AR and OR system was determined by imaging a 100 nm gold nanoparticle (742031, Sigma Aldrich). To determine the resolution of the AR-PAM system, a single nanoparticle was scanned with a step size of 5 microns. Similarly, the nanoparticle was scanned with a step size of 0.5 microns in order to find the resolution of the OR-PAM system. The photoacoustic amplitude along the central lateral direction of the nanoparticle image was fitted to a Gaussian function. The full width at half maximum (FWHM) of the Gaussian fit was considered the lateral resolution. Theoretically, the optical diffraction-limited lateral resolution for the OR-PAM was calculated from 0.51 λ/NA, where λ was the laser wavelength, and NA was the numerical aperture of the objective. Similarly, the theoretical lateral resolution for the AR-PAM was determined using the equation 0.72 λ/NA, where λ was the central acoustic wavelength, and NA was the numerical aperture of the ultrasonic transducer. The photoacoustic axial spread profile from the nanoparticle was used to determine the axial resolution of the system. Both OR-PAM and AR-PAM share the same axial resolution since the same ultrasound transducer (and the focusing lens) was used in both systems. The axial resolution was determined by acoustic parameters according to 0.88 $c/\Delta f$, where c is the speed of sound in soft tissue, and Δf is the frequency bandwidth of the ultrasonic transducer. Since the size of the nanoparticle was much smaller than the axial resolution, the axial spread profile can be considered as axial point spread function of the imaging system. The FWHM of the envelope gives the axial resolution. The axial resolution was also calculated by numerically shifting and summing two A-line signals and by checking whether the two peaks could be differentiated in the envelope with a contrast-to-noise ratio (CNR) greater than 2. The CNR was plotted against the shift between the two impulse responses. The contrast was defined as the difference between the smaller of the two peaks in the photoacoustic envelope and the valley between the peaks. The noise was the standard deviation in the background photoacoustic signal.

3.2. *USAF Resolution Test Target Imaging*

The lateral resolution of the AR and OR system was further validated imaging a USAF 1951 test target (R1DS1P, Thorlabs). Initially, a 5 mm × 5 mm area (Group numbers 2 to 7) were scanned using AR-PAM. The scan step size was 10 µm in both X and Y directions. Similarly, a 1.3 mm × 1.3 mm area (Group numbers 4 to 7) was scanned using OR-PAM with a step size of 0.5 µm in both X and Y directions. Finally, a 0.3 mm × 0.3 mm area consisting of the smallest groups (Group Numbers 6 and 7) were scanned using OR-PAM imaging with a step size of 0.5 µm in both X and Y directions.

3.3. *Imaging Depth*

To determine the maximum imaging depth of both AR-PAM and OR-PAM, a black tape was inserted obliquely on a chicken tissue. A single B-scan image was captured using both AR-PAM and OR-PAM. The signal-to-noise ratio (SNR) was also determined at the maximum imaging depth. SNR is defined as V/n, where V is the peak-to-peak PA signal amplitude, and n is the standard deviation of the background noise.

3.4. *In Vivo Imaging of Mouse Ear Blood Vasculature*

To demonstrate in vivo imaging using the combined system, the ears of 4-week-old female mice with body weights of 25 g, procured from InVivos Pte. Ltd. (Singapore), were used. Animal experiments were performed according to the approved guidelines and regulations by the institutional Animal Care and Use committee of Nanyang Technological University, Singapore (Animal Protocol Number ARF-SBS/NIE-A0263). The animal was anesthetized using a cocktail of ketamine (120 mg/kg) and xylazine (16 mg/kg) injected intraperitoneally (dosage of 0.1 mL/10 g, body weight). After removing hair from the ear, the mouse was positioned on a platform that also has a miniature plate to position the ear. The animal was further anesthetized with vaporized isoflurane system (1 L/min oxygen and 0.75% isoflurane) during the imaging period. The imaging region was placed into contact with the polyethylene membrane using ultrasound gel. Using AR-PAM, a large area (9 mm × 7 mm) of the ear was first imaged, using a step size of 15 µm in the Y direction and 30 µm in the X direction. The same area (4.5 mm × 5 mm) was scanned using OR-PAM with a step size of 2 µm in the Y direction and 3 µm in the X direction.

4. Results and Discussion

4.1. *Spatial Resolution of the Imaging System*

The lateral resolution of the AR-PAM is shown in Figure 2a. The measured lateral resolution is 45 µm determined by FWHM. Similarly, lateral resolution of OR-PAM is shown in Figure 2b. The measured lateral resolution determined from the FWHM is 4.2 µm. The inset of the figures shows the corresponding PAM image of the gold nanoparticle.

Figure 2c shows the axial spread profile of the averaged PA signal from the gold nanoparticle and its envelope. The axial resolution was measured to be 33 μm. The experimentally determined axial resolution matches closely to the theoretical axial resolution of 29 μm. The simulated results in Figure 2d show that we can distinguish the two absorbers separated by 16.5 μm with a CNR of 2. Figure 2e shows the plot of CNR versus axial shift.

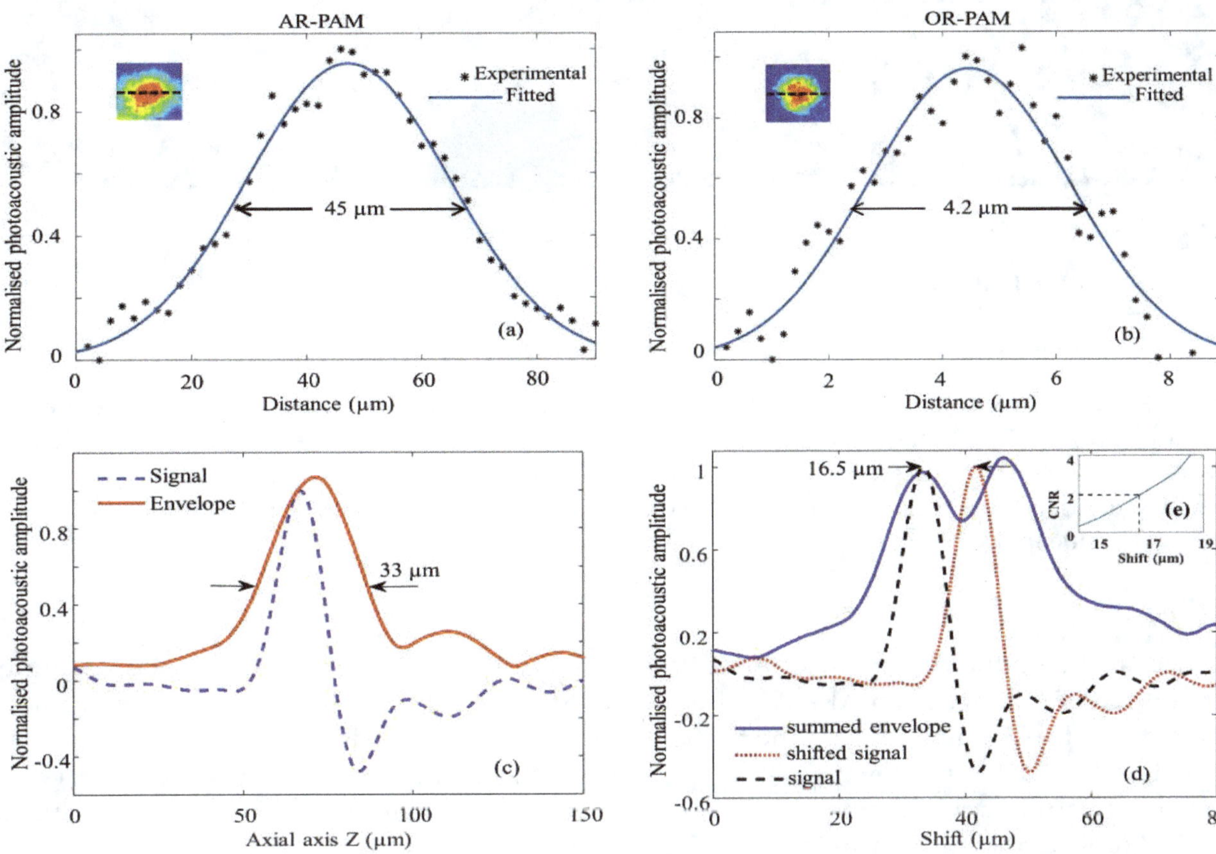

Figure 2. Spatial resolution test of the AR-OR-PAM system: Lateral resolution estimated by imaging gold nanoparticles ~100 nm diameter, Black (*) dots: photoacoustic signal; blue line: Gaussian-fitted curve; (**a**) AR PAM; (**b**) OR-PAM. The inset shows the representative AR-PAM image in (**a**) and OR-PAM image in (**b**) of the single gold nanoparticle; (**c**) Photoacoustic axial spread profile and its envelope; (**d**) Simulated photoacoustic shift-and-sum A-line signals. The dashed line and dotted line indicate two photoacoustic signals 16.5 μm apart. The solid line indicates the summed envelope of the two shifted signals; (**e**) Contrast-to-noise ratio (CNR) versus the shift distance between the two signals.

4.2. USAF Resolution Test Target Imaging

MAP AR-PAM image of a USAF resolution test target is shown in Figure 3a. From Figure 3a,d, we can see that the AR-PAM system is capable of resolving 49.61 μm line pairs (Group 3, Element 3) with a modulation transfer function (MTF) of 0.28. Figure 3b is a MAP OR-PAM image done on the red dotted area shown in Figure 3a.

Figure 3c shows the MAP OR-PAM image done on the yellow dotted area on Figure 3b. From Figure 3c,d, we can see that the OR-PAM system can clearly resolve 3.91 μm line pairs (Group 7, Element 1) with an MTF of 0.64. Theoretically, the optical diffraction-limited lateral resolution for the OR-PAM is 2.6 μm. The experimentally measured lateral resolution was poorer than the diffraction-limit estimate, which might be due to wavefront aberrations. Similarly, the theoretical lateral resolution for the AR-PAM is 46 μm. The theoretical resolution agrees well with our experimental data.

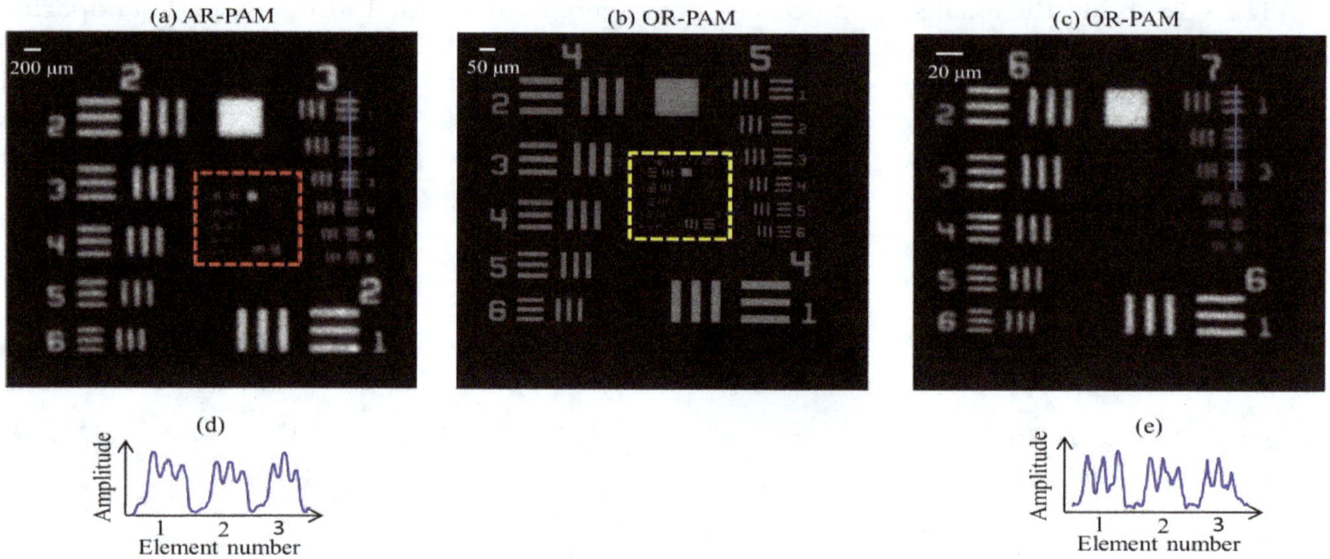

Figure 3. Lateral resolution test of the AR-OR-PAM system: (**a**) AR-PAM image of an air force resolution test target; (**b**) OR-PAM image of the red dotted area; (**c**) OR-PAM image of the yellow dotted region of the test target; (**d**) The cross-sectional profile of the first two elements in Group 3 of the resolution target, blue line in (**a**); (**e**) The cross-sectional profile of the first three elements in Group 7 of the resolution target, blue line in (**c**).

4.3. Imaging Depth

Figure 4a shows the schematic of a black tape obliquely inserted on chicken tissue. Figure 4b shows the B-scan PA image from AR-PAM. It is evident that the AR-PAM system can clearly image the black tape down to ~7.6 mm beneath the tissue surface. Similarly, using the OR-PAM system, we can clearly image the black tape down to ~1.4 mm beneath the tissue surface. For AR-PAM, the SNR at 4.6 mm and 7.6 mm imaging depth were 2.5 and 1.4, respectively. In case of OR-PAM, the SNR of the target object (black tape) at 1.4 mm imaging depth was 1.5.

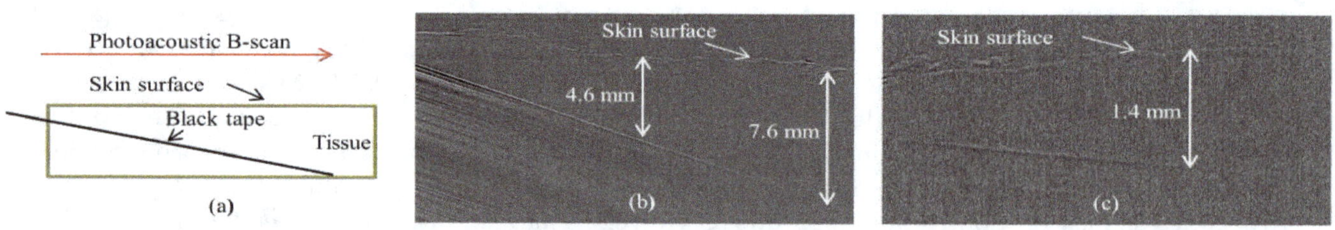

Figure 4. Single B-scan PA image of a black tape inserted obliquely in a chicken tissue. (**a**) Schematic diagram; (**b**) AR-PAM image; (**c**) OR-PAM image.

4.4. In Vivo Imaging of Mouse Ear Blood Vasculature

Figure 5a shows the photograph of the mouse ear vasculature. A unidirectional B-scan imaging of 9 mm × 7 mm area using AR-PAM took 10 min to complete. The MAP image of AR-PAM is show in Figure 5b. Figure 5c shows the zoomed out image of the white dotted region in Figure 5b. The same area as in Figure 5b (4.5 mm × 5 mm) was scanned using OR-PAM (imaging time 50 min). The MAP image of the OR-PAM is shown in Figure 5d. Figure 5c,d are the same region scanned with AR-PAM and OR-PAM. We can see OR-PAM can clearly resolve single capillaries that AR-PAM cannot resolve. AR-PAM can resolve deep vessels thicker than 45 μm. Figure 5e shows the zoomed out area (white dotted region in Figure 5d). Due to the high resolution of the OR-PAM, the region appears clearer, and smaller structures are also visible.

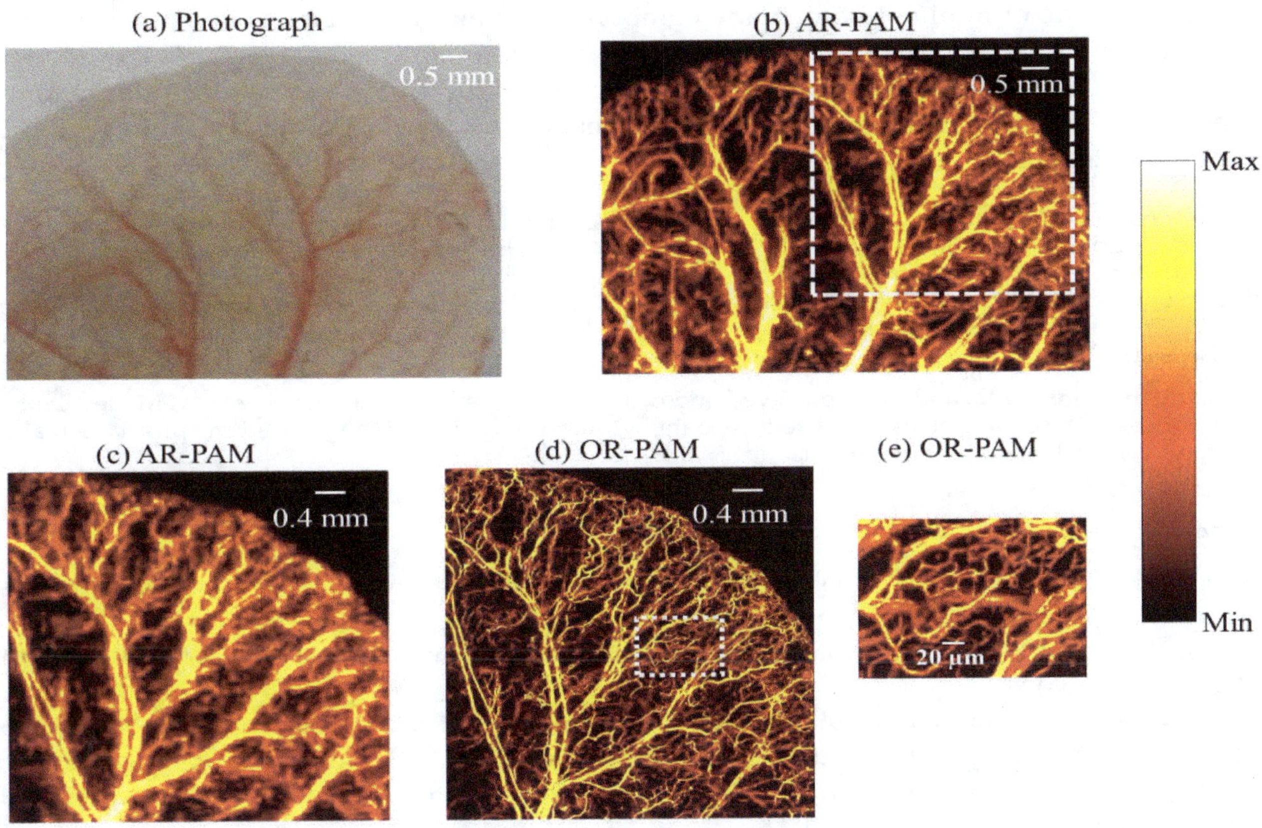

Figure 5. In vivo photoacoustic image of mouse ear: (**a**) photograph of the mouse ear vasculature; (**b**) AR-PAM image; (**c**) close up of the region of interest (ROI) in (**b**) as shown by white dash line; (**d**) OR-PAM image of the same ROI; (**e**) close up of the region of interest in (**d**) as shown by white dotted line.

In summary, a switchable AR-OR-PAM system that can achieve high-resolution imaging utilizing optical focusing as well as deep tissue imaging using dark field illumination and acoustic focusing was developed. This combined photoacoustic microscopy system can provide high spatial resolution, which makes the system important for applications including imaging of angiogenesis and drug response, where imaging single capillaries as well as deep vasculatures will be important. Further improvement in the system can be done by replacing the switchable plate with a 10 cm traveling motorized stage (y-axis). Wavefront aberration corrections for the OR-PAM will improve the lateral resolution further. Delivering higher pulse energy to the AR-PAM will improve the SNR and imaging depths as well. The limitations of the proposed technique include the scanning speed. Currently longer scanning time is required, which can be further reduced by acquiring data in both directions during imaging. High speed imaging using OR-PAM was reported by the use of a high repetition rate laser and a water immersible MEMS (microelectromechanical system) mirror [32]. Simultaneous image acquisition using both AR-PAM and OR-PAM is not possible at the moment. Developing a system that can do simultaneous data acquisition using OR-PAM and dark field AR-PAM would have been more advantageous.

5. Conclusions

A switchable acoustic resolution and optical resolution photoacoustic microscopy system that can achieve both high-resolution imaging at lower imaging depth and lower resolution imaging at higher imaging depth was developed. This is the first combined system using the same laser, which can be easily switched between OR-PAM and dark field AR-PAM. The combined system will have a 4.2 μm resolution with a 1.4 mm imaging depth, as well as a 45 μm resolution with a 7.6 mm imaging depth.

The system is made of minimal homemade components, making it easier to assemble, align, and build. Using the combined system, in vivo imaging was successfully demonstrated. The developed system can be used for pre-clinical imaging. Major preclinical applications include imaging of angiogenesis, microcirculation, tumor microenvironments, drug response, brain functions, biomarkers, and gene activities.

Acknowledgments: The authors would like to acknowledge the financial support from Tier 2 grant funded by the Ministry of Education in Singapore (ARC2/15: M4020238). The authors would like to thank Benjamin Tay Wee Ann for Labview programming and Chow Wai Hoong Bobby for machine shop help. The authors would also like to thank Lidai Wang (City University of Hong Kong), Liang Song (Shenzhen Institute of Advanced Technology, Chinese Academy of Science), Junjie Yao (Duke University), and Song Hu (University of Virginia) for useful discussions.

Author Contributions: M.M. and M.P. conceived and designed the system and experiments. M.M. developed the system; performed the experiments; analyzed the data; wrote the paper. M.P. supervised the project. All authors contributed to critical reading of the manuscript.

References

1. Wang, L.V.; Yao, J. A practical guide to photoacoustic tomography in the life sciences. *Nat. Methods* **2016**, *13*, 627–638. [CrossRef] [PubMed]
2. Zhou, Y.; Yao, J.; Wang, L.V. Tutorial on photoacoustic tomography. *J. Biomed. Opt.* **2016**, *21*, 061007. [CrossRef] [PubMed]
3. Yao, J.; Wang, L.V. Photoacoustic Brain Imaging: From Microscopic to Macroscopic Scales. *Neurophotonics* **2014**, *1*, 011003. [CrossRef] [PubMed]
4. Wang, L.V.; Hu, S. Photoacoustic Tomography: In Vivo Imaging from Organelles to Organs. *Science* **2012**, *335*, 1458–1462. [CrossRef] [PubMed]
5. Beard, P. Biomedical photoacoustic imaging. *Interface Focus* **2011**, *1*, 602–631. [CrossRef] [PubMed]
6. Pan, D.; Pramanik, M.; Senpan, A.; Allen, J.S.; Zhang, H.; Wickline, S.A.; Wang, L.V.; Lanza, G.M. Molecular photoacoustic imaging of angiogenesis with integrin-targeted gold nanobeacons. *FASEB J.* **2011**, *25*, 875–882. [CrossRef] [PubMed]
7. Pan, D.; Pramanik, M.; Senpan, A.; Ghosh, S.; Wickline, S.A.; Wang, L.V.; Lanza, G.M. Near infrared photoacoustic detection of sentinel lymph nodes with gold nanobeacons. *Biomaterials* **2010**, *31*, 4088–4093. [CrossRef] [PubMed]
8. Wang, L.V. Multiscale photoacoustic microscopy and computed tomography. *Nat. Photonics* **2009**, *3*, 503–509. [CrossRef] [PubMed]
9. Zhang, E.Z.; Laufer, J.G.; Pedley, R.B.; Beard, P.C. In vivo high-resolution 3D photoacoustic imaging of superficial vascular anatomy. *Phys. Med. Biol.* **2009**, *54*, 1035–1046. [CrossRef] [PubMed]
10. Park, S.; Lee, C.; Kim, J.; Kim, C. Acoustic resolution photoacoustic microscopy. *Biom. Eng. Lett.* **2014**, *4*, 213–222. [CrossRef]
11. Zhang, H.F.; Maslov, K.; Stoica, G.; Wang, L.V. Functional photoacoustic microscopy for high-resolution and noninvasive in vivo imaging. *Nat. Biotechnol.* **2006**, *24*, 848–851. [CrossRef] [PubMed]
12. Maslov, K.; Stoica, G.; Wang, L.V. In vivo dark-field reflection-mode photoacoustic microscopy. *Opt. Lett.* **2005**, *30*, 625–627. [CrossRef] [PubMed]
13. Zhang, C.; Maslov, K.; Wang, L.V. Subwavelength-resolution label-free photoacoustic microscopy of optical absorption in vivo. *Opt. Lett.* **2010**, *35*, 3195–3197. [CrossRef] [PubMed]
14. Kim, J.Y.; Lee, C.; Park, K.; Lim, G.; Kim, C. Fast optical-resolution photoacoustic microscopy using a 2-axis water-proofing MEMS scanner. *Sci. Rep.* **2015**, *5*, 07932. [CrossRef] [PubMed]
15. Matthews, T.P.; Zhang, C.; Yao, D.K.; Maslov, K.; Wang, L.V. Label-free photoacoustic microscopy of peripheral nerves. *J. Biomed. Opt.* **2014**, *19*, 016004. [CrossRef] [PubMed]
16. Hai, P.; Yao, J.; Maslov, K.I.; Zhou, Y.; Wang, L.V. Near-infrared optical-resolution photoacoustic microscopy. *Opt. Lett.* **2014**, *39*, 5192–5195. [CrossRef] [PubMed]
17. Danielli, A.; Maslov, K.; Garcia-Uribe, A.; Winkler, A.M.; Li, C.; Wang, L.; Chen, Y.; Dorn, G.W., 2nd; Wang, L.V. Label-free photoacoustic nanoscopy. *J. Biomed. Opt.* **2014**, *19*, 086006. [CrossRef] [PubMed]

18. Zhang, C.; Maslov, K.; Hu, S.; Chen, R.; Zhou, Q.; Shung, K.K.; Wang, L.V. Reflection-mode submicron-resolution in vivo photoacoustic microscopy. *J. Biomed. Opt.* **2012**, *17*, 020501. [CrossRef] [PubMed]
19. Hu, S.; Maslov, K.; Wang, L.V. Second-generation optical-resolution photoacoustic microscopy with improved sensitivity and speed. *Opt. Lett.* **2011**, *36*, 1134–1136. [CrossRef] [PubMed]
20. Maslov, K.; Zhang, H.F.; Song, H.; Wang, L.V. Optical-resolution photoacoustic microscopy for in vivo imaging of single capillaries. *Opt. Lett.* **2008**, *33*, 929–931. [CrossRef] [PubMed]
21. Nedosekin, D.A.; Galanzha, E.I.; Dervishi, E.; Biris, A.S.; Zharov, V.P. Super-resolution nonlinear photothermal microscopy. *Small* **2014**, *10*, 135–142. [CrossRef] [PubMed]
22. Yao, J.; Wang, L.; Li, C.; Zhang, C.; Wang, L.V. Photoimprint Photoacoustic Microscopy for Three-Dimensional Label-Free Subdiffraction Imaging. *Phys. Rev. Lett.* **2014**, *112*, 014302. [CrossRef] [PubMed]
23. Upputuri, P.K.; Krishnan, M.; Pramanik, M. Microsphere enabled sub-diffraction limited optical resolution photoacoustic microscopy: A simulation study. *J. Biomed. Opt.* **2017**, *22*, 045001. [CrossRef] [PubMed]
24. Upputuri, P.K.; Wen, Z.-B.; Wu, Z.; Pramanik, M. Super-resolution photoacoustic microscopy using photonic nanojets: A simulation study. *J. Biomed. Opt.* **2014**, *19*, 116003. [CrossRef] [PubMed]
25. Strohm, E.M.; Moore, M.J.; Kolios, M.C. Single Cell Photoacoustic Microscopy: A Review. *IEEE J. Sel. Top. Quant. Electron.* **2016**, *22*, 6801215. [CrossRef]
26. Allen, T.J.; Berendt, M.O.; Spurrell, J.; Alam, S.U.; Zhang, E.Z.; Richardson, D.J.; Beard, P.C. Novel Fibre Lasers as Excitation Sources for Photoacoustic Tomography and Microscopy. *Proc. SPIE* **2016**, *9708*, 97080W-1.
27. Estrada, H.; Turner, J.; Kneipp, M.; Razansky, D. Real-time optoacoustic brain microscopy with hybrid optical and acoustic resolution. *Laser Phys. Lett.* **2014**, *11*, 045601. [CrossRef]
28. Xing, W.; Wang, L.; Maslov, K.; Wang, L.V. Integrated optical- and acoustic-resolution photoacoustic microscopy based on an optical fiber bundle. *Opt. Lett.* **2013**, *38*, 52–54. [CrossRef] [PubMed]
29. Jeon, S.; Kim, J.; Kim, C. In Vivo Switchable Optical- and Acoustic-Resolution Photoacoustic Microscopy. *Proc. SPIE* **2016**, *9708*. [CrossRef]
30. Madsen, E.L.; Zagzebski, J.A.; Banjavie, R.A.; Jutila, R.E. Tissue mimicking materials for ultrasound phantoms. *Med. Phys.* **1978**, *5*, 391–394. [CrossRef] [PubMed]
31. American National Standard for Safe Use of Lasers. *ANSI Standard Z136.1–2000*; Laser Institute of America: Orlando, FL, USA, 2000.
32. Yao, J.; Wang, L.; Yang, J.M.; Maslov, K.I.; Wong, T.T.W.; Li, L.; Huang, C.H.; Zou, J.; Wang, L.V. High-speed label-free functional photoacoustic microscopy of mouse brain in action. *Nat. Methods* **2015**, *12*, 407–410. [CrossRef] [PubMed]

12

Blood Vessel Imaging at Pre-Larval Stages of Zebrafish Embryonic Development

Alexander S. Machikhin [1], Mikhail V. Volkov [2], Alexander B. Burlakov [3], Demid D. Khokhlov [1,*] and Andrey V. Potemkin [2]

1 Laboratory of Acousto-optical Spectroscopy, Scientific and Technological Center of Unique Instrumentation, Russian Academy of Sciences, 117342 Moscow, Russia; machikhin@ntcup.ru
2 Department of Applied Optics, University ITMO, 190000 Saint Petersburg, Russia; ph-m.volkov@yandex.ru (M.V.V.); appanpotemkin@gmail.com (A.V.P.)
3 Department of Ichthyology, Faculty of Biology, Lomonosov Moscow State University, 119991 Moscow, Russia; alexander_burl08@rambler.ru
* Correspondence: khokhlov.dd@ntcup.ru

Abstract: The zebrafish (*Danio rerio*) is an increasingly popular animal model biological system. In cardiovascular research, it has been used to model specific cardiac phenomena as well as to identify novel therapies for human cardiovascular disease. While the zebrafish cardiovascular system functioning is well examined at larval stages, the mechanisms by which vessel activity is initiated remain a subject of intense investigation. In this research, we report on an in vivo stain-free blood vessel imaging technique at pre-larval stages of zebrafish embryonic development. We have developed the algorithm for the enhancement, alignment and spatiotemporal analysis of bright-field microscopy images of zebrafish embryos. It enables the detection, mapping and quantitative characterization of cardiac activity across the whole specimen. To validate the proposed approach, we have analyzed multiple data cubes, calculated vessel images and evaluated blood flow velocity and heart rate dynamics in the absence of any anesthesia. This non-invasive technique may shed light on the mechanism of vessel activity initiation and stabilization as well as the cardiovascular system's susceptibility to environmental stressors at early developmental stages.

Keywords: zebrafish; embryonic development; cardiovascular system; in vivo imaging; optical mapping; non-invasive measurements

1. Introduction

The zebrafish has emerged to become a common and useful vertebrate animal model for cardiovascular research in recent years [1–4]. It is a powerful genetic system to study cardiac function due to several advantages. The ability to implement the main modern genome editing tools and techniques, including engineered nucleases (meganucleases, zinc-finger nucleases, transcription activator-like effector nucleases) and CRISPR gene editing, have been demonstrated for *Danio rerio* [5–8]. Various zebrafish transgenic lines can be used to enhance the visualization contrast of different transformation processes [9–11]. The use of the zebrafish as a model organism is of particular interest for the analysis of innate immunity [12] and for the study of viral [13–15], bacterial [16,17] and fungal infections [18,19].

Small size, ease of maintenance, short reproduction cycle with multiple (up to 2000) embryos and short period (3 days) of embryonic development make *Danio rerio* a convenient object for continuous observation and experimental research of the mechanisms by which genetic and disease-related modifications are being passed to the offspring.

Cardiovascular system functional characteristics of zebrafish are well studied in various conditions and in the whole life cycle. Their accurate analysis and patterning may indicate developmental disorders and presence of pathology at the very early stages. Detailed studies of cardiovascular system function are of great value for understanding cardiac failures and identifying novel therapies for human cardiovascular disease [20–22].

Zebrafish embryos develop in the external environment and are relatively small-sized and transparent in the optical wavelength range. These features allow one to easily visualize the circulatory system structure [23,24], observe heart and blood vessel formation and development, and simulate cardiovascular diseases [25–28]. While the zebrafish cardiovascular system functioning is well examined at larval stages [24,29–31], the mechanisms by which the vessel activity is initiated under natural conditions remain a subject of intense investigation. At the pharyngula stage (24–40 hpf) that precedes hatching [32], invasive procedures (excising, fixation, sectioning and staining) are not effective for real-time monitoring due to the fast-changing and vulnerable state of the emerging cardiovascular system.

Thus, biomedical optical imaging techniques are remaining promising in the field of in vivo zebrafish studies [2,33]. Though heart function analysis from bright field time-lapse image sequences [31,33–35] as well as quantitative research of zebrafish heartbeat initiation and stabilization [36] have been reported, blood vessel imaging during early embryonic development has not been carried out. Due to constant embryo motion within the shell, conventional processing algorithms based on image subtraction are inefficient and require precise initial image stabilization. In this research, we show that a combination of time-lapse bright-field microscopy and an advanced image processing technique represents an effective approach to in vivo stain-free cardiac activity mapping across the whole specimen and quantitative analysis of cardiovascular performance even at pre-larval developmental stages in the absence of any anesthesia.

2. Materials and Methods

2.1. Experimental Animals

Zebrafish embryos were from an existing stock at the Biological Faculty of Lomonosov Moscow State University. Before embryo collection, single species groups of males and females were kept by local aquarists in isolated 10 L glass aquaria at a temperature of 26 °C with the aquaria illumination turned on for 12 h daily. The selected groups were fed three times a day ad libitum on flake and *Artemia*. For embryo collection, males and females were placed together in a breeding tank and the embryos were collected immediately post-fertilization. A mixture of individuals from several different breeding groups was used during the experiment to maximize genetic variation among embryos. The two-cell development stage was used as initial time point during observation because the exact time of fertilization was difficult to determine. The development, survival rate and morphology of the collected embryos was not affected in comparison to the control group not subjected to the study.

2.2. Experimental Setup

The conventional off-the-shelf trinocular transmitted light bright-field microscope is the basis of the experimental setup (Figure 1). A Koehler system was implemented to achieve uniform illumination of the object. Images were formed by an optical system assembled of a flat field corrected apochromatic objective (10× NA 0.25) and a standard tube lens. To acquire the digital images, the complementary metal-oxide-semiconductor active-pixel image sensor (IDS uEye UI-3060CP-M-GL Rev.2, 1/1.2″, 1936 × 1216 pixels) was installed onto the camera tube. The image sensor was connected to the PC for raw data acquisition and storage. The image processing and data analysis pipeline is described in Section 2.3.

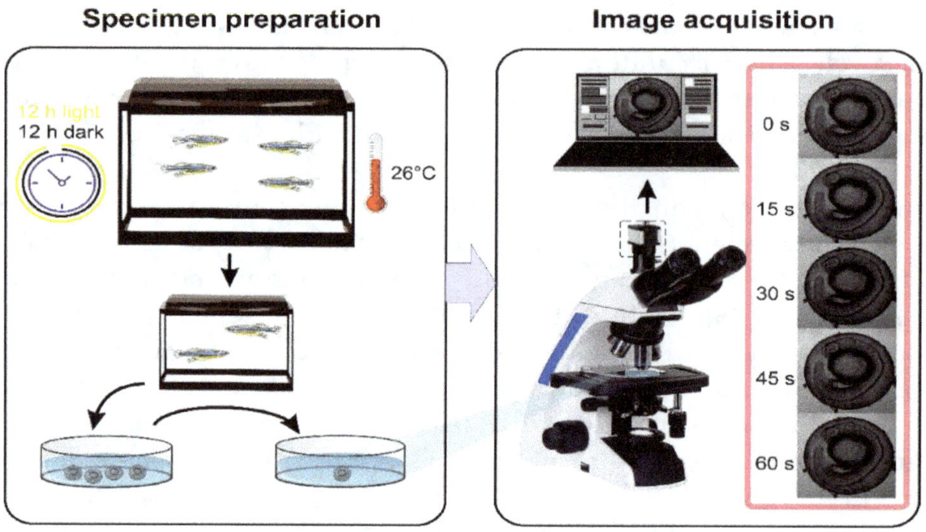

Figure 1. Experimental protocol.

2.3. Experimental Protocol

The single experimental dataset contained 3000 12-bit grayscale digital images with 1200 × 1200 pixel resolution obtained during a 60-s time series (50 fps). For preliminary geometrical calibration of the imaging setup, the images of the test chart were captured before the experimental dataset acquisition. The geometrical calibration procedure is an essential step for the magnification determining and estimation of the real image distortions. During image acquisition, the inspected embryo may move and rotate within the shell, and illumination conditions and background characteristics may also vary. Data analysis procedures require pre-processing of raw images to crop the region of interest, compensate for movement and eliminate the illumination non-uniformity (Figure 2). After these procedures, we obtained the well-matched and intensity-corrected spatiotemporal data cube $I(x,y,t)$ including time-domain dependences $I(t)$ for each image pixel with spatial coordinates x,y.

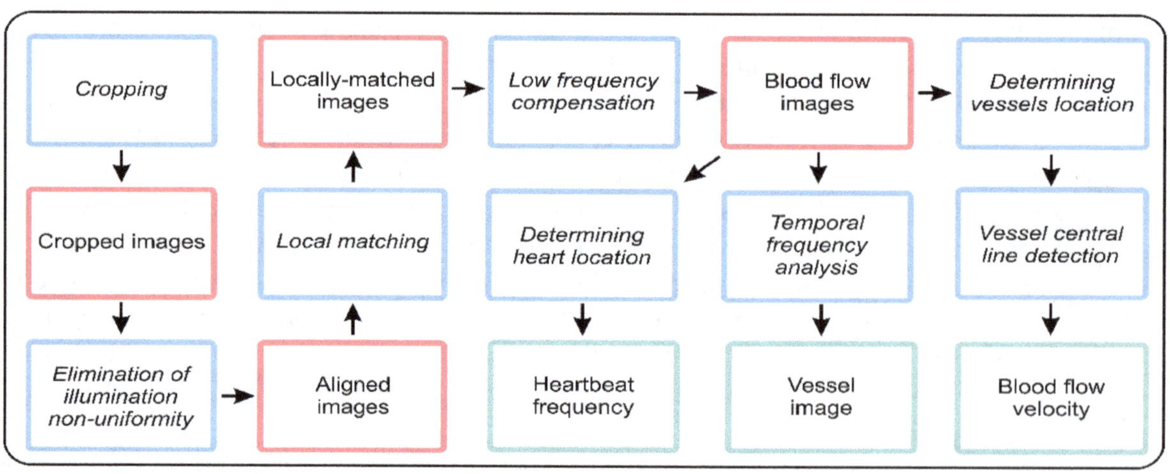

Figure 2. Image processing pipeline.

Figure 3 illustrates the main image pre-processing stages shown in pink color in Figure 2. First, the microscopic images of 26 hpf unhatched zebrafish embryo in a lateral position were to be cropped down to the embryo dimensions (Figure 3a). Second, to compensate for illumination non-uniformity and align the average intensity of all images in a series, we subtracted a smoothed image and constant term 127 (Figure 3b). Third, to ensure pixel-to-pixel matching of all images, we calculated local motion vectors and matched the images with respect to their directions and lengths. Figure 3c shows a locally matched image with crosses indicating the positions of each grid knot in the first (black) and the last (white) image of the sequence. Shape and intensity of the temporal signal $I(t)$ in each pixel of the obtained data cube $I(x,y,t)$ characterizes morphogenetic events occurring during embryonic development. The blood flow changes may be detected by the periodic variations of the transmitted light intensity since blood cells absorb light more strongly than the surrounding tissues [37]. Plotting the spectrum of the temporal signal using Fourier transform allowed detection of the dominant frequencies, which corresponded to the cardiovascular activity. After obtaining the intensity deviation values in each image pixel, we could subtract the blood-free background and consider only the pixels with blood flow related to significant intensity oscillations. Thus, we obtained a series of well-matched blood flow images ready for cardiac activity analysis (Figure 3d). The blood circulation was clearly visible throughout the full cardiac cycle (Supplementary Video).

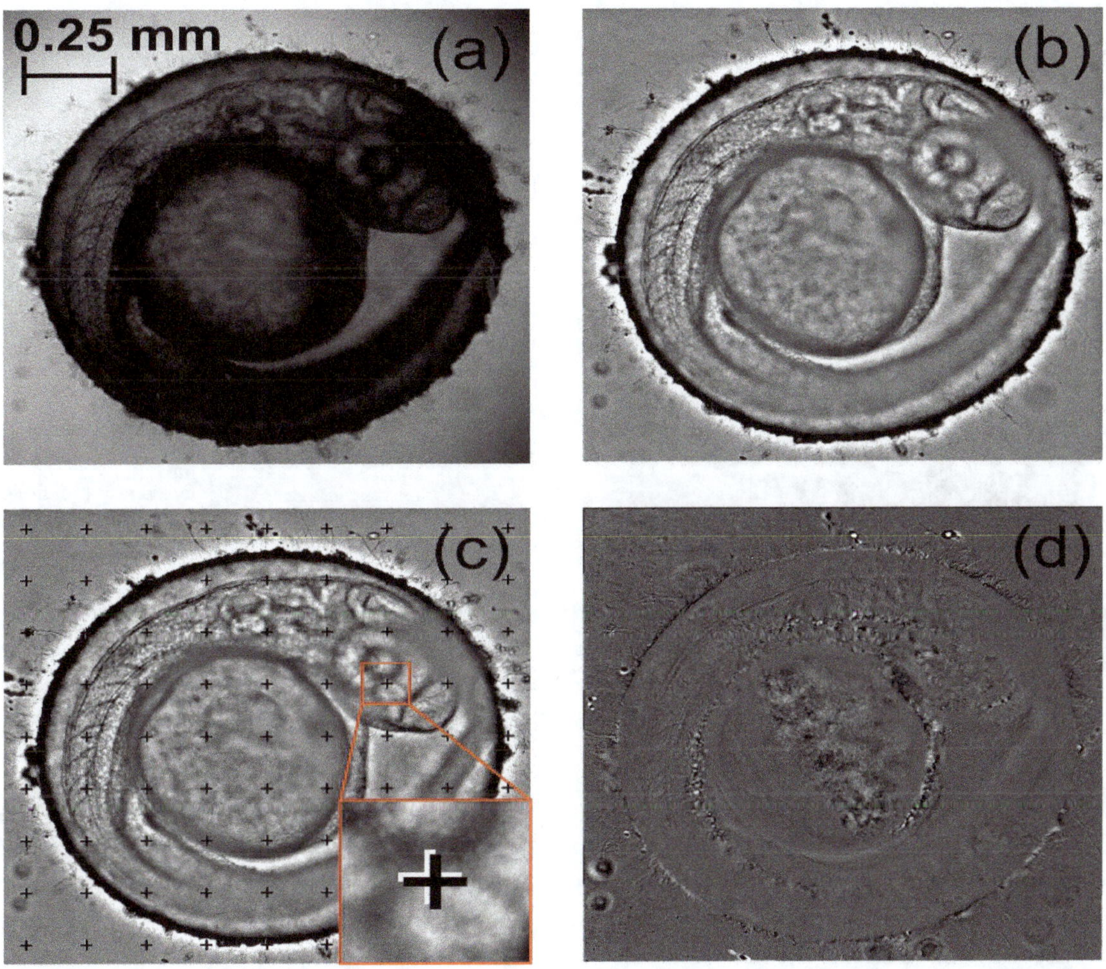

Figure 3. Stages of image pre-processing: (**a**) cropped image, (**b**) aligned image, (**c**) locally matched image and (**d**) blood flow image.

3. Results

From the series of blood flow images (Figure 4a), we could calculate the intensity of blood volume changes as the ratio of high- and low-frequency spectral components in the Fourier spectrum. Thus, we obtained the vessel image. It vividly depicts the tissues associated with cardiac activity, i.e., the spatial structure of the cardiovascular system existing at this developmental stage (Figure 4b). The heart and the system of vessels that carry blood throughout the embryo's body may be clearly identified on the blood-free background [32,38,39]. The calculated vessel image in Figure 4b demonstrates the efficiency of the proposed processing algorithm and shows the main elements of the existing cardiovascular system. Vessels are named according to commonly used classification [40]: ACeV—anterior cerebral vein; BA—basilar artery; CA—caudal artery; CaDI—caudal division of the internal carotid artery; CCV—common cardinal vein; CV—caudal vein; DA—dorsal aorta; MsA—mesencephalic artery; MsV—mesencephalic vein; PCV—posterior cardinal vein; PHBC—primordial hindbrain channel; PHS—primary head sinus; PICA—primitive internal carotid artery; PMBC—primordial midbrain channel; PMsA—primitive mesencephalic artery; PPrA—primitive prosencephalic artery.

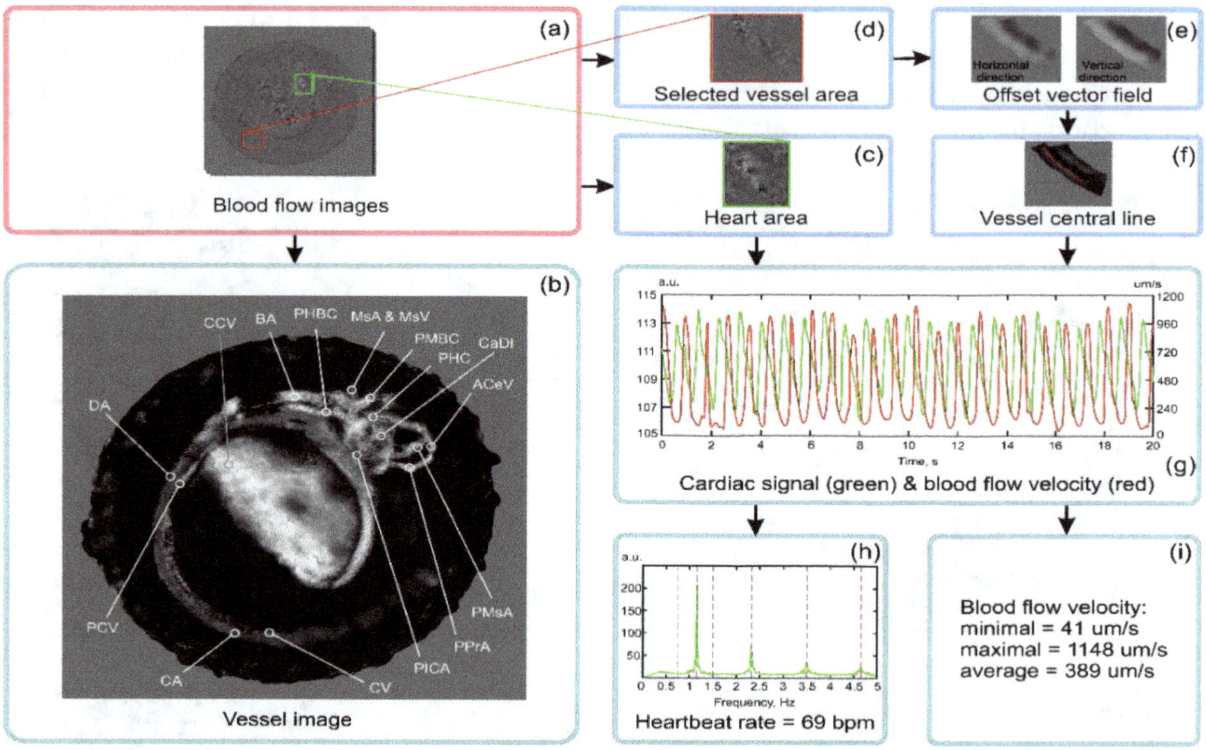

Figure 4. Example of cardiovascular data extraction using the proposed algorithm: (**a**) blood flow images, (**b**) vessel image, (**c**) the selected heart area, (**d**) the selected vessel area, (**e**) offset vector field examples, (**f**) the detected vessel central line, (**g**) cardiac signal and blood flow velocity examples, (**h**) cardiac signal spectrum, (**i**) blood flow velocity range and average value.

Besides the two-dimensional mapping of cardiac activity, the obtained spatiotemporal data cube $I(x,y,t)$ allowed calculation of the heartbeat rate and blood flow velocity—quantitative parameters characterizing cardiovascular functioning. The heart location (Figure 4c) could be detected automatically as the image pixel group demonstrating the most intensive and constant oscillations. Heart area detection in the blood flow images allowed accurate cardiac beat detection and heart rate monitoring. The obtained temporal signals in the heart area had the correct shape and spectrum [30,34]. In the experiment shown in Figure 4, the measurement result for the heart rhythm was 69 bpm (Figure 4h), which is in good agreement with the values obtained in other studies for this stage of zebrafish development [36,41].

Pulsatile flow of blood cells could be easily detected in zebrafish embryo blood vessels from the beginning of circulation at 24 hpf. To demonstrate blood flow velocity measurement, we selected one of the vessel areas (Figure 4d) and carried out its morphological analysis in order to detect the offset vector field (Figure 4e) and central line of the vessel (Figure 4f) and to calculate normal direction at each point. Implementation of this procedure allowed the alignment of the pixels corresponding to the blood vessel into a straight line [42] to calculate the blood flow velocity. Since the blood vessel pixels were aligned, the relative shift between consequent images could be estimated. Then the blood flow velocity could be determined as the ratio of this shift to the time interval between the moments of image acquisition. The obtained blood flow velocity signal was compared with the temporal signal in the heart area to validate the proposed velocity measurement technique. In the diagram in Figure 4g, the curves corresponding to these signals are superimposed so that their mean values are equal. Heart area temporal signal and blood flow velocity signal had the same period of 0.86 s and a constant relative temporal shift of 0.35 s. Average blood flow velocity was 389 μm/s, which is close to the value measured using quantitative fluorescent imaging at the larval stage (Figure 4i) [24].

We implemented the described image processing algorithms in C++ using parallel computing on multiple CPU cores. The software includes modules for camera control and image acquisition, preprocessing and data analysis. The total processing time of 3000 12-bit monochrome images with 1200 × 1200 resolution was about 12 min using Intel's 8th generation 4-core processor. The most time-consuming processes were local matching (18 min) and vessel image calculation (1 min). Further optimization may be related to GPU computing.

Figure 5 illustrates the vessel activity across the whole embryo and the heart rate at the stages from 22 hpf to 27 hpf. Due to the absence of anesthesia, embryos moved and were randomly oriented in chorions. For this reason, the viewing angle and orientation of the embryos differed. Figure 5 shows temporal dynamics of the key features indicating the state of the embryos and suitability for non-invasive measurements at early developmental stages. The experiments demonstrated a continuous increase of the heartbeat rate and gradual activation of vasculature initiated by the heart functioning. Such measurements are important for predicting the further development of the embryo, in particular the time of its hatching.

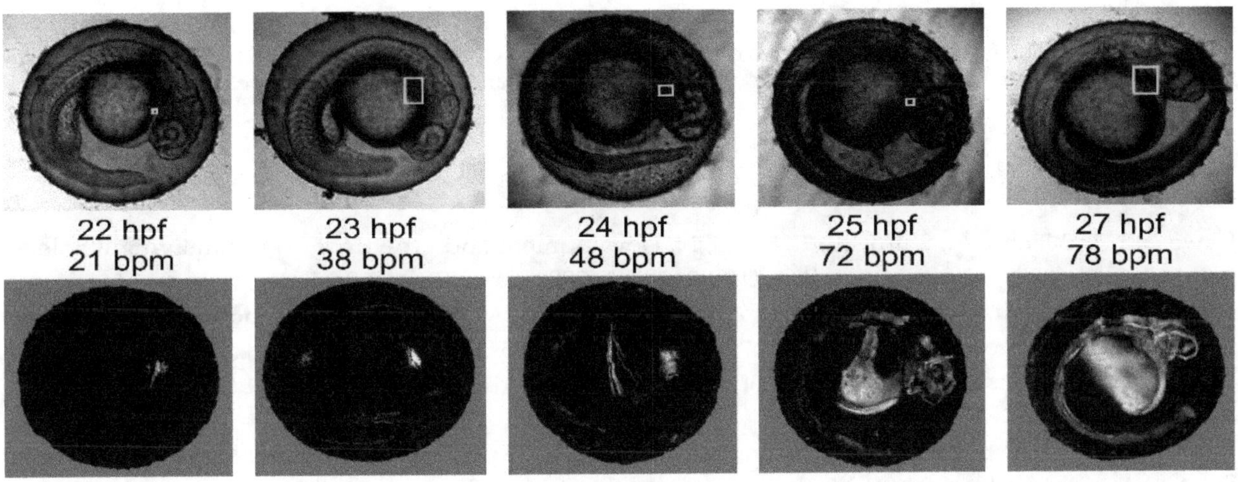

Figure 5. Calculated vessel images (green rectangles indicate the detected heart area).

4. Discussion

As a model biological system, the zebrafish possesses numerous advantages: rapid embryonic development, fully sequenced genome, low cost, etc. This organism also has a unique collection of features at pre-larval developmental stages: large size, optical transparency of the embryo's interior and relatively slow embryo movements inside the shell. This makes zebrafish an attractive model for in vivo study of the formation and functioning of its cardiovascular system using optical imaging techniques.

In this study, we have demonstrated that time-lapse bright-field microscopy and digital signal processing allow blood vessel imaging of a living embryo as well as heartbeat and blood flow velocity measurements without any anesthesia. In contrast to straightforward approaches based on image subtraction, the described pre-processing procedure enables the compensation of shifts and rotations between images and their pixel-to-pixel matching necessary for accurate quantitative characterization of cardiac activity.

The proposed algorithm is applicable for processing the images obtained by various microscope setups widely used for in vivo studies of zebrafish embryos. It can complement optical coherence tomography, acoustic microscopy and other imaging techniques by adding cardiac activity mapping capability.

5. Conclusions

The presented algorithm does not require the use of contrast agents and may be used to visualize cardiac morphology and measure dynamics in zebrafish embryos without anesthesia. We believe that it may help to shed light on the mechanisms by which the cardiovascular system's activity is initiated under natural conditions. Continuous study of the heart function and vessel structure transformation using the proposed algorithm may contribute to recognizing possible warning signs of developmental disorders at the very early stages and understanding the symptoms of various diseases, i.e., help to improve the techniques for their correct diagnosis and timely treatment.

Further development of this technique may include the interactive analysis of vessel structure and function in both normal and pathological condition at embryonic stages, as well as detecting and studying the changes in zebrafish cardiovascular system initiation, development and functioning induced by various environmental stressors.

Author Contributions: A.S.M. and A.B.B. conceived and designed the project; M.V.V. and D.D.K. acquired data; A.S.M., M.V.V. and A.V.P. analyzed data; A.S.M. drafted the article; and A.B.B., M.V.V. and D.D.K. revised it critically for important intellectual content. All authors gave final approval of the version to be published and agreed to be accountable for all aspects of the work. All authors have read and agreed to the published version of the manuscript.

Acknowledgments: The experiments were carried out on the base of the Center for Collective Use of the Scientific and Technological Center of Unique Instrumentation of the Russian Academy of Sciences.

References

1. Kawasaki, T.; Maeno, A.; Shiroishi, T.; Sakai, N. Development and growth of organs in living whole embryo and larval grafts in zebrafish. *Sci. Rep. UK* **2017**, *7*, 16508. [CrossRef] [PubMed]
2. Yalcin, H.C.; Amindari, A.; Butcher, J.T.; Althan, A.; Yacoub, M. Heart function and hemodynamic analysis for zebrafish embryos. *Dev. Dynam.* **2017**, *246*, 868–880. [CrossRef] [PubMed]
3. Lawson, N.D.; Weinstein, B.M. Arteries and veins: Making a difference with zebrafish. *Nat. Rev. Genet.* **2002**, *3*, 674–682. [CrossRef] [PubMed]
4. Konno, M.; Asai, A.; Kitagawa, T.; Yabumoto, M.; Ofusa, K.; Arai, T.; Hirotsu, T.; Doki, Y.; Eguchi, H.; Ishii, H. State-of-the-Art Technology of Model Organisms for Current Human Medicine. *Diagnostics* **2020**, *10*, 392. [CrossRef]
5. Soroldoni, D.; Hogan, B.M.; Oates, A.C. Simple and efficient transgenesis with meganuclease constructs in zebrafish. *Methods Mol. Biol.* **2009**, *546*, 117–130. [CrossRef]
6. Foley, J.E.; Maeder, M.L.; Pearlberg, J.; Joung, J.K.; Peterson, R.T.; Yeh, J.R. Targeted mutagenesis in zebrafish using customized zinc-finger nucleases. *Nat. Protoc.* **2009**, *4*, 1855–1867. [CrossRef]
7. Hwang, W.Y.; Peterson, R.T.; Yeh, J.R. Methods for targeted mutagenesis in zebrafish using TALENs. *Methods* **2014**, *69*, 76–84. [CrossRef] [PubMed]
8. Du, X.; Xu, B.; Zhang, Y.; Du, J. A transgenic zebrafish model for in vivo long-term imaging of retinotectal synaptogenesis. *Sci. Rep. UK* **2018**, *8*, 14077. [CrossRef] [PubMed]
9. Marquart, G.D.; Tabor, K.M.; Brown, M.; Strykowski, J.L.; Varshney, G.K.; LaFave, M.C.; Mueller, T.; Burgess, S.M.; Higashijima, S.; Burgess, H.A. A 3D searchable database of transgenic zebrafish Gal4 and Cre lines for functional neuroanatomy studies. *Front. Neural Circuits* **2015**, *9*, 78. [CrossRef] [PubMed]
10. Mathias, J.R.; Perrin, B.J.; Liu, T.X.; Kanki, J.; Look, A.T.; Huttenlocher, A. Resolution of inflammation by retrograde chemotaxis of neutrophils in transgenic zebrafish. *J. Leukoc. Biol.* **2006**, *80*, 1281–1288. [CrossRef]
11. Ellett, F.; Pase, L.; Hayman, J.W.; Andrianopoulos, A.; Lieschke, G.J. mpeg1 promoter transgenes direct macrophage-lineage expression in zebrafish. *Blood* **2011**, *117*, e49–e56. [CrossRef] [PubMed]
12. Novoa, B.; Figueras, A. Zebrafish: Model for the study of inflammation and the innate immune response to infectious diseases. *Adv. Exp. Med. Biol.* **2012**, *946*, 253–275. [CrossRef] [PubMed]

13. Gabor, K.A.; Goody, M.F.; Mowel, W.K.; Breitbach, M.E.; Gratacap, R.L.; Witten, P.E.; Kim, C.H. Influenza A virus infection in zebrafish recapitulates mammalian infection and sensitivity to anti-influenza drug treatment. *Dis. Model. Mech.* **2014**, *7*, 1227–1237. [CrossRef]
14. Burgos, J.S.; Ripoll-Gomez, J.; Alfaro, J.M.; Sastre, I.; Valdivieso, F. Zebrafish as a new model for herpes simplex virus type 1 infection. *Zebrafish* **2008**, *5*, 323–333. [CrossRef]
15. Ding, C.B.; Zhang, J.P.; Zhao, Y.; Peng, Z.G.; Song, D.Q.; Jiang, J.D. Zebrafish as a potential model organism for drug test against hepatitis C virus. *PLoS ONE* **2011**, *6*, e22921. [CrossRef]
16. Prajsnar, T.K.; Cunliffe, V.T.; Foster, S.J.; Renshaw, S.A. A novel vertebrate model of Staphylococcus aureus infection reveals phagocyte-dependent resistance of zebrafish to non-host specialized pathogens. *Cell. Microbiol.* **2008**, *10*, 2312–2325. [CrossRef] [PubMed]
17. Bernut, A.; Dupont, C.; Sahuquet, A.; Herrmann, J.L.; Lutfalla, G.; Kremer, L. Deciphering and Imaging Pathogenesis and Cording of Mycobacterium abscessus in Zebrafish Embryos. *J. Vis. Exp.* **2015**, *103*, 53130. [CrossRef] [PubMed]
18. Brothers, K.M.; Wheeler, R.T. Non-invasive imaging of disseminated candidiasis in zebrafish larvae. *J. Vis. Exp.* **2012**, *65*, e4051. [CrossRef]
19. Voelz, K.; Gratacap, R.L.; Wheeler, R.T. A zebrafish larval model reveals early tissue-specific innate immune responses to Mucor circinelloides. *Dis. Models Mech.* **2015**, *8*, 1375–1388. [CrossRef]
20. Brown, D.R.; Samsa, L.A.; Qian, L.; Liu, J. Advances in the study of heart development and disease using zebrafish. *J. Cardiovasc. Dev. Dis.* **2016**, *3*, 13. [CrossRef]
21. Bakkers, J. Zebrafish as a model to study cardiac development and human cardiac disease. *Cardiovasc. Res.* **2011**, *91*, 279–288. [CrossRef]
22. Asnani, A.; Peterson, R.T. The zebrafish as a tool to identify novel therapies for human cardiovascular disease. *Dis. Models Mech.* **2014**, *7*, 763–767. [CrossRef] [PubMed]
23. Major, R.J.; Poss, K.D. Zebrafish heart regeneration as a model for cardiac tissue repair. *Drug Discov. Today Dis. Model.* **2007**, *4*, 219–225. [CrossRef] [PubMed]
24. Watkins, S.C.; Maniar, S.; Mosher, M.; Roman, B.L.; Tsang, M.; St Croix, C.M. High resolution imaging of vascular function in zebrafish. *PLoS ONE* **2012**, *7*, e44018. [CrossRef]
25. Mably, J.D.; Childs, S.J. Developmental physiology of the zebrafish cardiovascular system. *Fish Physiol.* **2010**, *29*, 249–287. [CrossRef]
26. Liu, J.; Stainier, D.Y. Zebrafish in the study of early cardiac development. *Circ. Res.* **2012**, *110*, 870–874. [CrossRef]
27. Giardoglou, P.; Beis, D. On zebrafish disease models and matters of the heart. *Biomedicines* **2019**, *7*, 15. [CrossRef] [PubMed]
28. Gut, P.; Reischauer, S.; Stainier, D.Y.R.; Arnaout, R. Little fish, big data: Zebrafish as a model for cardiovascular and metabolic disease. *Physiol. Rev.* **2017**, *97*, 889–938. [CrossRef]
29. Pylatiuk, C.; Sanchez, D.; Mikut, R.; Alshut, R.; Reischl, M.; Hirth, S.; Rottbauer, W.; Just, S. Automatic zebrafish heartbeat detection and analysis for zebrafish embryos. *Zebrafish* **2014**, *11*, 379–383. [CrossRef]
30. De Luca, E.; Zaccaria, G.M.; Hadhoud, M.; Rizzo, G.; Ponzini, R.; Morbiducci, U.; Santoro, M.M. ZebraBeat: A flexible platform for the analysis of the cardiac rate in zebrafish embryos. *Sci. Rep. UK* **2014**, *4*, 4898. [CrossRef]
31. Kang, C.P.; Tu, H.C.; Fu, T.F.; Wu, J.M.; Chu, P.H.; Chang, D.T. An automatic method to calculate heart rate from zebrafish larval cardiac videos. *BMC Bioinform.* **2018**, *19*, 169. [CrossRef] [PubMed]
32. Kimmel, C.B.; Ballard, W.W.; Kimmel, S.R.; Ullmann, B.; Schilling, T.F. Stages of embryonic development of the zebrafish. *Dev. Dynam.* **1995**, *203*, 253–310. [CrossRef] [PubMed]
33. Weber, M.; Huisken, J. In vivo imaging of cardiac development and function in zebrafish using light sheet microscopy. *Swiss. Med. Wkly.* **2015**, *145*, w14227. [CrossRef] [PubMed]
34. Chan, P.K.; Lin, C.C.; Cheng, S.H. Noninvasive technique for measurement of heartbeat regularity in zebrafish (*Danio rerio*) embryos. *BMC Biotechnol.* **2009**, *9*, 11. [CrossRef] [PubMed]
35. Machikhin, A.; Burlakov, A.; Volkov, M.; Khokhlov, D. Imaging photoplethysmography and videocapillaroscopy enable non-invasive study of zebrafish cardiovascular system functioning. *J. Biophotonics* **2020**, *13*, e202000061. [CrossRef]

36. Gierten, J.; Pylatiuk, C.; Hammouda, O.T.; Schock, C.; Stegmaier, J.; Wittbrodt, J.; Gehrig, J.; Loosli, F. Automated high-throughput heartbeat quantification in medaka and zebrafish embryos under physiological conditions. *Sci. Rep. UK* **2020**, *10*, 2046. [CrossRef] [PubMed]
37. Moraes, J.L.; Rocha, M.X.; Vasconcelos, G.G.; Vasconcelos Filho, J.E.; de Albuquerque, V.H.C.; Alexandria, A.R. Advances in photopletysmography signal analysis for biomedical applications. *Sensors* **2018**, *18*, 1894. [CrossRef]
38. Gore, A.V.; Monzo, K.; Cha, Y.R.; Pan, W.; Weinstein, B.M. Vascular development in the zebrafish. *Cold Spring Harb. Perspect. Med.* **2012**, *2*, a006684. [CrossRef]
39. Kunz, Y. *Developmental Biology of Teleost Fishes*; Springer: Dordrecht, The Netherlands, 2004. [CrossRef]
40. Isogai, S.; Horiguchi, M.; Weinstein, B.M. The vascular anatomy of the developing zebrafish: An atlas of embryonic and early larval development. *Dev. Biol.* **2001**, *230*, 278–301. [CrossRef]
41. Ibrahim, M.; Balakrishnan, A.; Prakash, S.; Lee, H.J. Effect of ethanol exposure on heart development in zebra fish (*Danio rerio*) embryos. *Int. J. Anat. Sci.* **2014**, *5*, 26–33.
42. Volkov, M.V.; Margaryants, N.B.; Potemkin, A.V.; Volynsky, M.A.; Gurov, I.P.; Mamontov, O.V.; Kamshilin, A.A. Video capillaroscopy clarifies mechanism of the photoplethysmographic waveform appearance. *Sci. Rep. UK* **2017**, *7*, 13298. [CrossRef]

13

Optical Methods in Fingerprint Imaging for Medical and Personality Applications

Chia-Nan Wang [1,*], Jing-Wein Wang [2,*], Ming-Hsun Lin [1,*], Yao-Lang Chang [1,*] and Chia-Ming Kuo [1]

1 Industrial Engineering and Management, National Kaohsiung University of Applied Sciences, Kaohsiung 80778, Taiwan; chungys@fotech.edu.tw

2 Institute of Photonics and Communications, National Kaohsiung University of Applied Sciences, Kaohsiung 80778, Taiwan

* Correspondence: cn.wang@kuas.edu.tw (C.-N.W.); jwwang@kuas.edu.tw (J.-W.W.); newfife711365@gmail.com (M.-H.L.); kc88899@gmail.com (Y.-L.C.)

Abstract: Over the years, analysis and induction of personality traits has been a topic for individual subjective conjecture or speculation, rather than a focus of inductive scientific analysis. This study proposes a novel framework for analysis and induction of personality traits. First, 14 personality constructs based on the "Big Five" personality factors were developed. Next, a new fingerprint image algorithm was used for classification, and the fingerprints were classified into eight types. The relationship between personality traits and fingerprint type was derived from the results of the questionnaire survey. After comparison of pre-test and post-test results, this study determined the induction ability of personality traits from fingerprint type. Experimental results showed that the left/right thumbprint type of a majority of subjects was left loop/right loop and that the personalities of individuals with this fingerprint type were moderate with no significant differences in the 14 personality constructs.

Keywords: personality traits; fingerprint classification; fingerprint types

---

1. Introduction

Understanding the personality traits of one's self and others contributes to harmonious interpersonal relationships. However, getting to know one's self and others in a short period of time is not an easy task, and inducing the personality traits of others is an even more difficult undertaking. In the Western world, studies on personality traits have a long and broad history [1]. Many related studies have since followed, but the number of proposed personality characteristics has remained high. It was for this reason that Cattell [2] converted these characteristics into 16 types of personality factor questionnaires. Later, Fiske [3] performed a follow-up verification of Cattell's research and derived the "Big Five" personality dimensions. In 1963, Norman [4] verified Cattell's procedures and announced that the five major factors constituted a reasonable method of personality classification.

Research on personality traits is core to many major disciplines, such as medicine, psychology and corporate management, whether for theoretical investigation or practical application [5]. Personality traits stem from a consistent behavioral model and internal processes within each individual, allowing the individual to identify with a consistent behavioral model in different situations. The internal processes of personality traits include emotions, motivation and cognition. Although these processes occur at a deep level, they influence human behavior and feelings [6]. Additionally, other studies have attempted to classify individuals into different personality types [7]. For hundreds of years, the Chinese people have used physiognomy, palmistry (the ridges on the skin of the palm), bone reading and other methods related to physiological features to divulge an individual's personality traits and fortune. To date, however, there are no studies that support a relationship between personality traits and fingerprints, which are an individually unique physiological feature.

Two features of fingerprints that are particularly important: (1) fingerprints do not change with time; and (2) every individual's fingerprints are unique [8]. Due to the above-described two characteristics, fingerprints have long been used for identification purposes [9,10]. Medina-Pérez proposed a new feature representation containing clockwise-arranged minutiae without a central minutia, a new similarity measure that shifted the triplets to find the best minutiae correspondence, and a global matching procedure that selected the alignment by maximizing the amount of global matching minutiae [11]. In comparison with six verification algorithms, the proposed method achieved the highest accuracy in the lowest matching time. Ballan and Gurgen [12] presented a method for fingerprint recognition based on principal component analysis and point patterns (minutiae) obtained from the directional histograms of a fingerprint. This study gave the same performance as that of the uncompressed data, but reduced computation. Yang et al. used fusion to enhance the biometric performance in template-protected biometric systems [13]. They investigated several scenarios (multi-sample, multi-instance, multi-sensor, multi-algorithm and their combinations) on the binary decision level and evaluated the performance and fusion efficiency on a multi-sensor fingerprint database with 71,994 samples. Fingerprint image quality improvement was proposed in [14]. The algorithm consists of two stages. The first stage is decomposing the input fingerprint image into four sub-bands by applying the two -dimensional discrete wavelet transform. At the second stage, the compensated image is produced by adaptively obtaining the compensation coefficient for each sub-band based on the referenced Gaussian template. The method concluded an improved clarity, quality and continuity of ridge structures, and therefore, the accuracy is also increased. Background and the blurred region of fingerprint images are also removed. Bartunek et al. [15] presented several improvements to an adaptive fingerprint enhancement method that is based on contextual filtering. Based on the global analysis and the matched filtering blocks, different forms of order statistical filters were applied. These processing blocks yield an improved and adaptive fingerprint image processing method. Yang et al. [16] proposed a novel and effective two-stage enhancement scheme in both the spatial domain and the frequency domain by learning from the underlying images. They first enhanced the fingerprint image in the spatial domain with a spatial ridge-compensation filter by learning from the images. With the help of the first step, the second stage filter, i.e., a frequency band-pass filter that was separable in the radial and angular frequency domains was employed. The experimental result showed that their algorithm is able to handle various input image contexts and achieves better results compared with some state-of-the-art algorithms over public databases and is able to improve the performances of fingerprint-authentication systems.

Fingerprints are closely related to genetics [17]; however, in the fields of biostatics and psychology, there are currently no studies indicating any relationship between fingerprints and personality traits. Therefore, using fingerprints to induce personality traits is an undeveloped area in scientific research. If the corresponding relationship between fingerprints and personality traits could be determined, this would be an important contribution to science. Since personality traits have a certain degree of stability, continuity and uniqueness and the left/right hand fingerprints of each person are unique, the relationship between these two features is a worthwhile topic for in-depth research. The Big Five personalities have generated substantial interest among personality researchers [3]. The Big Five is a model based on common language descriptors of personality. When factor analysis (a statistical technique) is applied to personality survey data, some words used to describe aspects of personality are often applied to the same person. These five factors are openness to experience (inventive/curious), conscientiousness (efficient/organized), extraversion (outgoing/energetic), agreeableness (friendly/compassionate) and neuroticism (sensitive/nervous).

The purpose in this study is to evaluate the generalizability of Big Five personality factor inventories as inducers of a common set of criteria, criteria representing classes of left and right thumb fingerprints. By assessing people using multiple criterion variables to measure the Big Five personality constructs, the same measure results normally will have the same personality constructs. If the Big Five inventories are all designed to measure equivalent dimensions of personality, then they should show a nontrivial amount of agreement in the variables they are able to induce. Constructing valid measures of personality variables should induce fingerprint classes, assuming those classes have personality determinants. This is especially true of Big Five inventories because those factors are presumed to account for most of the personality-based variation in fingerprints.

This study used classification technology to derive eight fingerprint types and combined these with questionnaire survey results to construct a new "System for Induction of Personality Traits from Fingerprints". Following the research of Costa and McCare [18], this study also summarized 14 personality constructs with Eigen values greater than one from the "Big Five" personality factors. We performed a principal components analysis of the data and found 14 components with Eigen values larger than one. Then, we created 14 scales each comprised of one of the 14 groups of items indicating the 14 components with Eigen values larger than one. The prototype of this system was modified and completed based on the fingerprints and questionnaire feedback of 362 test subjects. This study recruited a separate group of 351 subjects for the live testing of the system. The experimental results showed that the thumbprint types of the left and right hands were correlated with personality traits. Subjects in the left loop/right loop fingerprint category accounted for the largest group (41.8%). The second largest group was the S-type/S-type (twin loop/twin loop) type (13.5%), followed by the eddy/eddy type (12.1%). The personality traits of the latter two groups showed significant differences in some constructs.

Whilst better known in medication, double blind experiments are adopted in this paper. Surveys with questionnaires are used to keep credibility so the chance of observer's bias can be minimized. The framework of the following sections in this paper is as follows: Section 2: research framework and flow figure, expansion of the "Big Five" personality factors into 14 constructs, design of the personality traits questionnaire and the "System for Induction of Personality Traits from Fingerprints"; Section 3: statistical analysis and post-test verification of the survey results on the relationship between personality traits and finger classification; Section 4: conclusions.

2. Research Methods

2.1. Research Framework

The "Big Five" personality factors are advanced global factors that describe human personality, and the 16 personality factors are basic primary factors. This study summarized the questionnaire results after analysis of both global and primary factors. From these data, 14 personality constructs appropriate for describing the personalities of the test subjects were designed. A questionnaire was designed based on the 14 personality constructs. Along with the implementation of the questionnaire survey, an optical fingerprint machine of SecuGen Hamster Plus [19] was used to capture the left/right thumbprints of the test subjects. The fingerprint sensor features smart capture technology and switches on the scanner whenever it detects a finger. Thumb samples of both hands are collected, where 282 participants are mostly university students, and their ages are within the interval from 18 to 50 years old. The biometric data were collected in different periods within 3 months. A new fingerprint classification algorithm was used for fingerprint categorization. After relationship analysis of fingerprint types and the 14 personality constructs, this study compiled a table of associations between the eight fingerprint types and the 14 personality constructs. To verify the accuracy of the association table, this study performed post-testing with different subjects. After the questionnaire survey and fingerprinting had been re-conducted, this study modified the content of the association table. The conclusions of this study were formed after discussion of the pretest and posttest results. Figure 1 illustrates the framework and flow of this research.

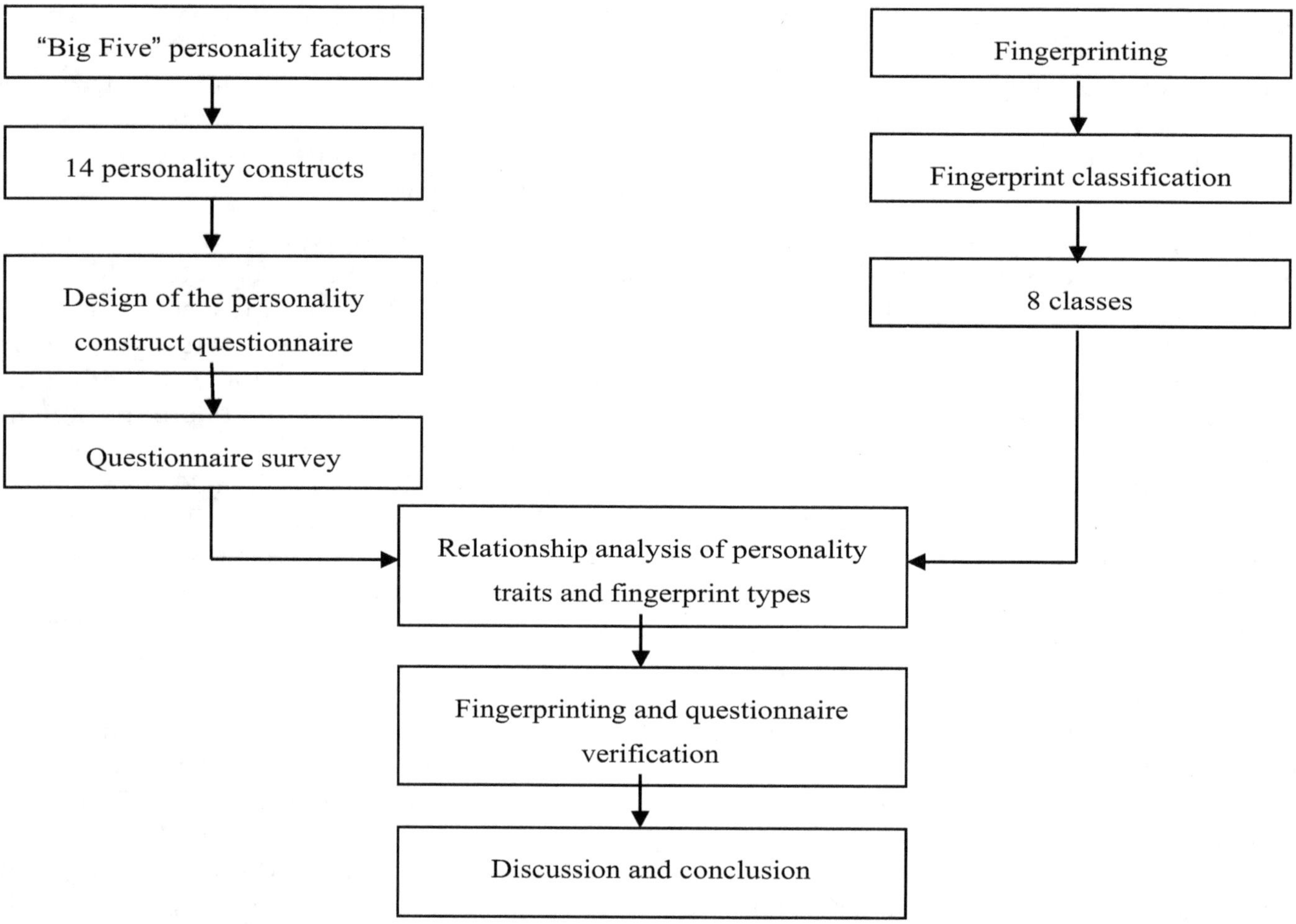

Figure 1. Research framework and flowchart.

2.2. The 14 Constructs of Personality

The "Big Five" personality factors, which have been analyzed and verified by Norman [4], Goldberg [20] and McCrae and Costa [21], are as follows: neuroticism, extraversion, openness, agreeableness and conscientiousness. This study referred to the Big Five personality factors and the 16 personality factors, summarized the questionnaire results according to the personality scores of test subjects and designed a personality trait questionnaire composed of the 14 personality constructs. Neuroticism is the tendency of an individual to experience anxiety or nervousness. This study sub-divided neuroticism into sentimentalism, impulsiveness and strong self-esteem. Extraversion refers to the characteristics and strength of an individual in interpersonal interaction. This study sub-divided extraversion into activeness and passivity. Openness refers to the degree of risk that an individual can accept with regard to new things. This study sub-divided openness into enthusiastic attitude and good money concept. Agreeableness refers to the cognition, affection and attitude displayed by an individual toward various situations or matters. This study sub-divided agreeableness into socially harmonious methods of operation, concern for others' well-being and impatience. Conscientiousness refers to the determination and self-discipline of an individual. This study sub-divided conscientiousness into strong sense of responsibility, slow method of operation, focused attention and strong leadership ability. Table 1 describes the 14 personality constructs in detail.

Table 1. Fourteen constructs of personality.

14 Constructs of Personality	Description of Constructs
Sentimentalism	Emotionally sensitive and easily becomes sentimental; emotionally vulnerable to external stimuli and reveals true feelings.
Impulsiveness	The link that precedes the conversion of one's feelings, perception and thoughts into actions: the desire before the action. The word 'rash' is commonly used to describe such actions that were not previously thought out.
Strong self-esteem	Maintains self-respect and dignity; does not allow discrimination, stigmatization or attack from others.
Liveliness	Refers to the *qi* (energy flow or vitalism) exhibited by an individual; lively people drive the surrounding atmosphere, influence people around them and attract more attention in a group.
Passivity	Always keeps personal opinions and decisions to one's self; does not take the initiative to directly express one's self, but is always waiting for the other person to ask.
Positive attitude	Enthusiasm is a type of outward manifestation of desire; whether the job is actually well done is considered secondary. It is a type of zeal, an attitude of full immersion without distraction.
Good money concept	Ensures that expenditure matches income and avoids debt; considers one's status and position when spending money to select products that are appropriate for one's self.
Socially harmonious method of operation	Behaves appropriately, does not openly offend others, is concerned that matters reach a socially harmonious and satisfactory conclusion.
Concern for others' well-being	Puts one's self in others' shoes and considers others in any situation; an attitude of "not doing unto others what you would not want done unto yourself".
Impatience	Unsettled and irritable behavior when facing situations that require waiting or delay.
Strong sense of responsibility	Fulfills one's obligations regarding any matter; is always aware of possible consequences no matter how great or small the matter and is able to assume one's proper responsibility.
Slow method of operation	Is slow and calm in any situation; gives others the impression of a slow and unconcerned attitude.
Focused attention	Is not easily influenced by the external environment when working or engaging in various matters.
Strong leadership ability	Plays the role of a leader in groups; is good at organizing/assigning tasks and coordinating interpersonal relationships; provides a team with sufficient centripetal force.

2.3. Fingerprint Classification

The actual number of different types of human fingerprints is currently unknown; however, a majority of studies use the five main categories proposed by Henry [22]: Right loop, left loop, tented arch, arch and whorl. This study used an optical fingerprinting machine to capture original images of fingerprints. These original images are often accompanied by deformation caused by problems such as dry, wet, damaged or scarred fingerprints and uneven application of force by the fingerprinting machine when capturing the image. Therefore, enhancement of the images is essential [23]. Fingerprint classification is a coarse level method of partitioning a fingerprint database into smaller subsets, which reduces the search space of a large database. To determine the class of the query fingerprint, only search templates with the same class as the query were used. Inputs are the fingerprint impressions from right and left thumb fingers of an individual. If the size of the database is n and c is the number of classes, the search space without classification is n^2. With fingerprint classification, the search space with classification is n/c. We made an extensive study of the occurrence of fingerprints and indexed them into eight major classes as shown in Figure 2.

After using histogram specification and ridge/valley energy analysis, this study performed energy image projection analysis in eight different directions at an angle of 45° to capture fingerprint regions of interest (ROI). Through the above-described methods, this study classified fingerprint into four categories. They are whorl (plain whorl), S-type (double-loop whorl), eddy (accidental whorl) and balloon (central pocket loop whorl). To accurately trace flow lines to determine fingerprint type, this study used the Poincare index-based modified hierarchical singularity detection algorithm after orientation field estimation to detect the location of singularity. The three-stage pyramid singularity detection algorithm designed by this study can accurately locate the point of singularity through progressively narrowing the detection range. Lastly, after initial type selection had been performed based on the number and type (delta, core point) of the singular points, fingerprint classification was conducted by tracing the flow of the orientation field surrounding the point of singularity and establishing related rules of judgement. This study is interested in finding the exact location of the core point defined by the Henry system and therefore traces the skeletonized ridge curves with 8-adjacency to explore wavelet extrema at one-pixel increments by starting at 10 pixels apart from two sides. The highest extrema in the ridge curve corresponds to the candidate of the core point. We devise two 8-adjacency grids to locate the wavelet extrema. Beginning from two opposite ends and moving toward the center of the sub-region, the black-color pixel of each grid is designated as the central point to trace. Based on this central point, the moving guideline is as follows: if the gray-level of the adjacent pixel is 0, then move toward that pixel, where the number shown in the grid indicates the moving sequence. This method makes it possible to follow the real track of the ridge curve. Whenever a singularity is detected, its location is noted. It is common to have multiple findings of the core point candidate with small vertical displacements, and the area underneath the lowest ridge curve is circumscribed for locating the core point. In the Henry system, the exact core point location can be performed as follows: (a) locate the topmost extrema in the innermost ridge curve, if there is no rod; (b) otherwise, locate the top of the rods. The final eight categories derived are as follows (see Figure 2): right loop, left loop, arch, tented arch, whorl (plain whorl), S-type (double-loop whorl), eddy (accidental whorl) and balloon (central pocket loop whorl).

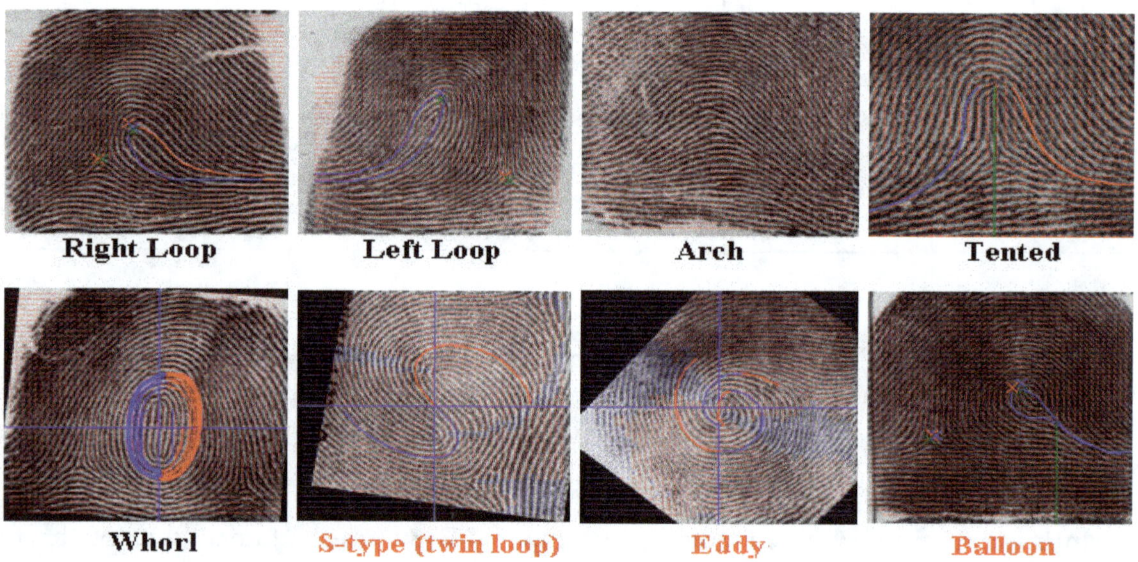

Figure 2. The eight fingerprint types.

2.4. *Questionnaire Design and Survey*

This study designed a questionnaire with 74 closed questions since there is no measure of personality and fingerprint available. Since the 74 closed questions are many, this study does not provide all question items in this study. The 74 questions followed the 14 different personality constructs [18]. Each construct had at least 3 questions prepared by this study to confirm the results of respondents. However, this study also designed the reliability analysis and validation analysis for verifying the questionnaire design and post-test verification for final result checking. Based on reliability analysis and validation analysis, we confirmed that our questionnaire has the right dimensionality and composition. After factor analysis, the recovered questionnaire data were used to develop 14 personality constructs. The information collected from the questionnaire, along with the left/right thumbprints taken from the test subjects, was used in conjunction with the personality constructs to derive the relationship between fingerprint type and personality traits. A 5-point Likert scale was used for the personality trait questionnaire; 1–5 points were respectively assigned to the options of strongly disagree, disagree, neither agree, nor disagree, agree and strongly agree.

Sampling in this study was conducted via the following steps:

1. Research targets: The use of fingerprints involves personal privacy issues, and the agreement of the respondent with regard to using his/her fingerprints for research is difficult to obtain. Thus, for the sake of convenience in collecting information, this study used non-probability proportional sampling methods and selected the National Kaohsiung University of Applied Sciences at Taiwan as the site for questionnaire distribution. The main respondent targets were students in the Department of Industrial Management, Continuing Education Division.
2. Questionnaire response process: The process of filling out the questionnaires proceeded according to classes (as units) and was arranged according to students' class hours. After the left/right thumbprints of the respondents had been collected into the fingerprint classification system, the questionnaires were filled out.
3. Results: This study distributed 362 questionnaires. After the questionnaires had been collected and any invalid questionnaires removed, the number of valid questionnaires was 282, resulting in a valid recovery rate of 75.4%. After the average value of the questions in each construct had been processed, these data were used for the final score of each respondent.

2.5. Statistical Analysis and Testing

Reliability analysis: This study used Cronbach's α [24] to measure the reliability of the questionnaire. According to the research of DeVellis [25], a reliability coefficient value of 0.7 and up is acceptable. The overall Cronbach's α value for the 74 items in this questionnaire was 0.799, indicating that this questionnaire had high reliability. The Cronbach's α value for the 14 constructs also exceeded 0.7, indicating the reliability of the data. The Cronbach's α value of individual constructs of sentimentalism, impulsiveness, strong self-esteem, liveliness, passivity, positive attitude, good money concept, socially harmonious method of operation, concern for others' well-being, impatience, strong sense of responsibility, slow method of operation, focused attention and strong leadership ability are 0.797, 0.786, 0.793, 0.771, 0.829, 0.770, 0.792, 0.783, 0.764, 0.795, 0.776, 0.808, 0.804 and 0.771, respectively.

Validity analysis: Validity is the degree to which the questionnaire accurately measures what it is intended to measure; in other words, the degree to which it reaches the goals of measurement. This study used factor analysis to obtain the total variance explained by the questionnaire, and this value was used to measure validity. However, Sharma [26] advised against relying solely on the results of Bartlett's test of sphericity to determine whether data are suitable for factor analysis, because the validity of Bartlett's test of sphericity is easily influenced by sample size. Therefore, this study mainly used the Kaiser–Meyer–Olkin (KMO) measure and Bartlett's test of sphericity to determine whether the data were suitable for factor analysis. The KMO coefficient was used to measure whether each variable had sampling adequacy. A KMO coefficient of 0.9 and up was considered upper level, 0.8–0.89 was considered moderate level and lower than 0.5 was an unacceptable level. The KMO and Barlett test results show that KMO = 0.536, indicating that the data in this study were in an acceptable range with regard to sampling adequacy. Bartlett's test of sphericity also reached a level of significance ($p < 0.001$), indicating that the data were suitable for factor analysis. The number of factors in factor analysis could have been determined by the relationship of the 74 questionnaire items. This study used principal component analysis for repeated estimation until the estimation of commonalities converged. Varimax was then used for rotation. The analysis results showed that the Eigen value of 14 questions exceeded 1, and the total explainable variance was 74.75%, surpassing the minimum requirement of 50%. Therefore, this study used these 14 factors as personality constructs.

3. Experimental Results

This study recovered 282 valid questionnaires. Initial results indicated that in left/right hand fingerprint types, the right hand fingerprints did not show arch type; arch type was also not found in some of the left hand fingerprints. Among the fingerprint types, the left loop/right loop type accounted for the largest group of test subjects (118 subjects), followed by the S-type/S-type (38 subjects), eddy/eddy type (34 subjects) and whorl/whorl type (28 subjects). The summary of type numbers is shown in Table 2 and Figure 3. In the questionnaire, 1–5 points each were assigned to the Likert scale options (strongly disagree, disagree, neither agree, nor disagree, agree, strongly agree). This study calculated the mean and standard deviation of each of the 14 personality constructs. Based on the responses on Likert items, this study derived the interrelationship between fingerprint type and personality construct; for details, please see Table 3.

Table 2. Fingerprint type number summary.

Fingerprint Type	Left Loop	Right Loop	Tent	Arch	Whorl	Eddy Loop	S-type	Balloon
Left Loop	2	118	2	0	6	2	6	0
Right Loop	0	0	0	0	2	0	0	0
Tent	0	0	0	0	0	0	0	0
Arch	0	0	0	0	2	0	0	2
Whorl	0	2	0	0	28	2	0	0
Eddy loop	0	4	0	0	10	34	0	0
S-type	0	2	0	0	0	14	38	2
Balloon	0	0	0	0	0	0	0	4

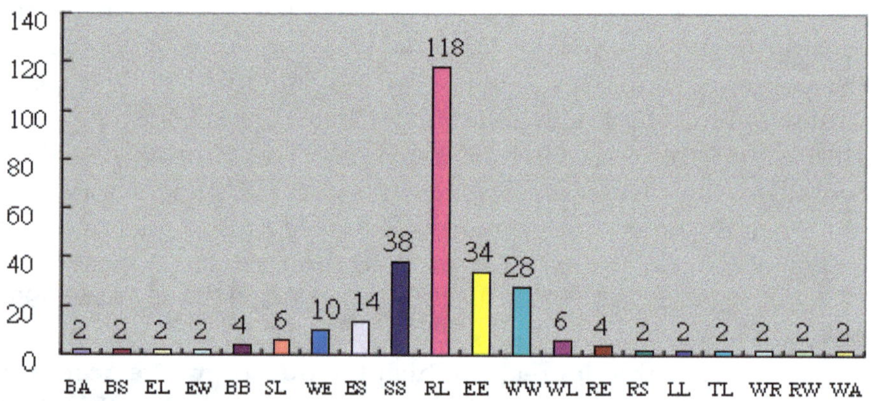

Figure 3. Fingerprint type statistics. BA: Balloon/Arch; BS: Balloon/S-type; EL: Eddy Loop/Left Loop; EW: Eddy Loop/Whorl; BB: Balloon/Balloon; SL: S-type/Left Loop; WE: Whorl/Eddy Loop; ES: Eddy Loop/S-type; SS: S-type/S-type; RL: Right Loop/Left Loop; EE: Eddy Loop/Eddy Loop; WW: Whorl/Whorl; WL: Whorl/Left Loop; RE: Right Loop/Eddy Loop; RS: Right Loop/S-type; LL: Left Loop/Left Loop; TL: Tent/Left Loop; WR: Whorl/Right Loop; RW: Right Loop/Whorl; WA: Whorl/Arch.

Table 3 shows that S-type/right Loop had the highest overall average in the 14 constructs, indicating that subjects with this fingerprint type demonstrated significant inclination in personality traits. The overall average of arch/whorl was the second highest in the 14 constructs, particularly with regard to the traits of "socially harmonious method of operation", "concern for others' well-being", "enthusiastic attitude" and "strong sense of responsibility"; the overall average in terms of these four constructs even exceeded that of S-type/right loop. This indicated that individuals with this fingerprint type have outstanding leadership qualities. Additionally, to summarize the distribution trend of fingerprint type and personality constructs, a sample distributed clustering image of fingerprint type and personality traits is shown in Figure 4, using four of the fingerprint types that accounted for a higher number of subjects and two personality traits. This is a sample distributed chart of personality traits based on fingerprint type, using four of the fingerprint types that accounted for a number of subjects and two personality traits (1–5 points each were assigned to the Likert scale options).

Table 3. Fingerprint types and personality constructs.

Fingerprint Type/Personality	Socially Harmonious Method of Operation	Sentimentalism	Liveliness	Concern for Others' Well-Being	Strong Self-Esteem	Impatience	Impulsiveness	Positive Attitude	Strong Sense of Responsibility	Slow Method of Operation	Passivity	Focused Attention	Strong Leadership Ability	Good Money Concept
Left Loop/Right Loop	△	△	△	△	△	△	△	△	△	△	△	△	△	△
Whorl/Right Loop	X	X	○	△	△	△	X	X	△	X	△	X	X	○
Eddy/Right Loop	X	○	X	△	○	○	△	X	X	○	○	△	○	○
S-type/Right Loop	○	○	△	○	○	○	○	○	○	○	○	○	○	○
Left Loop/Left Loop	○	△	X	△	○	X	X	○	○	X	○	X	X	X
Left Loop/Tent	X	X	○	△	○	△	○	X	X	○	○	X	X	○
Right Loop/Whorl	X	○	X	X	△	△	○	X	X	○	○	X	X	○
Left Loop/Whorl	○	△	△	○	△	△	X	○	△	○	△	X	○	X
Arch/Whorl	○	△	○	○	○	○	X	○	○	X	X	○	○	X
Whorl/Whorl	△	○	△	△	X	△	○	○	△	△	X	X	△	○
Eddy/Whorl	○	△	X	△	○	△	△	○	○	○	X	○	○	△
Left Loop/Eddy	△	△	○	○	○	△	○	△	X	X	X	X	○	X
Whorl/Eddy	X	○	X	△	○	○	X	△	X	X	△	△	X	○
Eddy/Eddy	○	X	○	△	○	△	△	X	○	△	○	△	△	X
S-type/Eddy	△	△	○	△	△	○	△	△	△	X	△	X	△	○
Left Loop/S-type	X	△	X	X	X	△	○	X	X	△	△	X	X	○
S-type/S-type	△	X	△	△	△	△	△	△	△	X	X	△	△	○
Arch/Balloon	△	△	○	X	○	○	X	X	△	○	○	X	△	○
S-type/balloon	△	X	X	X	○	X	X	△	△	X	○	○	△	X
Balloon/Balloon	X	○	X	X	○	X	X	X	X	X	△	X	X	X

△ = within the interval; X = left of the interval (less than 3.6169); ○ = right of the interval (more than 3.8215).

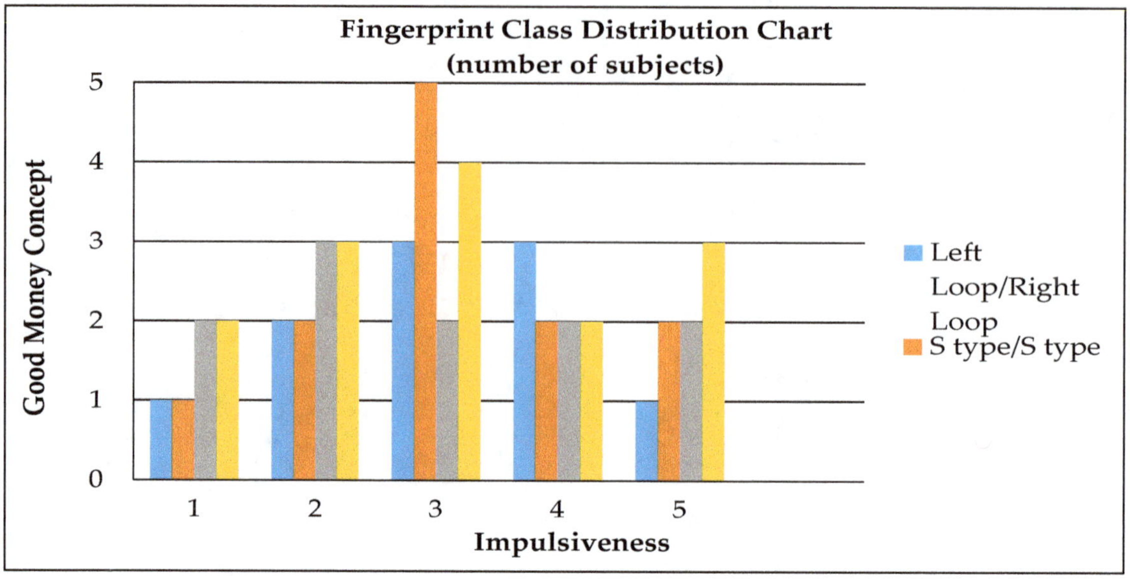

Figure 4. A sample distributed chart of personality traits.

4. Discussions

This study used the statistical concept of interval estimation to determine the personality traits corresponding to different fingerprint types. Using the construct of "socially harmonious method of operation" as an example: this study first calculated the average ($\overline{X} = 3.721$) and standard deviation ($S = 0.6307$) of this construct in the 282 questionnaires collected and then calculated the 95% confidence interval for the mean: $3.6169 \leq \mu \leq 3.8215$. The researchers then determined whether the average of the personality traits corresponding to each fingerprint type fell within the interval. The results of the interval estimation are shown in Table 3.

4.1. Post-Test Verification I

The purpose of verifying the questionnaire was to test the accuracy level of the system. Verification of the questionnaire consisted of three parts: The first part was a simple personality trait questionnaire consisting of 15 questions; the second part was fingerprinting; and the third part was the test subjects' rating of the accuracy level of the system. The assessment options were extremely inaccurate to extremely accurate (1–10 points). The process of questionnaire verification was as follows: After test subjects had filled in the personality trait questionnaire, their left/right thumbprints were taken. Fingerprint classification was used to determine personality constructs. Test subjects then rated the accuracy level of the system according to their personality construct placement. This study distributed 56 verification questionnaires in total and recovered 45 valid questionnaires, making a recovery rate of 80.34%. Initial results showed that only 12 fingerprint types had been obtained, among which left loop/right loop accounted for the highest proportion. The number summary of fingerprint type is shown in Table 4. Table 4 shows that the left loop/right loop accounted for the highest proportion (14 subjects), followed by eddy/eddy (nine subjects), S-type/S-type (six subjects) and whorl/whorl (five subjects). This study used the concept of interval estimation on the fingerprint type data collected, to determine the relationship between fingerprint type and personality constructs, as shown in Table 5.

Table 4. Fingerprint types number summary and proportions.

Fingerprint Type	Amount	Fingerprint Type	Amount	Fingerprint Type	Amount
Left Loop/Right Loop	14	Left Loop/Whorl	2	S-type/Eddy	1
Whorl/Right Loop	1	Whorl/Whorl	5	Left Loop/S-type	1
Eddy/Right Loop	2	Eddy/Whorl	2	S-type/S-type	6
Left Loop/Tent	1	Eddy/Eddy	9	Balloon/Balloon	1

Table 5. Relationship between fingerprint type and personality traits.

	Socially Harmonious Method of Operation	Sentimentalism	Liveliness	Concern for Others' Well-Being	Strong Self-Esteem	Impatience	Impulsiveness	Positive Attitude	Strong Sense of Responsibility	Slow Method of Operation	Passivity	Focused Attention	Strong Leadership Ability	Good Money Concept
Left Loop/Right Loop	△	△	△	△	△	△	△	○	△	△	△	△	△	X
Whorl/Right Loop	X	X	○	X	X	△	○	X	○	X	△	X	X	○
Eddy/Right Loop	○	△	△	○	X	△	○	X	X	△	○	△	X	○
Left Loop/Tent	△	○	○	X	○	△	○	△	○	△	X	X	△	○
Left Loop/Whorl	○	△	△	X	X	X	○	○	△	X	X	X	○	X
Whorl/Whorl	△	○	△	△	○	○	○	○	△	△	X	X	X	△
Vortex/Whorl	X	△	X	X	○	△	△	○	X	△	○	△	△	○
Vortex/Vortex	○	X	○	△	○	X	△	X	○	△	○	△	△	△
S-type/Eddy	○	X	△	○	○	△	△	△	○	△	X	○	△	○
Left Loop/S-type	○	○	△	X	X	X	X	X	X	X	○	○	X	X
S-type/S-type	△	X	X	△	△	△	△	△	△	△	X	△	△	○
Balloon/Balloon	X	○	△	○	○	△	○	△	X	○	X	X	X	○

Discrepancy between pre-test and post-test shown in the highlighted cell, △ = within the interval; X = left of the interval; ○ = right of the interval.

Table 5 shows that some of the verification questionnaire results regarding personality traits that correspond to fingerprint types differ from the pre-test questionnaire results (Table 3). There are some discrepancies between pre-test and post-test. We amended the legend as the discrepancy between pre-test and post-test shown in the highlighted cell. Possible reasons for these differences are summarized below:

1. Insufficient sample number (subjects): Obtaining test subjects for the post-test verification was difficult, resulting in a small sample number. This may have caused some errors in the process of using interval estimation to determine corresponding personality traits, producing some differences in the results.
2. Insufficient number of samples for different fingerprint types: This study noticed that the number of samples for certain fingerprint types, such as whorl/right loop and left loop/S-type, was very few. The pre-test results and the verification results show that the number of samples obtained for some fingerprint types was very few; this insufficient sample number may have produced error in the process of summarizing results. By contrast, the amount of samples collected in the pre-test and verification processes for certain fingerprint types such as left loop/right loop, whorl/whorl and eddy/eddy, is significantly higher than others. In the verification process, the results of personality traits corresponding to these four fingerprint types were significantly more consistent as compared to other fingerprint types.

This study used the mean confidence interval to determine whether the differences between the pre-test results and those of post-test verification were significant. In view of the individual uniqueness of fingerprints, this study assumed that fingerprint types were mutually independent. Below is a simple explanation using the fingerprint type left loop/right loop and the construct "socially harmonious way of operation":

Pre-test questionnaire: $n_1 = 59$, $\overline{X_1} = 3.65$, $S_1 = 0.665$; verification questionnaire: $n_2 = 14$, $\overline{X_2} = 3.44$, $S_2 = 0.8644$; these data were used for a mean difference test ($\alpha = 0.05$). The resulting mean difference confidence interval was $[-0.2736, 0.6936]$, and the 95% confidence interval included zero; therefore, we can assume that there is no significant difference between the pre-test and post-test results for the fingerprint type left loop/right loop and the construct "socially harmonious method of operation".

4.2. Post-Test Verification II

This study randomly sampled interested participants as subjects for this test. Following the test, participants filled out an accuracy questionnaire on their degree of satisfaction with using fingerprint types to analyze personality traits. There were 306 participants in this test. With the inclusion of the 45 valid questionnaires recovered from Post-Test Verification I, this totals to 351 results for the accuracy survey. The average was 7.1268, and the mode was eight. This means that subjects rated the accuracy of the system developed by this study at more than 70%. The results of the accuracy survey are shown in Table 6. This study used the above data for hypothesis testing. Because researchers wished to determine whether the outcome significantly exceeded the median (5), the null hypothesis was H0: $\mu \leqq 6$, and the alternative hypothesis was H1: $\mu > 6$. The test result was 9.7. At the $\alpha = 0.001$ level of significance, the mean was shown to significantly exceed six. Therefore, we can infer that the results obtained from this system were very accurate.

Table 6. Results of the accuracy survey.

Mean	7.126801153	Minimum	1
Standard error	0.116532499	Maximum	10
Standard deviation	2.170759935	Total	2473
Variance	4.712198697	Number of results	351
Mode	8	Median	8

5. Conclusions

Analysis and accurate induction of personality traits is extremely valuable in both daily life and academic research. This study designed 14 personality constructs and implemented the questionnaire survey and fingerprinting through innovative fingerprint classification technology. Through comparison of pre-test and post-test results, this study realized the induction ability of personality traits from fingerprint type. Detailed conclusions are as follows:

1. Validity and reliability analysis showed that personality traits and fingerprint type are statistically correlated. Additionally, more than 70% of subjects were satisfied with the accuracy of the results of personality trait induction.
2. The results of the relationship between personality trait and fingerprint type showed that subjects with the left loop/right loop fingerprint type accounted for the largest proportion and were more moderate in terms of personality traits. In other words, subjects with this fingerprint type did not exhibit any especially prominent personality trait in the 14 constructs. The overall average of S-type/left loop was the highest among the 14 personality constructs, indicating that subjects with this fingerprint type had generally obvious personality traits. Arch/whorl had the second highest overall average in the 14 personality constructs, particularly in the constructs of "socially harmonious method of operation" (5.00), "strong sense of responsibility" (4.83), "enthusiastic attitude" (4.50) and "concern for others' well-being" (4.11). In these four constructs, the overall average of arch/whorl exceeded that of S-type/right loop, indicating that subjects with this fingerprint type had strong leadership qualities.
3. Among the 20 left/right fingerprint types derived from fingerprint classification, four fingerprint types accounted for a majority of subjects. The type accounting for the highest proportion was left loop/right loop (pre-test: 42%, Post-Test Verification I: 34%), followed by eddy/eddy (pre-test: 14.29%, Post-Test Verification I: 12%); S-type/S-type (pre-test 13.74%, Post-Test Verification I: 13%) and whorl/whorl (pre-test: 10.44%, Post-Test Verification I: 10%).
4. In the process of investigating fingerprint type, this study found an additional three fingerprint types apart from the five known types: S-type, eddy and balloon. This is a new discovery in fingerprint classification. With regard to accuracy, the classification accuracy of the eight fingerprint types reached 89.76%.

Research on personality traits, whether in terms of theoretical or practical application, is a key topic in modern research domains. Accurate induction of personality traits is a field of human research that not only urgently requires development, but also offers high practical value in such circumstances as schools selecting suitable students or corporations recruiting suitable personnel. Fingerprints are a unique human biological characteristic. This study is the first to propose a method of using fingerprint type to induce personality traits, as well as to verify the effectiveness of this method. Future research can build on the results of this study and expand research on fingerprint type to other areas, such as the relationship between fingerprint type and learning ability or the industries to which individuals with different fingerprint types are more suited. Moreover, more samples need to be prepared to study in this field to verify the original results and discover new findings.

Acknowledgments: This research was supported in part by MOST 106-2221-E-151-030 from the ministry of Sciences and Technology. The authors also appreciate the support from National Kaohsiung University of Applied Sciences in Taiwan.

Author Contributions: Chia-Nan Wang guided the research direction and found the solutions. Jing-Wein Wang conducted the fingerprint hardware, software and designed the experiments. Ming-Hsun Lin summarized the data and edited the paper. Yao-Lang Chang contributed to software coding. Chia-Ming Kuo worked on the experiment and analyzed the results. All authors contributed to produce the results.

References

1. Barrick, M.R.; Mount, M. The big five personality dimensions and job performance: A meta-analysis. *Pers. Psychol.* **1991**, *44*, 1–26. [CrossRef]
2. Cattell, R.B. The description of personality: Basic trait resolved into clusters. *J. Abnorm. Soc. Psychol.* **1943**, *38*, 476–506. [CrossRef]
3. Fiske, D.W. Consistency of the factorial structures of personality ratings from different source. *J. Abnorm. Soc. Psychol.* **1947**, *44*, 329–344. [CrossRef]
4. Norman, W.T. Toward an adequate taxonomy of personality attributes: Replicated factor structure in peer nomination personality ratings. *J. Abnorm. Soc. Psychol.* **1963**, *66*, 574–583. [CrossRef] [PubMed]
5. Burger, J.M. *Personality*; CENGAGE Learning: Boston, CT, USA, 2015.
6. Hill, C.W.; Jones, G.R.; Schilling, M.A. *Strategic Management Theory: An Integrated Approach*; CENGAGE Learning: Boston, CT, USA, 2015.
7. Kretschmer, E. *Physique and Character*; Dick Press: London, UK, 2007.
8. Edward, H. *Classification and Uses of Finger Prints*; George Rutledge & Sons: London, UK, 1900.
9. Jain, A.; Hong, L.; Bolle, R. On-line fingerprint verification. *IEEE Trans. Pattern Anal. Mach. Intell.* **1997**, *19*, 302–314. [CrossRef]
10. Ratha, N.K.; Bolle, R. *Automatic Fingerprint Recognition Systems*; Springer: New York, NY, USA, 2004.
11. Medina-Pérez, M.A.; García-Borroto, M.; Gutierrez-Rodríguez, A.E.; Altamirano-Robles, L. Improving fingerprint verification using minutiae triplets. *Sensors* **2012**, *12*, 3418–3434. [CrossRef] [PubMed]
12. Ballan, M.; Gurgen, F. On the principal component based fingerprint classification using directional images. *Math. Comput. Appl.* **1999**, *4*, 91–97. [CrossRef]
13. Yang, B.; Busch, C.; Groot, K.; Xu, H.; Veldhuis, R.N.J. Performance evaluation of fusing protected fingerprint minutiae templates on the decision level. *Sensor* **2012**, *12*, 5246–5272. [CrossRef] [PubMed]
14. Wang, J.W.; Le, N.T.; Wang, C.C.; Lee, J.S. Enhanced ridge structure for improving fingerprint image quality based on a wavelet domain. *IEEE Signal Process. Lett.* **2015**, *22*, 390–394. [CrossRef]
15. Bartunek, J.S.; Nilsson, M.; Sallberg, B.; Claesson, I. Adaptive fingerprint image enhancement with emphasis on preprocessing of data. *IEEE Trans. Image Process.* **2013**, *22*, 644–656. [CrossRef] [PubMed]
16. Yang, J.; Xiong, N.; Vasilakos, A.V. Two-stage enhancement scheme for low-quality fingerprint images by learning from the images. *IEEE Trans. Hum. Mach. Syst.* **2013**, *43*, 235–248. [CrossRef]
17. Warman, P.H.; Ennos, A.R. Fingerprints are unlikely to increase the friction of primate fingerpads. *J. Exp. Biol.* **2009**, *212*, 2016–2022. [CrossRef] [PubMed]
18. Costa, P.T.; McCare, R.R. Four ways five factors are basic. *Pers. Individ. Differ.* **1992**, *13*, 653–665. [CrossRef]
19. SecuGen Hamster Plus. Available online: http://secugen.com/products/php.htm (accessed on 3 July 2016).
20. Goldberg, L.R. Language and individual differences: The search for universals in personality lexicons. *Rev. Pers. Soc. Psychol.* **1981**, *2*, 141–165.
21. McCrae, R.R.; Costa, P.T., Jr. *Personality in Adulthood: A Five-Factor Theory Perspective*; Guilford Press: New York, NY, USA, 2003.
22. Henry, E.R. *Classification and Uses of Fingerprints*; Routledge: London, UK, 1990.
23. Wang, J.W. Classification of fingerprint based on traced orientation flow. In Proceedings of the IEEE International Symposium on Industrial Electronics, Bari, Italy, 9–12 December 2010; pp. 1585–1588. [CrossRef]
24. Cronbach, L.J. Coefficient alpha and the internal structure of tests. *Psychometrika* **1951**, *16*, 297–334. [CrossRef]
25. DeVellis, R.F. *Scale Development: Theory and Application*; Sage Publications: London, UK, 2003.
26. Sharma, S. *Applied Multivariate Techniques*; John Wiley and Sons: New York, NY, USA, 1996.

14

Body Weight Estimation for Dose-Finding and Health Monitoring of Lying, Standing and Walking Patients Based on RGB-D Data

Christian Pfitzner [1,2,*], Stefan May [1] and Andreas Nüchter [2,*]

1 Department of Electrical Engineering, Precision Engineering, Information Technology at the Techniche Hochschule Nürnberg Georg Simon Ohm; Keßlerplatz 12, 90489 Nuremberg, Germany; stefan.may@th-nuernberg.de

2 Department of Informatics VII: Robotics and Telematics at the Julius-Maximilians University Würzburg, Am Hubland, 97074 Wuerzburg, Germany

* Correspondence: christian.pfitzner@th-nuernberg.de (C.P.); andreas.nuechter@uni-wuerzburg.de (A.N.)

Abstract: This paper describes the estimation of the body weight of a person in front of an RGB-D camera. A survey of different methods for body weight estimation based on depth sensors is given. First, an estimation of people standing in front of a camera is presented. Second, an approach based on a stream of depth images is used to obtain the body weight of a person walking towards a sensor. The algorithm first extracts features from a point cloud and forwards them to an artificial neural network (ANN) to obtain an estimation of body weight. Besides the algorithm for the estimation, this paper further presents an open-access dataset based on measurements from a trauma room in a hospital as well as data from visitors of a public event. In total, the dataset contains 439 measurements. The article illustrates the efficiency of the approach with experiments with persons lying down in a hospital, standing persons, and walking persons. Applicable scenarios for the presented algorithm are body weight-related dosing of emergency patients.

Keywords: image processing; machine learning; perception; sensor fusion; segmentation; RGB-D; thermal camera; kinect; human body weight; stroke

---

1. Introduction

When it comes to the treatment of ischemic stroke patients, it is crucial to solve the blood clot in the brain vessel as fast as possible. For the treatment of ischemic strokes, the medicament rtPA was approved in 1996 by the U.S. Food and Drug Administration [1]. The medicine has to be given with a dosage of 0.9 mg per kilogram of the patient's body weight. Furthermore, a maximum dose of 90 mg is specified for patients weighing more than 100 kilograms. It is best used within the first hour after the appearance of stroke symptoms. After three hours, side effects can prevail over the solving of the blood clot. Because of this narrow time window, physicians are in a hurry for treatment. Weighing a patient on a common standing scale is often not possible because the patient is in pain or is not able to stand due to other symptoms of stroke, e.g., paralysis. The obvious way to determine the body weight of someone quickly is to ask the person. However, if it comes to stroke, only half of the patients are knowledgeable and are not handicapped by stroke symptoms [2]. Additionally, elderly patients might suffer from dementia and cannot provide a reliable value for their body weight. Furthermore, relatives who could be asked might not be available in the trauma room or do not know the body weight of the patient. In addition, anthropometric methods exist, where lengths and circumferences of body parts are measured with a measuring tape. Based on an empirical equation, e.g., the equation for stroke patients presented by Lorenz et al. [3], gives an estimation of body weight.

The disadvantage of those anthropometric methods is that the patient has to be moved and the measuring is time-consuming.

Therefore, visual estimation of the patient's body weight by the attending physician in the emergency room has become routine worldwide. In a registry with 27,910 stroke patients, only 14.6 percent were weighed [4]. However, several studies [5–7] illustrate that such a weight estimation by a visual guess from a physician is often not sufficient for dosing: Every third patient receives a dosage out of the ± 10 percent bound. This result can be improved if the average estimation of several persons from medical staff is taken. Furthermore, the estimations from nursing staff are more reliable than the visual guesses by physicians [2].

The observation of body weight is also essential in elder care: People with a healthy weight can recover better from sickness than people who are underweight or obese. However, older people often have a reduced appetite, coupled with a decline in biological and physiological functions [8]. In elder care, people are weighed on common standing scales to observe changes in body weight. Multiple approaches with 3D sensors are being tested in the field of elder care, especially since the release of the low-cost Microsoft Kinect camera [9]. Some applications of these approaches are fall detection or the monitoring of breathing [10,11]. The contact-less body weight approach can be combined in context with these other approaches to monitor changes in body weight to improve elder care.

In contrast to the scenario of patients being measured on a stretcher, the weighing of standing people can be easily done on a spring scale. However, the automatic weighing of several people in a short time can bring a benefit in some applications: Since 2017, the Finnish airline Finnair weighs passengers to determine the total weight of an airplane for take-off. While the weight of baggage is measured with a scale, the weight of the passengers is only roughly rated with standardized weights [12]. The precise knowledge about the weight gives possibilities to optimize fuel requirements and therefore operating costs [13]. In 1985, a McDonnell Douglas DC-8 jetliner crashed with 256 people on board. One reason for the crash might have been the underestimated onboard weight, which was mentioned in the occurrence report [14]. Furthermore, the motivation for a visual weight system is gained as objects that the subject is wearing or carrying, e.g., a backpack, can be filtered out for weight estimation.

The presented approach is an extension of Pfitzner et al. [15]: While this previous work had the clear focus on clinical use, the work presented here extends the approach towards standing and walking people. First, this article contributes a summary about the visual body weight estimation for various situations. The settings for the different approaches are compared, as well as the results of the experiments. Second, the article shows that the feature set from previous work is also suitable for body weight estimation of standing or walking subjects. To obtain the body weight of walking subjects, a clustering method is presented, combining the estimations from each frame, to a single and also a more robust estimation. Finally, the article provides the 3D data used for experiments so that other research groups can contribute to this topic.

The paper is structured as follows: First, the related work concerning the body weight estimation based on a camera system is presented, focusing on lying, standing, and walking people. Second, the here applied and published dataset for body weight estimation based on RGB-D-T (color, depth and thermal) data is explained. In the following section, the approach for body weight estimation is presented and separated for standing and walking persons. Experiments with the here applied dataset and a dataset from related work demonstrate the efficiency of the developed algorithm. The results are examined in comparison to other approaches for visual weight estimation from related work. Finally, the paper concludes with a discussion and plans for future work.

2. Related Work

The related work is subdivided for lying, standing and walking people and further provides a summary of weighing and estimation devices for clinical usage.

2.1. Common Weighing and Medical Estimation Devices

Scales come in a wide range. The most common type is standing scales. Analog scales use a reference weight or a spring to obtain the body weight, while modern digital scales use strain gauges and a change in resistance to get a value for body weight. In the clinical scenario, chair scales exist, so a patient does not need to stand for the process of weighing. Different types of bed scales are available to weigh patients who are lying down. First, scales can be designed as a single plate integrated into the floor where the bed is placed. Second, bed scales are available with multiple weighing devices, which are attached to each wheel. The sum of all weight is the total weight of the bed, including the patient. In both scenarios, the tare weight of the empty bed has to be known. Consequently, either the bed is weighed in advance without the patient or the tare weight of the bed has to be identified. Choosing the wrong type of bed can result in a high degree of error concerning the patient's weight. Furthermore, different attachments, such as medical devices or handrails, can cause a change in tare weight. In addition, it is possible to integrate multiple strain gauges directly into the mattress. This solves the issue of determining the tare weight of the bed. It is also possible to integrate weighing directly into the computer tomography to speed up the process of weight acquisition [16].

Furthermore, rulers exist to approximate body weight for medical usage: Approximation rulers are common to estimate the body weight of young children; the Broselow tape was developed in 1985 by James Broselow and Robert Luten. It provides nine different weight groups for children younger than 12. A colored scale on the measuring tape relegates to different medical sets, prepared for emergency treatment of the different weight groups in case of an emergency. Several studies illustrate that the Broselow tape is reliable for first aid personnel [17]. However, for children, the estimation of the parents can be even more reliable, if available [18].

2.2. Estimation from Lying People

The body weight estimation of lying people is important mainly in the scenario of clinical usage. Most patients are already lying on a stretcher or a bed. Furthermore, the here presented approaches are suitable for bedridden patients.

Pirker et al. [19] employed 16 stereo cameras around a stretcher. Additional projectors are needed for complete illumination. A parametric human model complements the back side of the body. Composed images are filtered for noise reduction and, finally, the volume is calculated with the help of cross-sections along the body. Because of the high amount of cameras around the patient's bed, physicians would be constricted during treatment.

The here presented algorithm for the estimation of lying, walking and standing people is the continuation of preceding work: In 2015, Pfitzner et al. [20] showed an approach for body weight estimation with a depth camera. The algorithm extracts only the volume of a subject lying on a medical stretcher, multiplying it with a fixed value for the density. Color and depth gradient achieve the segmentation. The focus of this application was set on the body weight estimation of stroke patients within the treatment process in the trauma room. Although the approach is straightforward, the system was more reliable than the visual guess performed by the medical staff: 79 percent of all patients received a sufficient body weight estimation, while the visual guess from a physician could only provide a sufficient estimation in 68 percent of patients.

Figure 1 shows the scene in the trauma room with a patient on the stretcher and the complete system, as presented in Pfitzner et al. [20]. The setup with the patient lying on a medical stretcher and the sensors integrated into the ceiling is the same as in the following previous work.

The approach was extended in 2016 by the work of Pfitzner et al. [15]. An additional thermal camera improves the segmentation, and the patient in the fused field of view can be clearly segmented from the mattress that the subject is lying on. Furthermore, this paper introduced an extended feature extraction, as well as a machine learning approach—here an ANN—to improve the outcome in body weight estimation, by minimizing outliers and improving the standard deviation for the relative error.

In total, 89.9 percent of all subjects received an estimate of ±10 percent. For this approach, a patent exists [21].

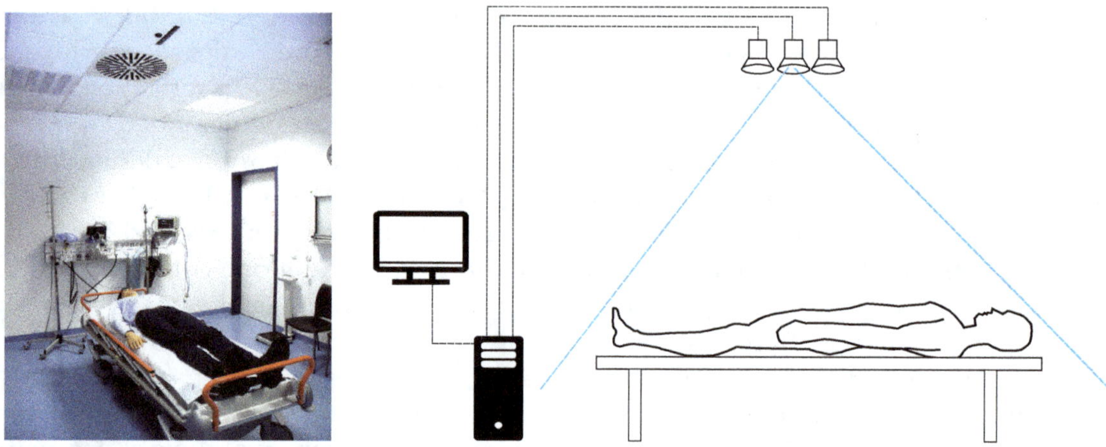

(**a**) (**b**)

Figure 1. Clinical integration of sensors into the trauma room, as shown in [15]. Within the scenario of trauma room in which physicians mostly treat emergency patients, the sensor system is integrated into the ceiling (**a**); The system does not hinder the physician while treating the patient, who is often lying on a medical stretcher. Besides the sensors in the ceiling, the system consists of a computer system—including a keyboard and a mouse for interaction, a monitor for visualization and a barcode scanner to identify patients with their ID (**b**). The connection between the sensors and the computer is achieved by USB cables. (**a**) Trauma room with sensors integrated into the ceiling; (**b**) Schematic of the sensor system and its connections to a computer.

Pfitzner et al. [22] presented a comparison of different depth sensors for the scenario of body weight estimation. In conclusion, the Kinect One can provide better results in body weight estimation—95.3 percent for the ±10 percent range—compared to the estimation based on the data of the Kinect with 94.8 percent. Additionally, this work also presents a correlation analysis of the extracted features, and how a different configuration of the available features can provide a reliable result.

2.3. Estimation from Standing People

In contrast to the estimation of lying people, the scenario for standing or walking people is more complex: The person is not aligned to a fixed surface on the back. Furthermore, the posture and the position of the subject changes in a sequence of frames.

Robinson and Parkinson [23] developed an approach for the body weight estimation of standing people. Here, anthropometric features are extracted from a scene's point cloud and the raw sensor data from an RGB-D sensor with a person standing in front of it can be seen. This approach also demonstrated that these raw features from the point cloud could lead to a bias because of un-calibrated sensor or noise. Furthermore, even thin clothes can confuse the extraction of the features, like the circumference of a body part, e.g., waist or hip circumference.

Cook et al. [24] presented a framework based on a structured light sensor for radiation dose estimation in CT examinations. In preliminary experiments, they showed results for five persons standing in front of a structured light sensor. The measured volume of the patient differs due to different positions of their arms.

With the help of skeleton tracking, Velardo and Dugelay showed a computer vision system to prove the health of a person with the help of a structured light sensor [25]. Apart from sensing the age of the subject, the sensor measures anthropometric features from arms, legs, and the body. The authors provide a trained statistical model from a medical database, containing anthropometric measurements from more than 28,000 subjects, as well as the ground truth body weight. This approach has the benefit of a large sample size for training. However, the estimation of the anthropometric features based on the RGB-D data is hard due to the sensor's noise. Additionally, the system provides information about obesity and nutrition to the user.

Based on a side-view feature, Nguyen et al. [26] developed a method to estimate the human body weight of standing people captured with an RGB-D camera. A model is trained based on regression. Together with handling the gender data, the algorithm can reach the mean average error of 5.20 kg over 300 subjects. In an additional experiment, the authors proved that the body weight estimation based on RGB-D data is more reliable compared with the human estimation. Furthermore, the utilized dataset with 300 subjects is published as an open-access source, containing the RGB-D data, the ground truth gender, and the ground truth body weight. This dataset is also applied to the following experiments.

2.4. *Estimation from Walking People*

Beside the body weight estimation from a single frame, it is also possible to estimate it by a sequence of sensor data. Labati et al. [27] developed a body weight estimation suitable for walking persons. The focus was set on a contact-less and low-cost method. The method is based on frame sequences from two cameras, which are placed to get a frontal and a side-view of the walking person. The feature vector consists of the height of a person, an approximation of the body volume, an approximation for the body shape and the walking direction. The extracted features are forwarded to an ANN to obtain body weight. Experiments are performed with 20 subjects, walking in eight different directions. A maximum absolute mean error was recorded with less than 2.4 kg.

Arigbabu et al. [28] demonstrated the extraction of soft biometrics, e.g., body height and weight, based on video frames from a single monocular camera. Due to a homogeneous background, the people's silhouette can be extracted easily with state of the art image processing techniques like background subtraction. The silhouette is converted into a binary mask, where 13 features are extracted depending on the pixel density in segmented regions. The feature vector is finally forwarded to an ANN to estimate the body weight. In experiments with 80 subjects, they reached a mean average error of 4.66 kg the estimation of body weight. The update rate of the extraction of all described soft biometrics was about 1 Hz. The approach was compared with the previously presented approach by Labati et al. [27] and Velardo and Dugelay [25].

Most of the approaches presented here use neural networks as a machine learning approach to generate a model for body weight estimation. The difference in the approaches can be found in the types of features forwarded to a neural network. In contrast to related work, the approach in this paper is not limited to a particular application. The selected features for machine learning are suitable for the scenarios of subjects who are lying, standing or walking. They can be used in general for the estimation of body weight. Furthermore, Table 1 compares the results of related work as a summary. The approaches presented by Nguyen et al. [26], Velardo and Dugelay [25], Labati et al. [27] and Arigbabu et al. [28] are compared in the experiment section.

Table 1. Results for contact-less human body weight estimation from related work in alphabetic order. The results are not directly comparable due to different evaluation metrics.

Method	Sensor	Approach	Constrains	Results
Cook et al. [24]	RGB-D structured light	image processing to reconstruct the volume	sample size 6 subjects	only volume estimation
Pirker et al. [19]	8 stereo cameras	image processing to reconstruct the volume	scene has to be known	only volume estimation
Nguyen et al. [26]	RGB-D structured light	machine learning with l2-regularization and support vector regression		5.2 kg MAE
Velardo and Dugelay [25]	RGB-D structured light	machine learning with multiple regression analysis	sample size 15 subjects	2.7 kg for a single subject
Pfitzner et al. [20]	RGB-D structured light	image processing to reconstruct the volume	person is lying on a flat surface	79.1 % within relative error of 10 %

Table 1. *Cont.*

Method	Sensor	Approach	Constrains	Results
Pfitzner et al. [15]	RGB-D structured light	machine learning with ANN	person is lying on a flat surface	89.6 % within relative error of 10 %
Pfitzner et al. [22]	RGB-D structured light and ToF	machine learning with ANN	person is lying on a flat surface	95.3 % within relative error of 10 %
Labati et al. [27]	2 RGB cameras	machine learning with ANN	sample size 20 subjects	2.3 kg std error
Arigbabu et al. [28]	RGB cameras	machine learning with ANN		4.66 kg MAE

3. Approach for Visual Body Weight Estimation

The algorithm is subdivided into sections for sensor fusion, segmentation, and feature extraction. It leads to a learning approach based on an ANN to obtain the body weight of a single person. Figure 2 illustrates the procedure in body weight estimation based on the previously segmented point cloud.

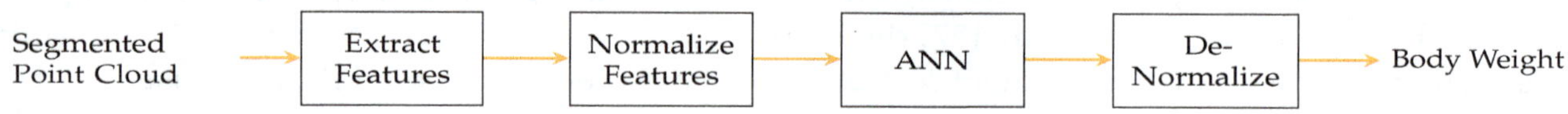

Figure 2. Process of body weight estimation.

3.1. System Description

The system uses different sensors, depending on the recorded dataset. It was developed for previous work [15,20] to be integrated into the clinical environment. There the system includes a Microsoft Kinect, a Microsoft Kinect One and an Optris PI400 thermal camera. A single depth sensor is sufficient for body weight extraction. However, the developed algorithm should not depend on the applied sensor. Therefore, experiments are performed with different sensors. Table 2 compares the sensors to each other.

Table 2. Property table of used sensors: The three sensors are selected for the body weight estimation because of their similar FOV, which provides a total view of the patient on the stretcher. For the 3D sensors, the measurement range is sufficient. The frame rate of at least 30 Hz is acceptable, while the thermal camera provides a frame rate of 80 Hz.

Model	Kinect	Kinect One	Optris PI400
Principle	Structured Light	Time-of-Flight	Thermal Camera
Resolution	320×240	512×424	382×288
Field of View	$57° \times 43°$	$70° \times 60°$	$62° \times 49°$
Frame rate	30 fps	30 fps	80 fps
Dimensions	$73 \times 283 \times 73$ mm^3	$249 \times 66 \times 67$ mm^3	$46 \times 56 \times 90$ mm^3
Weight	564 g	1400 g	320 g
Power consumption	12 W	32 W	<2.5 W via USB
Interface	USB 2.0	USB 3.0	USB 2.0
Price	$100	$200	$3500

Both the Kinect and the Kinect One are RGB-D cameras providing a color stream RGB, and a depth per pixel D. The first Kinect camera was released in 2011 bringing a low-cost consumer product into robotics. The sensor brought multiple applications and made an impact well beyond the gaming industry [29]. The Kinect holds a sensor for infrared (IR) and a sensor for color. Both sensors are calibrated to each other. The structured light principle obtains depth: A projector emits a known pattern in the environment. This pattern is seen by the IR sensor from a different pose to calculate the depth for an arbitrary pixel. Khoshelham and Elberink [30] illustrate the sensor's characteristics in image quality and noise.

In contrast to that, the Kinect One works by the Time-of-Flight (ToF) principle [31]: Having a highly precise measurement device for the time, it would be possible to calculate the distance between a light source and an object by measuring the time. The range of a given point can be calculated by the time t the light travels with the help of the speed of light c with $d = 0.5 \cdot t \cdot c$. Due to the fast traveling light, the distance measurement is obtained by modulated light: A source emits a light pulse towards an object. The frequency for modulation is known, and a phase shift can be measured from the reflected signal.

The here applied depth sensors differ not only in their resolution, but also the different principle provides a diverse characteristic of depth. Both sensors are compared to each other by Sarbolandi et al. [32]. Today, there exist various types of RGB-D sensors, which are suitable for the body weight estimation approach, e.g., Asus Xtion cameras from the Intel RealSense series [33]. The thermal camera is state of the art and is added to the sensor set to ease segmentation based on a simple thermal threshold. In this presented sensor configuration, the thermal camera is the most expensive part. It was used because it was already available from an earlier project. However, a cheaper thermal camera with a lower resolution and frame rate can be used for the segmentation. Pfitzner et al. [20] illustrated that the visual body weight estimation is possible without a thermal camera, but outliers due to insufficient segmentation can occur.

The algorithm—including the sensor fusion, the feature extraction and the forwarding to an artificial neural network—is implemented on a conventional desktop computer, which is installed in the trauma room. The computer in the trauma room, which is equipped with an Intel i7 of the 4th generation, can provide the result in body weight estimation within 300 ms, including the saving of the sensor data. The software does not rely on specialized hardware, like a high-end graphics card, although the processing speed could benefit from parallelization. For offline processing, a mobile computer (Dell M4800) is used, having a maximum power consumption of less than 80 Watt [34]. Therefore, the complete hardware could be designed with less than 100 W, including the mobile computer, the thermal camera (<2.5 Watt) and the Microsoft Kinect (12 Watt). Table 3 illustrates that the processing time for the desktop computer and the mobile computer is similar. A small experiment in our laboratory showed that the approach is also suitable for small size embedded computers, e.g., a Raspberry PI. With a reduced visualization, and without the saving of the sensor's data to the database, this configuration provided the estimation of body weight in around 5 s, see Table 3. The system is then limited in real-time visualization, as well as process time, and the estimation of the body weight is available with a higher delay. However, the embedded computer can have the benefit of lower power consumption and a smaller footprint, which provides easier integration in the clinical environment.

Table 3. Tested hardware including time measurements for the estimation: The biggest part of processing time is used to segment the patient from the environment. In contrast to that, the extraction of the features and the processing via an artificial neural network is small. The total time includes visualization and logging during the processing.

	Desktop Computer	Dell M4800 Mobile Computer	Raspberry PI 3	Asus Tinkerboard
Processor	Intel i7-4820K	Intel i7-4900MQ	ARM Cortex-A53	Rockchip RK3288
Nr. of Threads	8	8	4	4
max. Clock	3.90 GHz	3.80 GHz	1.2 GHz	1.8 GHz
TDP	130 W	47 W	<3.7 W	5 W
Time for Segmentation	239 ms	245 ms	5321 ms	2661 ms
Time for Estimation	22 ms	23 ms	267 ms	212 ms
Total Processing Time	263 ms	270 ms	5604 ms	2885 ms

3.2. Sensor Fusion

All applied projective depth, color, and thermal sensors are calibrated intrinsically based on the method presented by Zhang [35]. Therefore, a single calibration pattern is used, which is visible in depth, color, and thermal frame. Gonzalez-Jorge et al. [36] present different types of suitable calibration targets. The here applied calibration target consists of a metal plate on the back which is colored white and a black wooden plate on top. The wooden plate has holes in a circular pattern. The metal plate can be heated. Because of a space between the metal and the wood plate, a thermal gradient is visible, and the wholes appear to be warmer than the top surface. The circle pattern is therefore visible in the spectrum of the thermal camera [15].

The results of sensor fusion can be displayed in different settings. Besides the typical representation on the screen as a color image of the scene, the depth can be visualized by a color mapping. Furthermore, it is also possible to illustrate the scene as a false-color representation for temperature or fused with the color stream, similar to that presented by Vidas et al. [37]. This is achieved by comparing the color channel of every point in the cloud. Figure 3 illustrates the sensor fusion and its visualizations: In Figure 3c, the data from the color sensor of the Kinect camera is fused with its depth stream. In the fused image, the color stream provides the intensity of each pixel as a grayscale, while the color of a pixel arranges the depth in the scene, as shown in Figure 3b. In addition, the color data and the thermal data are aligned to be visible at the same time, see Figure 3d. From the given data, further data can be calculated to enhance the point cloud or the depth image, e.g., with normals.

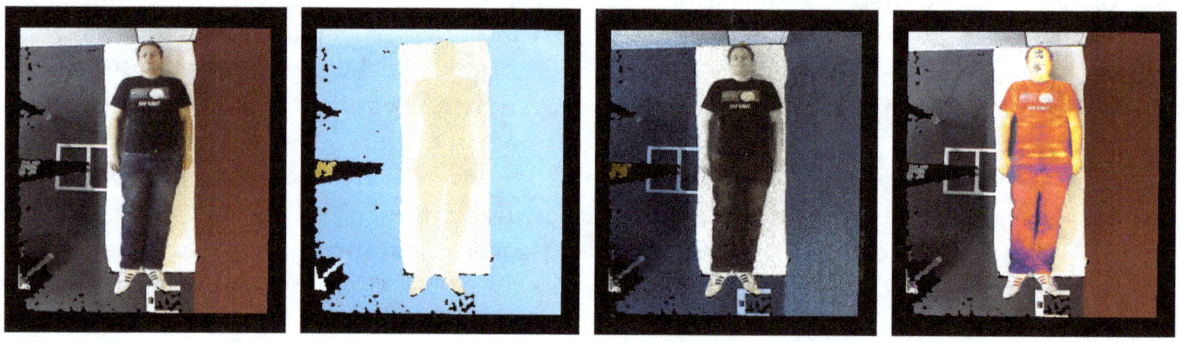

(**a**) Color (**b**) Depth (**c**) Color and Depth (**d**) Color and Therma

Figure 3. Visualization of sensor fusion: Figure (**a**) shows the raw color stream from an RGB-D camera. The depth stream can be visualized using a colormap, here drawing blue values for far objects and drawing white and orange for nearer objects (**b**). The stream from the thermal camera can be visualized in several ways: either it is drawn with false-color representation (**c**) or can be combined with other streams—here a combination of the color stream, highlighted with temperature (**d**). The here presented image-based sensor fusion is achieved by intrinsic and extrinsic camera calibration, which is presented in Figure 4.

Figure 4 presents the process of calibration for sensor fusion: The frames from the sensor are differentiated by indices, K for the Kinect, $K2$ for the Kinect One and T for the thermal camera. All three sensors are calibrated intrinsically. First, the raw streams from the sensors $\mathbf{I}$ are forwarded to rectification based on the determined intrinsic parameters $\mathbf{P}$ and $\mathbf{d}$ [35]. Second, the rectified images $\mathbf{I}$ are then calibrated extrinsically based on the previously estimated transformations $\mathbf{T}$. Third, the aligned data $\mathbf{I}$ is synchronized in time by the method presented by Lussier and Thrun [38] with $\Delta t_T, \Delta t_K, \Delta t_{K2}$. Finally, a point cloud $\mathcal{P} = (\mathbf{p}_1\ \mathbf{p}_2\ \dots\ \mathbf{p}_n)$ containing n points, can be generated with the help of the pinhole camera model.

The intrinsic calibration aims to remove the aberrations from the lens, bringing the image in the form of the pinhole camera model. For the intrinsic calibration, the projection matrix $\mathbf{P}$ has to be determined. The matrix contains the focal length , as well as the offset to the sensor's center. Therefore, based on the pinhole camera model, a point $\mathbf{p} = (x\ y\ z)^T \in \mathbb{R}^3$ can be projected onto the sensor as a pixel $\mathbf{q} = (u\ v)^T$. For the extrinsic calibration, the world frame's origin is set the same as the origin of the infrared sensor of the Kinect. The extrinsic factory calibration of both Kinect cameras is left as it is. The transformations between the two Kinect cameras and the thermal camera is estimated with the help of the same calibration pattern.

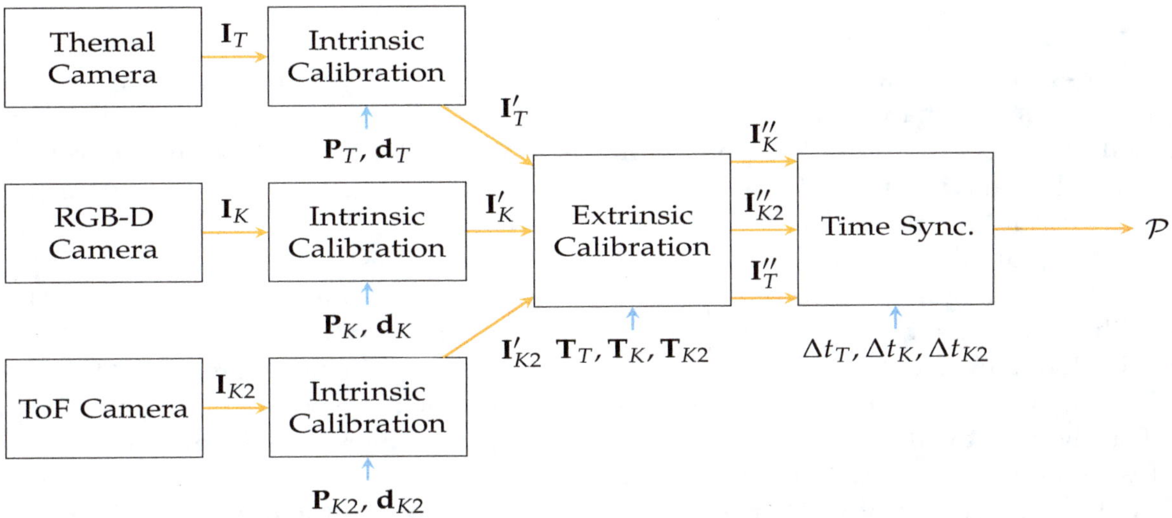

Figure 4. Process of sensor calibration: First, all projective sensors are calibrated intrinsically to remove distortions from the image and to obtain the projection matrix for each sensor $\mathbf{P}_T$, $\mathbf{P}_K$ and $\mathbf{P}_{K2}$. Furthermore, the coefficients for distortions $\mathbf{d} = (k_1\ k_2\ k_3\ p_1\ p_2)$ are necessary for rectification. The vector contains the parameters for radial distortion (k_1, k_2, k_3), as well as the parameters for tangential distortion (p_1, p_2) [35]. Second, the sensors are calibrated extrinsically, estimating the transformations between the sensors $\mathbf{T}$. The calibrated images are noted by $\mathbf{I}'_T$, $\mathbf{I}'_K$, and $\mathbf{I}'_{K2}$. Finally, the data from the sensors are synchronized in time based on $\Delta t_T, \Delta t_K, \Delta t_{K2}$. The synchronized images are noted by $\mathbf{I}''_K$, $\mathbf{I}''_{K2}$, and $\mathbf{I}''_T$. After this process of calibration, sensor fusion can be applied and data is converted towards a Cartesian point cloud $\mathcal{P} \in \mathbb{R}^3$.

Figure 5 illustrates the transformation between the sensors. The extrinsic parameters—the rotation $\mathbf{R}$ and the translation $\mathbf{t}$ —are combined to a pose ${}^{A}\xi_B$ describing the relative pose of $\{B\}$ with respect to $\{A\}$. After sensor fusion, every point can contain the Cartesian coordinates (x, y, z), color (rgb) and thermal data (t) with $\mathbf{p} = (x\ y\ z\ rgb\ t)^T$. For calibration and sensor fusion, OpenCV was applied [39].

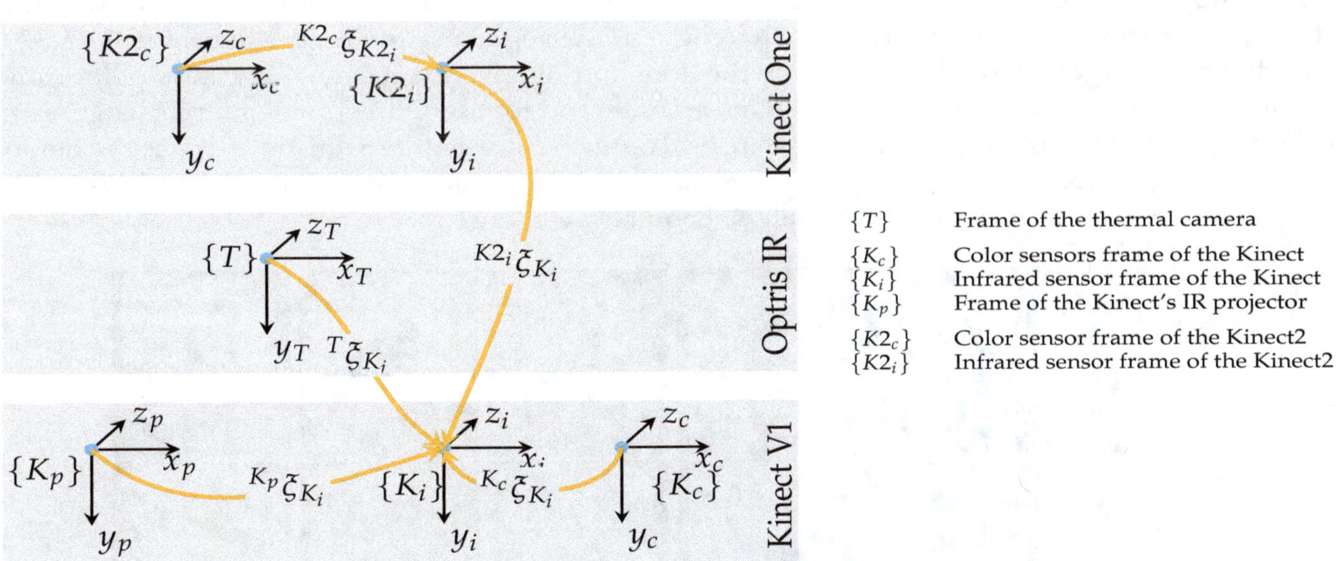

Figure 5. Transformation tree for the system's sensors: The infrared frame of the Kinect is used as reference for the world coordinate origin $\{0\}$. The manufacturer already calibrates the 3D sensor's own sensor frames. To obtain the transformation between the Kinect V1 and Kinect One, the IR sensors from both cameras are taken as a reference.

3.3. Segmentation

The process of segmentation differs with the scene: A patient lying on a medical stretcher with physicians on his side is harder to segment than someone standing in an empty room with a clear distance to the wall behind him. The point cloud $\mathcal{P}$ is segmented in a set belonging to the person $\mathcal{P}^p$ and a set for the environment $\mathcal{P}^E$ with $\mathcal{P} = \mathcal{P}^E + \mathcal{P}^p$. Therefore, a point can only belong to the person's point cloud, or the environment. The segmentation for clinical applications is described by Pfitzner et al. [15]. For the reader's convenience, it is also presented as follows: The patient is placed in a set range within the field of view (FOV) of the sensors mounted on the ceiling. This range is visible with markers on the floor. In an initial step, the amount of data in the point cloud is reduced. Therefore, the floor and all data outside the range of the markers on the floor is removed from the point cloud. After this step, the point cloud should contain mostly the patient and the stretcher he or she is lying on. Based on the available thermal data from the thermal camera, the segmentation can be done with a threshold in temperature. Points having a higher temperature than a fixed limit are included in the patient's point set $\mathcal{P}^p$. Physicians or family members close to the patient can be removed by finding the most significant contour easily under the assumption that the most significant part of the remaining scene is the patient and the stretcher. Based on the Random Sample Consensus (RANSAC) algorithm [40], the surface of the stretcher is obtained with a model for a plane. On one side, this is necessary to improve the outcome of segmentation. On the other side, the surface of the stretcher is necessary for the upcoming feature extraction. Morphological operations like erosion and dilation improve the outcome of segmentation [41]. Finally, the scene's point cloud $\mathcal{P}$ is segmented, and the patient's point cloud $\mathcal{P}^p$ is available. To check if a patient is within the FOV of the camera, state of the art algorithms like the histogram of oriented gradients can be used [42]. Further, the measurement can be started by the medical staff by pressing a button attached to the wall in the trauma room. The segmentation in this medical scenario is reliable and robust. The data from the thermal camera provides good results in segmentation, sufficient for feature extraction. However, also without a thermal camera, the segmentation can be achieved, but outliers can occur, as illustrated in previous work [20].

The segmentation of a standing or walking person is less complex: To segment the person from the background, a reference frame $\mathcal{P}_{\text{ref}}$ without the person is recorded in advance. The current frame containing the person is subtracted from the reference frame $\mathcal{P}^P = \mathcal{P} - \mathcal{P}_{\text{ref}}$. Due to the sensor's noise, a threshold in distance should be applied to get a good outcome of background subtraction. Furthermore, to improve the outcome of the segmentation on the floor, the RANSAC algorithm can be applied to detect points on the floor and remove them from the scene's point cloud. Therefore, the segmentation of the feet gets more accurate and robust. Outliers and jumping edge errors can be removed by morphological filters or statistical outlier filters. Figure 6 illustrates the segmentation based on background subtraction with a person walking towards the camera. This procedure is similar as presented in related work by Labati et al. [27] and Nguyen et al. [26].

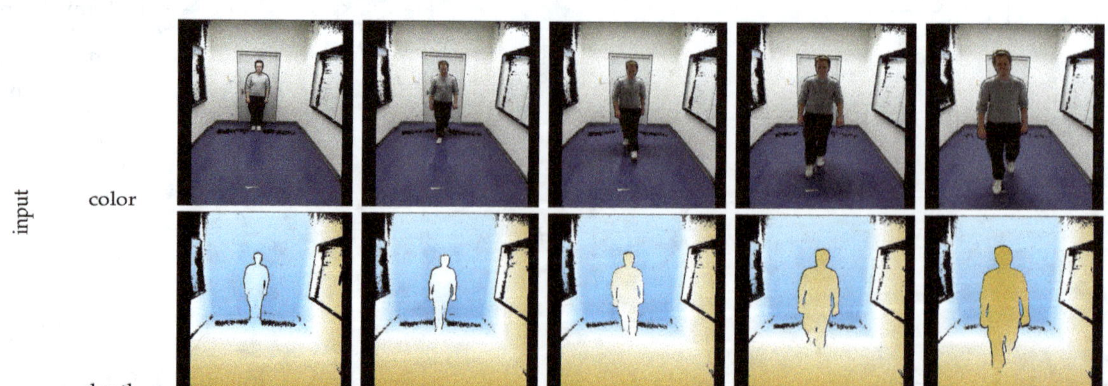

Figure 6. *Cont.*

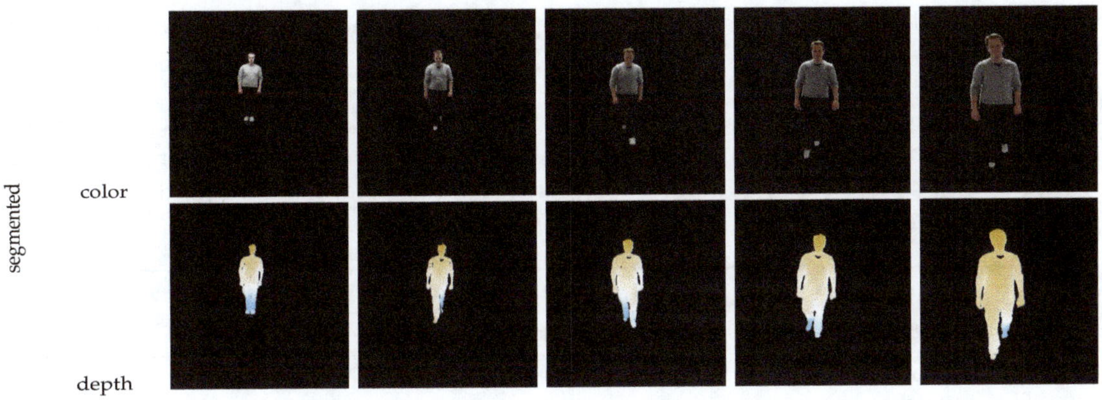

Figure 6. Sequence of someone walking towards the camera: The first two rows in the table illustrate the raw scene in color and depth representation, while the lower part of the table shows the segmented person. The sequence was recorded over four to five seconds. The scene is recorded with the Kinect One.

3.4. Feature Extraction

Based on the segmentation, features are obtained from the person's point cloud $\mathcal{P}^P$. The position of a patient does not vary much in the clinical scenario with the patient on a medical stretcher in a previously defined position of the bed and in a fixed distance from the sensors. In contrast to that, the pose of multiple persons standing in front of a camera can vary more; while walking the pose of the person changes from frame to frame. Therefore, it is necessary that the extracted features are robust against changes in scale, translation, and perspective. The difference in posture is small for most people standing in front of the camera or lying on a stretcher: most of them have their arms aside their body and a few have their arms crossed over their stomach.

The extracted features are presented in Table 4. The correlation of those features to the ground truth body weight is shown in Pfitzner et al. [22]. A good feature is invariant against scale (s), rotation (r), translation (t), perspective (pe) and posture of the person (po) in front of the camera. However, while most of the here presented features are invariant for scale, due to the applied 3D data, no feature is invariant against changes in posture. Therefore, the data applied for training the model should cover many different common postures for standing and walking people.

The features can be grouped: The features f_1 to f_4 are simple geometric features. The estimation of the volume is only possible due to the stretcher the patient is lying on. The volume is calculated based on a triangle mesh of the person's frontal surface s. The not visible surface on the back of the person is modeled by a single plane. The calculation of the volume is presented in detail in Pfitzner et al. [20]. Further, the triangle mesh is taken to calculate the frontal surface of a person. Although both features, the volume, and the surface, are only estimations and can be far from ground truth values, they can be a hint for an estimator: A person having a higher value for volume tends to be heavier compared to someone having a lower volume value. In addition, this first feature group contains the number of points belonging to the person's point cloud $|\mathcal{P}^P|$ and the calculated density of the scene, setting the number of points from the person in relation to the number of points of the whole scene $|\mathcal{P}|$.

The second group of features (f_5 to f_{10}) is based on eigenvalues and the eigenvalues itself: The normalized eigenvalues have the benefit that they are invariant against coordinate transformations like scale, rotation, and translation. Therefore, the features based on these eigenvalues — sphericity, flatness, and linearity — are also invariant against transformations.

The third group consists of features from statistics: Compactness and kurtosis are normalized and therefore invariant against scale, rotation, and translation.

Features from the silhouette of a person are grouped in the fourth section: The area and length of the contour and the convex hull are invariant against rotation, and translation, but not against scale. However, a small change in posture can change the outcome from the calculation of contour and convex hull.

Table 4. List of features for body weight estimation $\forall\, \mathbf{p}_j \in \mathcal{P}^P$. The table further lists the invariance of each feature by scale (s), rotation (r), translation (t), perspective (pe) and posture of the person (po) with + (invariant), 0 (invariant with limitations) and - (not invariant). The equations in the table are taken from the previous work [22].

	Feature	Invariance s	r	t	pe	po	Equation
f_1	volume	+	+	+	0	-	v
f_2	surface	+	+	+	0	-	s
f_3	number of patient's points	-	+	+	0	-	$\|\mathcal{P}^P\|$
f_4	density	-	+	+	0	-	$\|\mathcal{P}^P\|/\|\mathcal{P}\|$
f_5	1. eigenvalue	+	+	+	0	-	λ_1
f_6	2. eigenvalue	+	+	+	0	-	λ_2
f_7	3. eigenvalue	+	+	+	0	-	λ_3
f_8	sphericity	+	+	+	0	-	$\lambda_3/\sum_j \lambda_i$
f_9	flatness	+	+	+	0	-	$2\cdot(\lambda_2-\lambda_3)/\sum_i \lambda_i$
f_{10}	linearity	+	+	+	0	-	$(\lambda_1-\lambda_2)/\sum_i \lambda_i$
f_{11}	compactness	+	+	+	0	-	$\sqrt{1/n\sum_i(\mathbf{p}_j-\bar{\mathbf{p}})^2}$
f_{12}	kurtosis	+	+	+	0	-	$1/n\sum_j \|\|\mathbf{p}_j-\bar{\mathbf{p}}\|\|$
f_{13}	alt. compactness	+	+	+	0	-	$\sum_j(\mathbf{p}_j-\bar{\mathbf{p}})^4/f_9$
f_{14}	distance to person	+	+	+	+	0	d
f_{15}	contour length	-	+	+	-	-	l_c
f_{16}	contour area	-	+	+	-	-	a_c
f_{17}	convex hull length	-	+	+	-	-	l_h
f_{18}	convex hull area	-	+	+	-	-	a_h
f_{19}	gender	+	+	+	+	+	g

Related work showed that the body weight estimation could be improved if the gender is known [26]. The gender was here taken from ground truth, but could also be estimated by algorithm [26,43]. Apparently, the gender does not change in any way with applied transformation. Further, the cited algorithms are robust in detecting gender [43].

Table 5 demonstrates the changes in the feature values with different postures: The first scene shows a subject standing straight with the arms aside. The features are listed and calculated by the previously presented equations. In the second scene, the subject raises both hands a bit. The values for surface and density do not change much. In addition, the first eigenvalue nearly stays the same. However, the value for the third eigenvalue changes, due to the arms raised in front of the person. Flatness and sphericity—which correlate with the third eigenvalue—also change significantly. Compared to the third scene, where the subject stands with legs apart, the second eigenvalue changes most. Therefore, flatness and also linearity change. Comparing the first and the fourth scene, the subject crosses the arms: The surface lowers, as well as all features from contour and convex hull. The second eigenvalue lowers while the third eigenvalue increases. In the last scene, the subject is wearing a backpack. Comparing the features from this scene with the first scene, most of the features are within the same range. However, there are differences due to slight differences in posture. Apparently, the body weight estimation can ignore such objects as backpacks, if not visible to the sensor.

Concerning all the poses presented here, the features from contour and convex hull are able to vary the most: A subject having the arms aside can cause a much higher length in contour when there is a small gap between the body and the arm. However, as shown in [22], the length and area of the contour correlate with the body weight and therefore it can be useful to enclose such features for body weight estimation.

Table 5. Changes in features with different poses: Five different scenes illustrate the change in feature values depending on the posture.

Features	Scene 1	Scene 2	Scene 3	Scene 4	Scene 5
Surface	9.5×10^{-1}	9.7×10^{-1}	9.6×10^{-1}	8.6×10^{-1}	9.7×10^{-1}
Density	1.1×10^{-1}	1.1×10^{-1}	1.2×10^{-1}	1.0×10^{-1}	1.3×10^{-1}
1st eigenvalue	4.7×10^{3}	4.7×10^{3}	5.1×10^{3}	4.5×10^{3}	5.4×10^{3}
2nd eigenvalue	3.9×10^{2}	4.6×10^{2}	6.9×10^{2}	2.5×10^{2}	5.2×10^{2}
3rd eigenvalue	7.1×10^{1}	3.2×10^{2}	7.9×10^{1}	9.4×10^{1}	7.7×10^{1}
Sphericity	4.1×10^{-2}	1.8×10^{-1}	4.0×10^{-2}	5.8×10^{-2}	3.8×10^{-2}
Flatness	1.2×10^{-1}	5×10^{-2}	2.0×10^{-1}	6×10^{-2}	1.4×10^{-1}
Linearity	8.3×10^{-1}	7.7×10^{-1}	7.5×10^{-1}	8.8×10^{-1}	8.1×10^{-1}
Compactness	4.6×10^{-1}	4.6×10^{-1}	4.6×10^{-1}	4.7×10^{-1}	4.5×10^{-1}
Kurtosis	5.4×10^{3}	5.5×10^{3}	6.2×10^{3}	5.0×10^{3}	6.0×10^{3}
AltCompactness	8.6×10^{-1}	8.7×10^{-1}	8.6×10^{-1}	8.6×10^{-1}	8.7×10^{-1}
Contour length	1.0×10^{3}	1.4×10^{3}	1.4×10^{3}	1.1×10^{3}	1.4×10^{3}
Contour area	2.5×10^{4}	2.5×10^{4}	2.8×10^{4}	2.1×10^{4}	1.4×10^{3}
Convex hull length	8.2×10^{2}	8.3×10^{2}	9.3×10^{2}	8.0×10^{2}	8.8×10^{2}
Convex hull area	3.0×10^{4}	3.5×10^{4}	4.3×10^{4}	2.6×10^{4}	3.7×10^{4}
Distance	1.8	1.8	1.7	1.8	1.6
color	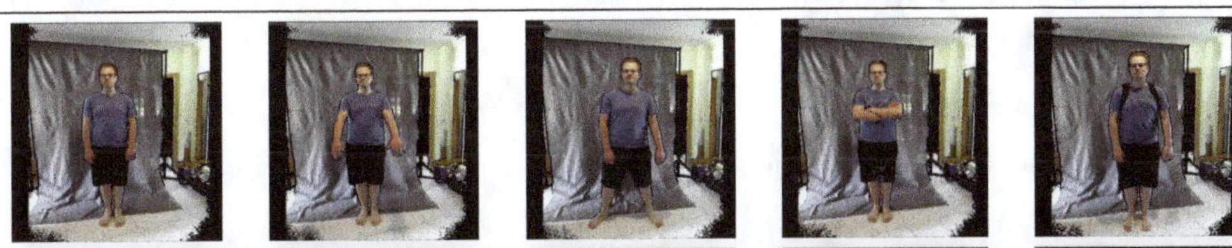				
segmented depth	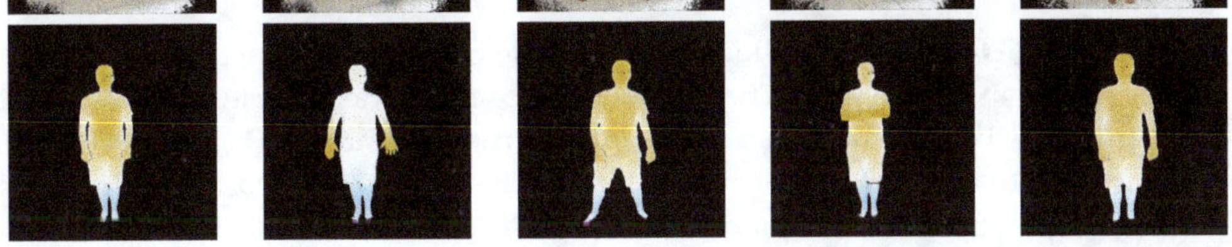				

Machine learning minimizes the invariances in selected features. However, a suitable set for training and testing should cover most of the various poses, especially when the subject is moving during body weight estimation.

3.5. Weight Estimation Based on a Single Frame

The previously extracted features are forwarded to an ANN. The network is designed as a three-layer feedforward network, having one layer as input, one hidden layer, and a single output layer. The output layer consists of a single neuron representing the body weight in kilograms. The number of input units is set by the number of features forwarded to the network. For every element of the feature vector, an input unit exists.

The network is trained with a subset of the available data. For the upcoming experiments, 70 percent of a dataset is forwarded to the neural network for training. The remaining 30 percent of each dataset is used to evaluate the network. Those data are never used for training so the network cannot overfit for the training data. Learning is achieved by resilient propagation [44]. Regularization is applied with weight decay to improve the outcome. First, the error of training and testing decreases. After a while the error in testing dataset increases while the training error is still decreasing. This is the moment to abort the training to prevent an over-fitting. Due to randomized starting points, the learning via the neural network approach can come to different solutions for every trial.

3.6. Estimation of a Sensor Stream

The FOV, the person's height, and the maximum distance for 3D data acquisition mark the starting and end markers on the floor, see Figure 7b. Figure 7a illustrates the poses of all people walking towards the camera. Due to different settings for the experiments, the path people tend to walk differs. Further, the camera did not always have the same orientation towards the floor and was not always mounted at the same height.

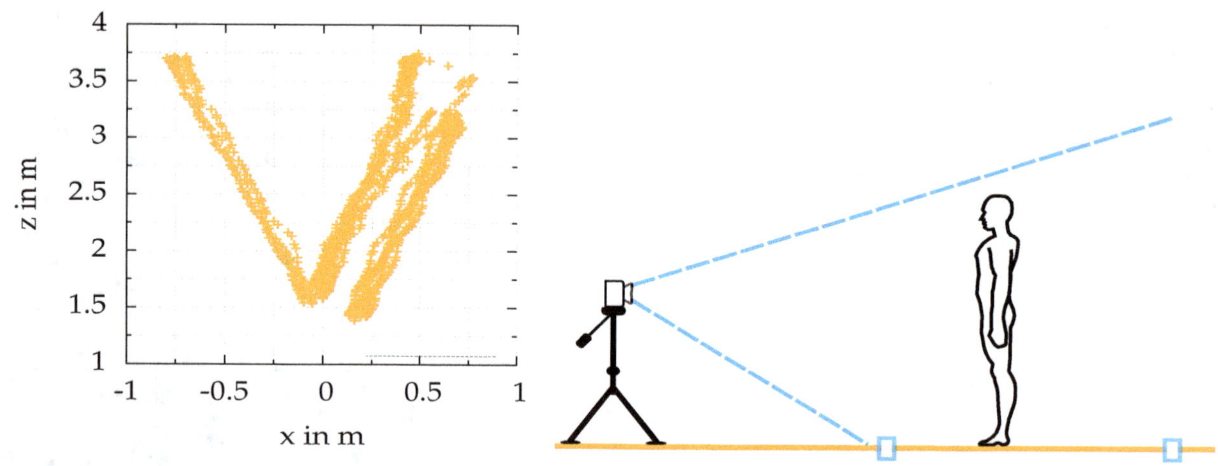

(**a**) Position of subjects while walking. (**b**) Setting for walking subjects.

Figure 7. Poses of people walking towards the camera (**a**): The complete datasets consist of several independent experiments. Therefore, the poses of the people walking differ, depending on the orientation of the camera. The people stand at the first marker (**b**). While walking towards the second marker close to the camera, every frame from the sensor is saved for offline processing. The recording is stopped when the second marker is reached.

First, the person is segmented from the background by the methods described in the previous section. Second, for every frame of the dataset, the body weight estimation is applied. In a scatter plot together with the ground truth body weight, a line becomes visible for every single person. Some of the estimations are close to the ground truth body weight. Even outliers of more than 30 percent occur. Therefore, taking an arbitrary frame from a person's dataset will likely lead to a close to random result. Third, a clustering method is applied, so not only an arbitrary frame from a person's dataset provides an estimation of the body weight. A Euclidean clustering method is applied to improve the outcome. The clustering is applied as follows: A dataset of a person $\mathcal{D}$ consists out of N frames from the sensor $D_0, D_1, \ldots, D_N$. Every frame consists of a point cloud $\mathcal{P}$.

1. For every frame in the dataset $D_i \in \mathcal{D}$ estimate the body weight based on the calculated features $w_i(D_i \rightarrow \mathbf{f})$.
2. Calculate the mean distance $\bar{d}$ for every estimation of a dataset $\mathcal{D}$ to all other estimations by

$$\bar{d}_i(D_i) = \frac{1}{N} \sum_{j=1}^{N} |w_i - w_j| \quad \text{where } i \neq j \tag{1}$$

   and store the calculated average distances in a vector $\bar{\mathbf{d}}$.
3. Sort the calculated distances in an ascending order $\bar{d}_0 \leq \bar{d}_1 \leq \ldots \leq \bar{d}_N$.
4. Remove values with the highest distances. Keep a fixed amount of distances, e.g., 20 percent.

5. Calculate the centroid of the remaining estimations containing $n_{0.2} = 0.2 \cdot N$ estimations

$$\bar{w} = \frac{1}{n_{0.2}} \sum_{i=1}^{n_{0.2}} w_i \tag{2}$$

which is the result of the body weight estimation based on a stream of data.

The principle in clustering is demonstrated in the upcoming section with experiments.

4. A Dataset for Body Weight Estimation

In addition to the here presented algorithm, a dataset is published to boost research in this field. Public datasets, as provided by Nguyen et al. [26] help to improve models for body weight estimation. Furthermore, developed algorithms and models can be applied to the dataset to generate comparable results. Depending on the recorded dataset, different sensors are used for recording. First, the Microsoft Kinect camera from the first generation of the XBox is used to obtain 3D data from the environment. Another sensor used for data acquisition is the second generation Kinect camera, the Kinect One. Additionally, a thermal camera is added and fused to the 3D data. This should ensure an easy segmentation approach based on a thermal threshold.

Table 6 illustrates the characteristics of the subjects in the dataset. The datasets are the following:

- **HospitalNoThermo**: From May 2014 to September 2014 a dataset was recorded from the Universitätsklinikum Erlangen, Germany, for preliminary testing. In this early dataset only RGB-D data is available without thermal data. The thermal camera was added after this experiment. The dataset contains 192 measurements.
- **Hospital**: This dataset includes feature values from trauma room patients from the Universitätsklinkum Erlangen, Germany. The dataset contains 127 measurements from people lying on a medical stretcher, recorded with a Microsoft Kinect. For this dataset a proper distribution is achieved consisting of people of different ages, body weights and shapes, see Table 4. Additionally, this dataset contains the patients' self-estimation, age, sex, as well as anthropometric features like body height, abdominal girth, and waist circumference. The distance between the sensors and the subjects was around 2 m.
- **Event**: The features from this dataset were recorded at a public event, called Long Night of Science in 2015 in Nuremberg, Germany. People in this dataset were visitors of the public event. This dataset contains 106 people. For this public event, it was not convenient to take anthropometric measurements. Ground truth was validated with a standard digital scale. The dataset consists of sensor values from Kinect and thermal camera. Additionally, this dataset includes point clouds from Microsoft Kinect One.
- **Walking**: Based on the results of the previous three datasets, experiments with people standing and walking in front of the camera are complemented. The dataset consists of 14 people, mostly employees, and students from the laboratory.

For the first three datasets, the camera is mounted over a stretcher. The stretcher at the event and the hospital datasets are different. Furthermore, the installation of the sensors did not pay attention to the same height or distance to the stretcher. Therefore, the distance to the stretcher differs between the datasets.

Table 6. Datasets applied for this article: The first two datasets are recorded in a trauma room of the University Hospital Erlangen, Germany. The third dataset is based on a public event in a laboratory, containing visitors of this event. The fourth set is recorded with employees and students of the laboratory. For comparison, the average body weight of the German population in 2009 is 73.9 kg [45]. This average value is close to the first three datasets. The last dataset W8-300 is recorded by [26], showing people standing in the front of a Kinect camera.

Dataset	Sensors	Scenario	Real Weight in kg				Gender		Total
			min	max	Mean	σ	Female	Male	
HospitalNoThermo	K	lying	48.8	165	78.3	17.3	93	99	192
Hospital	K, T	lying	48.6	129	77.8	17.1	72	55	127
Event	K, K2,T	lying	48.8	114	78.6	12.0	24	82	106
Walking	K2	walking	68	134	84.2	16.4	0	14	14
W8-300 [26]	K1	standing	40	104	67.2	14.7	97	207	299

Due to privacy issues, the datasets only contain the depth and the thermal information. The datasets are available via https://osf.io/rhq3m/ [46]. Each frame from the sensors is stored as a point cloud within the common PCD file format, used by the point cloud library [47]. An arbitrary point in the cloud contains the Cartesian coordinates **p** and three values for color—red, green and blue channel. The data can be enhanced with temperature values t.

The name of each frame contains the metadata of each person in front of the camera. The data name is structured as follows `GENDER_GROUNDTRUTH_PERSONID_FRAME_ID.pcd`. Besides the raw data from the sensors, an already segmented version of each frame exists within the repository. Furthermore, the parameters from intrinsic and extrinsic calibration are available. The authors gratefully acknowledge collaboration and joint work to improve the outcome of body weight estimation based on RGB-D data, especially for the clinical application.

5. Experiments and Results

For the upcoming section, the presented algorithm is evaluated for standing and walking people. Experiments for lying people are presented and discussed in the previous work [15,20].

The validate the experiments, different metrics are used for comparison: For each measurement the absolute error e can be calculated, having the ground truth value $\hat{x}$ as well as the estimated value $\tilde{x}$ by $e_i = \hat{x} - \tilde{x}$. The absolute error would be good to compare a group of people having the same body weight and differ only in their visual appearance. The here presented group of people for testing has a high variety of body weight and visual appearance. Therefore, the absolute error is not sufficient for comparison. Better for comparison of variant datasets is the relative error which is defined for an arbitrary dataset with

$$\epsilon = \frac{\hat{x}_i - \tilde{x}_i}{\hat{x}_i} = \frac{e_i}{\hat{x}_i} \tag{3}$$

Another way to prove and benchmark the body weight estimation approach is the mean absolute error (MAE). The absolute error of each dataset e_i is summed up and divided by the total number of datasets for benchmarking. It is defined by

$$e_{mae} = \frac{1}{N} \sum_{i=1}^{N} |e_i|. \tag{4}$$

Further, the mean square error (MSE) can be used for validation. Here the absolute error is squared before summation. It is defined by

$$e_{mse} = \frac{1}{N} \sum_{i=1}^{N} e_i^2. \tag{5}$$

Compared to the mean absolute error, outliers were weighted stronger.

5.1. Standing

In contrast to experiments for people who were lying down, the most correlating feature—the volume—cannot be used because no reference surface for the back of a person exists. Therefore, the body weight estimation has to rely on the remaining features. A previous experiment with the two datasets from a hospital and the event dataset illustrated that the body weight estimation gets worse if the volume is missing. Nevertheless, the decrease in accuracy can be sufficient for other applications.

For the experiment, the dataset W8-300 generated by Nguyen et al. [26] is applied. It contains 299 people standing in front of a Microsoft Kinect camera. The color and the depth frame are saved separately with a resolution for each channel of 8 bit. The segmentation has been done in advance based on ground detection with RANSAC model [40]: The images in the dataset are already segmented, only containing the person's data as a depth and color image; the background is not visible. The file name of each dataset contains first the gender, second the ground truth body weight, and lastly the surname of the person. The ground truth body weight varies within a range starting from 40 kg up to 104 kg. In the experiments, 202 males and 97 females participated.

Figure 8 illustrates the result from the dataset: First, the ground truth ordered datasets are shuffled. For training of the ANN, 70 percent of the dataset were used; the other 30 percent were applied for testing.

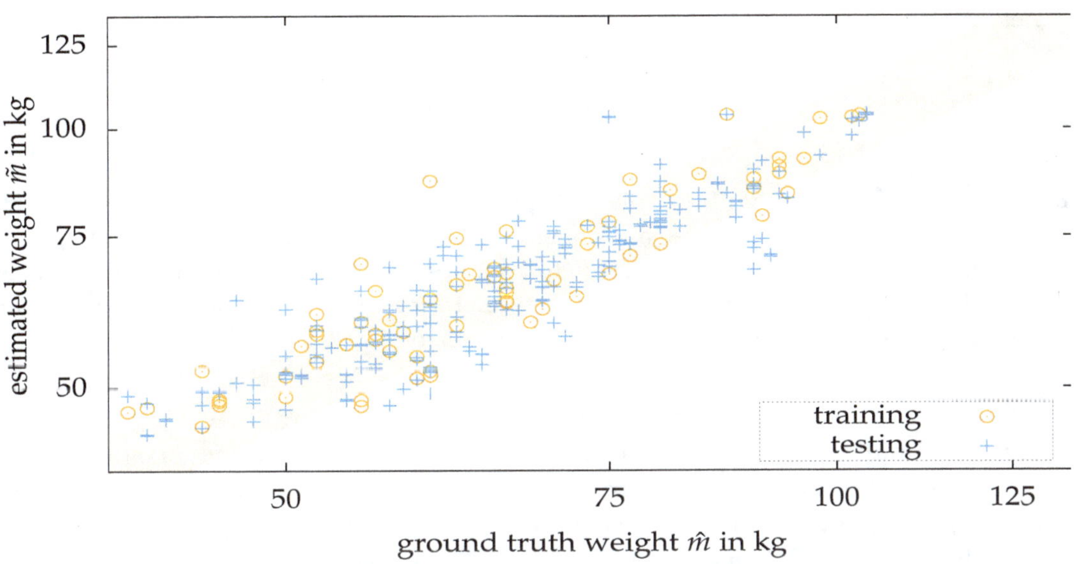

Figure 8. Results of the experiment with people standing in front of the camera based on the here proposed algorithm and the W-300 dataset contributed by Nguyen et al. [26]. The orange area marks the range for the relative error of ±10 percent.

All people were not told to hold a fixed posture but most of them were standing normally with their arms aside.

Nguyen et al. [26] compared the MAE in their publication: They reached a MAE of 4.62 kg for female and 5.59 kg for male persons. Without the discrimination in gender, the algorithm performs with a MAE of 5.20 kg. This experiment also includes the ground truth of the gender for the applied model. Compared to their results, the here performed experiment reaches an MAE of 4.3 kg. The approach presented by [25] can outperform the here presented results with a MAE of 2.7 kg. However, the sample size in the published article contains only six subjects.

5.2. Walking

In addition to the previous experiments, walking people should also be estimated for their body weight. Therefore, a dataset was recorded with students and employees of the Technische Hochschule Nürnberg, Georg Simon Ohm, walking in front of a Microsoft Kinect One. The person is walking towards the sensor, starting at a fixed distance. A marker on the floor shows the limitation of the recorded scene, due to the FOV of the sensor. The sensor is mounted on a tripod in a height of around 1.5 m.

The setting for this experiment is described in detail in the previous section. Figure 9 illustrates the results of this experiment as a scatter plot:

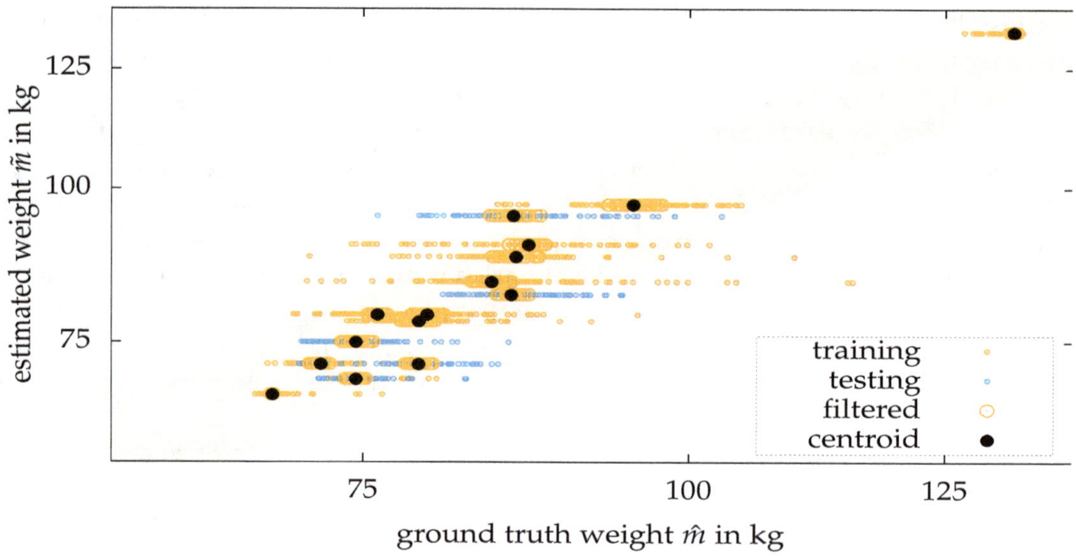

Figure 9. Results of the experiment with people walking towards the camera: The estimations for every frame for an arbitrary person generate a set of estimations, formed as a line together with the ground truth value in the scatter plot. Based on Euclidean clustering, 80 percent of the estimations are removed from the dataset. The final estimation is given based on the centroid of the remaining estimations. The orange area marks the range for the relative error of ± 10 percent.

The estimations for an arbitrary person lead in the scatter plot points, aligning on a horizontal line. Often, most of the estimations are outside of the ± 10 percent bound. However, some estimations appear to be more dense to other estimations than some outliers. The previously presented approach for clustering now minimizes the set of estimations of an arbitrary person (here marked in bigger points) and calculates the centroid of these sets. For this small sample size of 14 subjects, all of the final estimations were within a range of ± 10 percent.

The results provided by Labati et al. [27] outperform the here presented approach when comparing the standard deviation. In contrast to that, the proposed approach outperforms the estimation for walking people presented by Arigbabu et al. [28].

6. Discussion

All presented experiments rely on the same set of features. Table 7 compares the result from walking and standing people for body weight estimation: The estimation works best if the subject is lying on a medical stretcher, comparing the results for the relative error and the percentage of in range estimations. This result occurs because in this configuration the volume of the subject can be extracted easily. Further, the variety of posture and position of the subject is low in the overall datasets [22]. The algorithm works with different types of sensors, e.g., a structured light sensor (Kinect) as well as a time of flight sensor (Kinect One). Figure 10 illustrates the relative error in a cumulative plot for lying, standing and walking subjects.

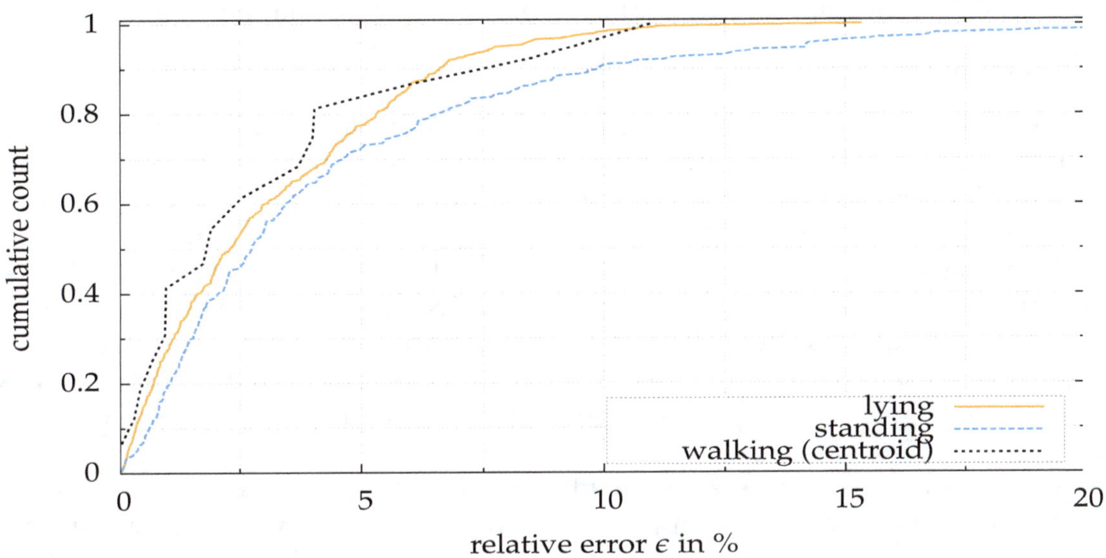

Figure 10. Comparison between the different settings for body weight estimation: Although the results for the estimation with standing people from the W8-300 dataset is the worst in this cumulative plot, the results can be sufficient for a certain applications. Due to the clustering approach, the estimation of walking subjects outperforms the other settings within the range of ±5 percent. The results for the lying patients are taken from Pfitzner et al. [22].

Table 7. Results from experiments for standing and walking people. Additionally, the results from Pfitzner et al. [22] are added for comparison. The lower part of the table illustrates the results from related work, when available in detail. The best result is marked in bold for each category.

	Dataset	Size	Relative Error in %				In Range in %			Error in kg / kg²	
			min	max	Mean	σ	5	10	20	MAE	MSE
Lying [22]	Event	106	−8.7	14.3	0.90	4.80	75.6	95.3	**100**	2.86	**13.8**
Standing	W8-300	299	−28.8	16.76	**−0.1**	5.80	70.5	91.3	99.3	4.31	33.5
Walking	Walking	14	**−6.7**	**9.38**	0.32	3.88	**78.5**	**100**	**100**	3.30	20.5
Nguyen et al. [26]	W8-300	299								5.2	
Velardo and Dugelay [25]		6			3.6					**2.7**	
Labati et al. [27]		20				**2.3**					
Arigbabu et al. [28]		13								4.66	

The results for subjects standing in front of a camera are less accurate in nearly every category. However, over 90 percent of the body weight estimation is within a range of ±10 percent. Comparing the here presented approach with the algorithm presented by Nguyen et al. [26], the experiment performs better for the dataset W8-300 with a MAE of 4.31 kg, facing 5.20 kg. In contrast to that, the estimation of subjects walking towards the camera is outstanding. However, the results rely on a small set of subjects. Therefore, the experiment is far from being statistically significant, but it proves the concept.

Although the system with its features is suitable for body weight estimation of lying, standing and walking subjects, there are some limitations. The previously trained ANN can only provide a sufficient result for the body weight estimation when a similar subject has been seen in advance, which is common for machine learning approaches. At a public laboratory event, children were estimated with relative errors in body weight of up to 50 percent—due to not being seen before. The used model was trained with patients from the hospital, where subjects younger than 18 years were excluded in the dataset. While the pose of the subjects lying in the clinical scenario is similar, the pose for walking subjects can vary strongly from frame to frame. For the here presented small experiment, all subjects are facing the camera and walking towards it. In a scenario with the people walking differently, e.g., walking sideways, the algorithms would not provide sufficient estimation results.

7. Conclusions and Future Work

This paper presented a novel approach for the estimation of body weight. In contrast to related work, the approach with its feature vector was tested for lying, standing and walking subjects. Experiments proved that the estimation is possible within a given range. The algorithm and the extracted features previously presented in [15] are also able to provide an estimation of standing and walking people. The missing volume—which correlates with the body weight the most [22]—is the reason the estimation for a single frame of a walking subject is worse than for a lying person. However, the estimation on a sequence of frames combined with the presented clustering provides a sufficient body weight estimation. In direct comparison with the approach for body weight estimation approach from Nguyen et al. [26], the approach presented here can outperform the results, while being applied to the same dataset.

For future work, it is the aim of the here presented project to obtain a bigger dataset: The estimation of standing people should be expanded to an approach where people do not need to face in the direction of the sensors. Further, the path for the estimation of walking people should be made more variable so people can move freely in front of the camera. This approach needs a higher demand for varying data. The authors gratefully acknowledge future joint work to improve the outcome of the algorithm and to develop a bigger dataset for experiments and modeling.

Author Contributions: Christian Pfitzner designed the algorithm and the experiments for the here presented multimodal sensor system; Stefan May and Andreas Nüchter contributed to the methology with conception and ideas for the experiment for the approach and experiments for visual body weight estimation. Furthermore, they improved the content of the article with their annotations.

Acknowledgments: Christian Pfitzner was supported by the BayWISS research training group "Digitization". This publication was funded by the German Research Foundation (DFG) and the University of Würzburg in the funding programme Open Access Publishing.

Abbreviations

The following abbreviations are used in this manuscript:

ANN	artificial neural network
FPV	field of view
IR	infrared
MAE	mean average error
MSE	mean square error
RANSAC	random sample consensus
RGB	red green blue
RGB-D	red green blue depth
RGB-D-T	red green blue depth thermal
PCD	point cloud data
rtPA	recombinant tissue plasminogen activator
TDP	thermal design power
ToF	time of flight

References

1. Zivin, J.A. Acute stroke therapy with tissue plasminogen activator (tPA) since it was approved by the U.S. Food and Drug Administration (FDA). *Annal. Neurol.* **2009**, *66*, 6–10. [CrossRef] [PubMed]
2. Breuer, L.; Nowe, T.; Huttner, H.B.; Blinzler, C.; Kollmar, R.; Schellinger, P.D.; Schwab, S.; Köhrmann, M. Weight Approximation in Stroke Before Thrombolysis The WAIST-Study: A Prospective Observational "Dose-Finding" Study. *Stroke* **2010**, *41*, 2867–2871. [CrossRef] [PubMed]

3. Lorenz, M.W.; Graf, M.; Henke, C.; Hermans, M.; Ziemann, U.; Sitzer, M.; Foerch, C. Anthropometric approximation of body weight in unresponsive stroke patients. *J. Neurol. Neurosurg. Psychiatry* **2007**, *78*, 1331–1336. [CrossRef] [PubMed]
4. Diedler, J.; Ahmed, N.; Glahn, J.; Grond, M.; Lorenzano, S.; Brozman, M.; Sykora, M.; Ringleb, P. Is the Maximum Dose of 90 mg Alteplase Sufficient for Patients With Ischemic Stroke Weighing >100 kg? *Stroke* **2011**, *42*, 1615–1620. [CrossRef] [PubMed]
5. Coe, T.; Halkes, M.; Houghton, K.; Jefferson, D. The accuracy of visual estimation of weight and height in pre-operative supine patients. *Anaesthesia* **1999**, *54*, 582–586. [CrossRef] [PubMed]
6. Cubison, T.; Gilbert, P. So much for percentage, but what about the weight? *Emerg. Med. J.* **2005**, *22*, 643–645. [CrossRef] [PubMed]
7. Menon, S.; Kelly, A.M. How accurate is weight estimation in the emergency department? *Emerg. Med. Australas.* **2005**, *17*, 113–116. [CrossRef] [PubMed]
8. Ahmed, N.N.; Pearce, S.E. Acute care for the elderly: A literature review. *Popul. Health Manag.* **2010**, *13*, 219–225. [CrossRef] [PubMed]
9. Webster, D.; Celik, O. Systematic review of Kinect applications in elderly care and stroke rehabilitation. *J. Neuroeng. Rehabil.* **2014**, *11*, 108. [CrossRef] [PubMed]
10. Gasparrini, S.; Cippitelli, E.; Spinsante, S.; Gambi, E. A Depth-Based Fall Detection System Using a Kinect® Sensor. *Sensors* **2014**, *14*, 2756–2775. [CrossRef] [PubMed]
11. Procházka, A.; Schätz, M.; Vyšata, O.; Vališ, M. Microsoft Kinect Visual and Depth Sensors for Breathing and Heart Rate Analysis. *Sensors* **2016**, *16*, 996. [CrossRef] [PubMed]
12. Publication, C.A.A. *Civil Aviation Safety Authority—Standard Passenger and Baggage Weights*; Civil Aviation Safety Authority: Woden Valley, Australia, 1990. Available online: https://www.casa.gov.au/file/104861/download?token=E70-zaqD (accessed on 19 April 2018)
13. Elliott, A.F. Why a Finnish Airline Is Weighing Passengers Before They Board, 2017. Available online: https://www.telegraph.co.uk/travel/news/why-a-finnish-airline-is-weighing-every-passenger-before-they-board/ (accessed on 2 April 2018).
14. Board, C.A.S. *Aviation Occurrence Report*; Arrow Air Inc. Douglas DC-8-63 N950JW; Gander International Airport: Gander, NL, Canada, 1988.
15. Pfitzner, C.; May, S.; Nüchter, A. Neural network-based visual body weight estimation for drug dosage finding. *Proceedings of the SPIE Medical Imaging 2016*; SPIE: San Diego, CA, USA, 2016.
16. Ragoschke-Schumm, A.; Razouk, A.; Lesmeister, M.; Helwig, S.; Grunwald, I.Q.; Fassbender, K. Dosage Calculation for Intravenous Thrombolysis of Ischemic Stroke: To Weigh or to Estimate? *Cerebrovas. Dis. Extra* **2017**, *7*, 103–110. [CrossRef] [PubMed]
17. Argall, J.A.W.; Wright, N.; Mackway-Jones, K.; Jackson, R. A comparison of two commonly used methods of weight estimation. *Arch. Dis. Child.* **2003**, *88*, 789–790. [CrossRef] [PubMed]
18. Krieser, D.; Nguyen, K.; Kerr, D.; Jolley, D.; Clooney, M.; Kelly, A.M. Parental weight estimation of their child's weight is more accurate than other weight estimation methods for determining childrens weight in an emergency department? *Emerg. Med. J.* **2007**, *24*, 756–759. [CrossRef] [PubMed]
19. Pirker, K.; Rüther, M.; Bischof, H.; Skrabal, F. Human Body Volume Estimation in a Clinical Environment, 2010. Available online: http://citeseerx.ist.psu.edu/viewdoc/download?doi=10.1.1.173.3803&rep=rep1&type=pdf (accessed on 2 January 2018).
20. Pfitzner, C.; May, S.; Merkl, C.; Breuer, L.; Braun, J.; Dirauf, F. Libra3D: Body Weight Estimation for Emergency Patients in Clinical Environments with a 3D Structured Light Sensor. In Proceedings of the IEEE International Conference on Robotics and Automation, Seattle, WA, USA, 26–30 May 2015.
21. Pfitzner, C.; May, S.; Merkl, C. Vorrichtung und verfahren zur optischen erfassung eines gewichtes einer person. Available online: https://patents.google.com/patent/DE102016103543A1/de (accessed on 5 January 2018).
22. Pfitzner, C.; May, S.; Nüchter, A. Evaluation of Features from RGB-D Data for Human Body Weight Estimation. In Proceedings of the 20th World Congress of the International Federation of Automatic Control (WC '17), Toulouse, France, 9–14 July 2017.
23. Robinson, M.; Parkinson, M.B. Estimating Anthropometry with Microsoft Kinect. In Proceedings of the 2nd International Digital Human Modeling Symposium, Ann Arbor, MI, USA, 11–14 June 2013.

24. Cook, T.S.; Couch, G.; Couch, T.J.; Kim, W.; Boonn, W.W. Using the Microsoft Kinect for Patient Size Estimation and Radiation Dose Normalization: Proof of Concept and Initial Validation. *J. Dig. Imaging* **2013**, *26*, 657–662. [CrossRef] [PubMed]
25. Velardo, C.; Dugelay, J.L. What can computer vision tell you about your weight? In Proceedings of the 20th European Signal Processing Conference EUSIPCO, Bucharest, Romania, 27–31August 2012.
26. Nguyen, T.V.; Feng, J.; Yan, S. Seeing Human Weight from a Single RGB-D Image. *J. Comput. Sci. Technol.* **2014**, *29*, 777–784. [CrossRef]
27. Labati, R.; Genovese, A.; Piuri, V.; Scotti, F. Weight Estimation from Frame Sequences Using Computational Intelligence Techniques. In Proceedings of the IEEE International Conference on Computational Intelligence for Measurement Systems and Applications (CIMSA), Tianjin, China, 2–4 July 2012; pp. 29–34.
28. Arigbabu, O.A.; Ahmad, S.M.S.; Adnan, W.A.W.; Yussof, S.; Iranmanesh, V.; Malallah, F.L. Estimating body related soft biometric traits in video frames. *Sci. World J.* **2014**, *2014*, doi:10.1155/2014/460973. [CrossRef] [PubMed]
29. Zhang, Z. Microsoft Kinect Sensor and Its Effect. *IEEE MultiMedia* **2012**, *19*, 4–10. [CrossRef]
30. Khoshelham, K.; Elberink, S.O. Accuracy and resolution of kinect depth data for indoor mapping applications. *Sensors* **2012**, *12*, 1437–1454. [CrossRef] [PubMed]
31. May, S. *3D Time-of-Flight Ranging for Robotic Perception in Dynamic Environments*; VDI-Verlag: Dusseldorf, Germany, 2009.
32. Sarbolandi, H.; Lefloch, D.; Kolb, A. Kinect range sensing: Structured-light versus Time-of-Flight Kinect. *Comput. Vis. Image Underst.* **2015**, *139*, 1–20. [CrossRef]
33. Draelos, M.; Qiu, Q.; Bronstein, A.; Sapiro, G. Intel realsense; Real low cost gaze. In Proceedings of the 2015 IEEE International Conference on Image Processing (ICIP), Quebec City, QC, Canada, 27–30 September 2015; pp. 2520–2524.
34. Winkler, T. Review Dell Precision M4800 Notebook. Available online: https://www.notebookcheck.net/Review-Dell-Precision-M4800-Notebook.104416.0.html (accessed on 3 April 2018).
35. Zhang, Z. A Flexible New Technique for Camera Calibration. *IEEE Trans. Pattern Anal. Mach. Intell.* **2000**, *22*, 1330–1334. [CrossRef]
36. Gonzalez-Jorge, H.; Rodríguez-Gonzálvez, P.; Martínez-Sánchez, J.; González-Aguilera, D.; Arias, P.; Gesto, M.; Díaz-Vilariño, L. Metrological comparison between Kinect I and Kinect II sensors. *Measurement* **2015**, *70*, 21–26. [CrossRef]
37. Vidas, S.; Moghadam, P.; Bosse, M. 3D thermal mapping of building interiors using an RGB-D and thermal camera. In Proceedings of the 2013 IEEE International Conference on Robotics and Automation, Karlsruhe, Germany, 6–10 May 2013; pp. 2311–2318.
38. Lussier, J.T.; Thrun, S. Automatic calibration of RGBD and thermal cameras. In Proceedings of the 2014 IEEE/RSJ International Conference on Intelligent Robots and Systems (IROS 2014), Chicago, IL, USA, 14–18 September 2014; pp. 451–458.
39. Bradski, G.; Kaehler, A. *Learning OpenCV*, 1st ed.; O'Reilly Media: Sebastopol, CA, USA, 2008.
40. Fischler, M.A.; Bolles, R.C. Random Sample Consensus: A Paradigm for Model Fitting with Applications to Image Analysis and Automated Cartography. *Commun. ACM* **1981**, *24*, 381–395. [CrossRef]
41. Szeliski, R. *Computer Vision: Algorithms and Applications*, 1st ed.; Springer: New York, NY, USA, 2010.
42. Dalal, N.; Triggs, B. Histograms of oriented gradients for human detection. In Proceedings of the IEEE Computer Society Conference on Computer Vision and Pattern Recognition, CVPR, San Diego, CA, USA, 20–25 June 2005; Volume I, pp. 886–893.
43. Linder, T.; Wehner, S.; Arras, K.O. Real-time full-body human gender recognition in (RGB)-D data. In Proceedings of the IEEE International Conference on Robotics and Automation, ICRA 2015, Seattle, WA, USA, 26–30 May 2015; pp. 3039–3045.
44. Riedmiller, M.; Braun, H. A Direct Adaptive Method for Faster Backpropagation Learning: The RPROP Algorithm. In Proceedings of the IEEE International Conference on Neural Networks, San Francisco, CA, USA, 28 March–1 April 1993; pp. 586–591.
45. Deutschland, S.B. Mikrozensus - Fragen zur Gesundheit 2009. Available online: https://www.destatis.de/DE/ZahlenFakten/GesellschaftStaat/Gesundheit/GesundheitszustandRelevantesVerhalten/Tabellen/GesundheitszustandBehandlungsanlaesse.pdf?__blob=publicationFile (accessed on 3 April 2018).

15

Scattering of Light from the Systemic Circulatory System

Sidra Batool [1,*], Mehwish Nisar [1,2], Fabio Mangini [3], Fabrizio Frezza [1] and Eugenio Fazio [2]

1 Department of Information Engineering, Electronics and Telecommunications, Sapienza University of Rome, Via Eudossiana 18, 00184 Rome, Italy; mehwish.nisar@uniroma1.it (M.N.); fabrizio.frezza@uniroma1.it (F.F.)
2 Department of Fundamental and Applied Sciences for Engineering, Sapienza University of Rome, Via A. Scarpa 16, 00161 Rome, Italy; eugenio.fazio@uniroma1.it
3 Department of Information Engineering, University of Brescia, Via Branze 59, 25123 Brescia, Italy; fabio.mangini@uniroma1.it
* Correspondence: sidra.batool@uniroma1.it

Abstract: There are many factors of methodological origin that influence the measurement of optical properties of the entire circulatory system which consists of blood as the basic component. The basic idea of this review article is to provide the optical properties of the circulatory system with all those factors of influence that have been employed in biomedical optics for different applications. We begin with the available optical properties, i.e., absorption, scattering and, reduced scattering coefficient, in general for any tissue inside the human body and prominent scattering theories (e.g., light, X-rays, neutrons) that are helpful in this regard. We have reviewed and compiled already available formulas and their respective available data for different human tissues for these optical properties. Then we have descended to the blood composition and to different scattering techniques available in the literature to study scattering and light propagation inside blood. We have reviewed both computational and theoretical scattering techniques.

Keywords: optical properties; scattering theories; circulatory system

---

1. Introduction

When light interacts with the human body, several phenomena take place depending on the type of tissue and on its biological composition [1], such as reflection, refraction, absorption, scattering or even emission. The different optical properties of the tissues influence the interaction with light and consequently the various diagnostic and therapeutic applications. The heterogeneity of the tissues increases the complexity of the analysis of interactions with light; therefore, following a methodological approach for further study, it is useful to first analyse the factors that influence the average optical properties on a macroscopic scale and then deal with the microscopic effects related to the heterogeneity of the individual structures. The optical properties that mainly describe the transport of light in the tissues are absorption and scattering. The absorption of light is due to the electronic transitions that can occur in the molecules that make up the tissues and whose selectivity, consequently, gives colour to the tissues (often the coloration of the fabric is identified with that part of the molecule responsible for absorption called chromophore, a word coming from the Greek term "chroma" which means colour) [2–5]. Electronic transitions typically have energies of the order of electronvolts and therefore occur in the optical band, i.e., partly in the UV, in the visible and partly in the IR too where the molecular transitions (rotations/vibrations/roto-vibrations) have more their characteristic energies. The scattering of light is instead due to fluctuations and discontinuities in the refractive index of the optical tissue due to the presence of cells, membranes, microstructures and sub-cellular components [6]. The most used technique for the characterization of the optical properties of matter is optical spectroscopy, with which it is possible to determine the light absorption and emission absorption properties. It is possible to carry out both absorption spectroscopy, revealing the spectral components of the sent light which have been absorbed or diffused due to absorption or scattering, and emission spectroscopy, in which case, given a high energy excitation, the spectral components of the radiation emitted by the material are measured [7–10]. In the next section, we shall describe the scattering and absorption of light by biological tissues.

2. Fundamental Optical Properties of Tissues

Tissues are generally characterized by structural inhomogeneities of very different dimensions, from tenths of nanometers to hundreds of micrometers [11]. For this reason, many different techniques are used for the microscopic and macroscopic characterization of the optical properties of the tissues, as shown in Figure 1 [12–15], and many different simulation models have been implemented to highlight the specific behaviour of the materials and the propagation of the light inside them. The light scattering from spherical particles is mainly described by the Rayleigh and Mie theories. The Rayleigh scattering indicates scattering by small particles or mass density variation much smaller than the wavelength of light, while the Mie scattering indicates the scattering by particles comparable to or larger than the wavelength of light [16–22]. One of the simplest and most used models for light scattering by biological tissues implements a Mie scattering procedure. Such a model represents a biological tissue as a mixture of particles of varying sizes dispersed within a host matrix with a different refractive index [23,24]. Mie scattering is defined as when the size of the object is larger than the wavelength of light. This type of model is certainly effective even, if the idealization of the sphericity of the scattering centers leads to results sometimes different from the real behaviours. An alternative approach to Mie scattering is represented by the continuum model, in which a tissue is modeled as a continuous medium where there are fluctuations in density and therefore in the refractive index, which can be described through an autocorrelation function [25]. The Wiener–Khintchine theorem, in general, relates the autocorrelation function to the corresponding spectrum of the scattered power [26].

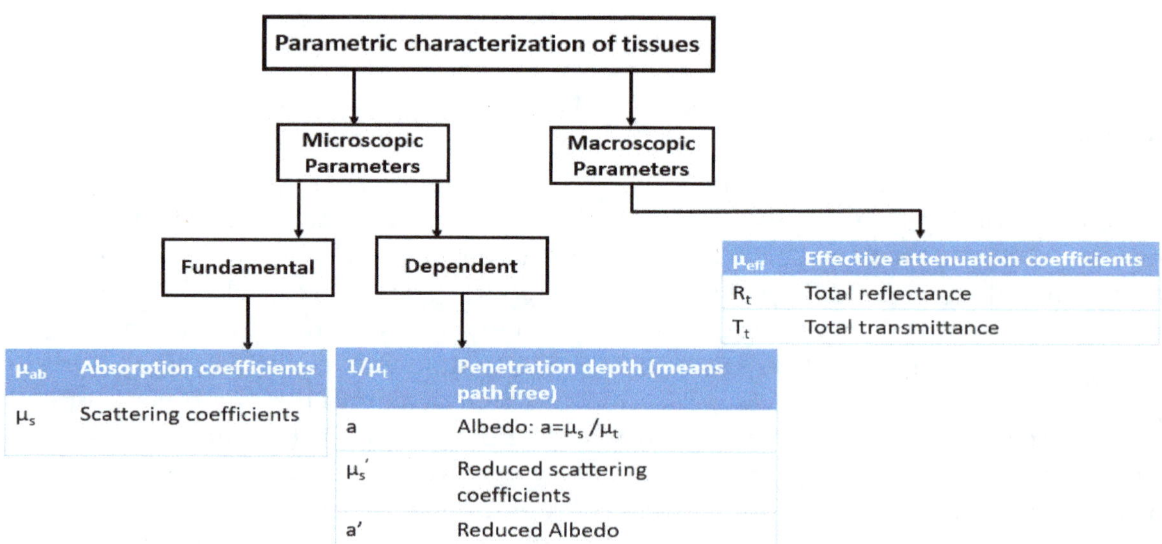

Figure 1. Parametric characterization of tissues on microscopic and macroscopic levels [27].

The popular scattering theories that have been employed in many fields of biomedical optics are Rayleigh and Mie scattering theories. The Rayleigh scattering indicates scattering by small particles or mass density variation much smaller than the wavelength of light, and Mie scattering indicates the scattering by particles comparable to or larger than the wavelength of light.

2.1. Absorption Coefficient

The absorption of light by an optimum volume of identical molecules can be expressed in terms of the absorption coefficient, which represents the probability that a photon is absorbed with respect to the medium according to its required path-length. Let us consider a homogeneous medium composed by absorbing molecules. The absorption coefficient is defined as the product between the probability that a photon is absorbed by a molecule (i.e., the cross-section a) and the density of the molecules present in the volume:

$$\mu_a = \rho_a \sigma_a \tag{1}$$

The absorption cross section measures the rate at which the photon energy is being absorbed from the light wave [27].

2.2. Scattering Coefficient

Similarly to absorption, the elastic scattering for single events (i.e., not for multiple scattering processes) in a certain medium can still be represented by a scattering coefficient s, that describes the probability of photon to be scattered during a unitary path-length. The reciprocal of s is called the scattering length of the object and denoted as the average distance traveled by a photon between consecutive scattering events (photon mean-free-path). Furthermore, the scattering coefficient may be defined as [28] as the product between the probability that a photon is diffused by a scattering center (i.e., the cross section s) and the density s of scatterers in the volume:

$$\mu_s = \rho_s \sigma_s \tag{2}$$

The scattering cross-section area is defined as the rate with which the power is removed from the initial S' direction towards the new S direction compatible with the medium, as shown in Figure 2. The probability that a photon is scattered within a certain solid angle is defined by the phase function p:

$$p = \frac{1}{\sigma_s} \frac{d\sigma_s}{d\Omega} \tag{3}$$

where the term $\frac{d\sigma_s}{d\Omega}$ represents the differential scattering cross section [29]. Both the scattering and the absorption coefficients depend on the light wavelength [30,31].

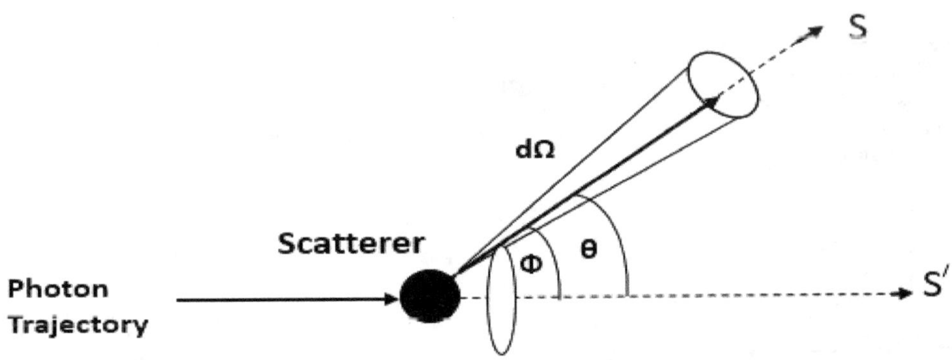

Figure 2. A photon initially traveling from S' is scattered into a differential solid angle $d\Omega$ along S. Here ϕ corresponds to the azimuthal angle from the scattered trajectory, and θ corresponds to the polar angle from the initial trajectory.

2.3. Reduced Scattering Coefficient

Instead of using the whole scattering theories, often an equivalent reduced scattering coefficient is used to describe both Mie and Rayleigh regimes. This reduced coefficient can effectively describe the dispersion properties of the main six different groups of tissues such as skin, breast, brain, bones, fibrous and fatty tissues. All of them are a set of small and large scatterers that act simultaneously. Its expression refers to the scattering efficiency at a reference visible wavelength 0 (usually the green @500 nm) according to the following wavelength-dependent expression:

$$\mu_s' = a\left(\frac{\lambda}{500\ (\text{nm})}\right)^{-b} \tag{4}$$

where a is the μ_s' value at the reference wavelength and b is the characteristic power dependence. A more explicit expression of the scattering coefficient separates the Rayleigh and the Mie contributions keeping the same wavelength-type dependence:

$$\mu_s' = a'\left(f_{Ray}\left(\frac{\lambda}{500\,\text{nm}}\right)^{-4} + (1 - f_{Ray})\left(\frac{\lambda}{500\,\text{nm}}\right)^{-b_{Mie}}\right) \tag{5}$$

where f_{Ray} and f_{Mie} represent the fraction of small and large scatterers, respectively and satisfy the conservation rule:

$$f_{Ray} + f_{Mie} = 1 \tag{6}$$

In Figure 3 the explicit expressions and values of μ_s' are reported for different tissues. All of them, as shown by the previous analytical expressions illustrated in Tables 1 and 2, have a hyperbolic decreasing dispersion increasing the wavelength, in the VIS-NIR spectral range [32–35].

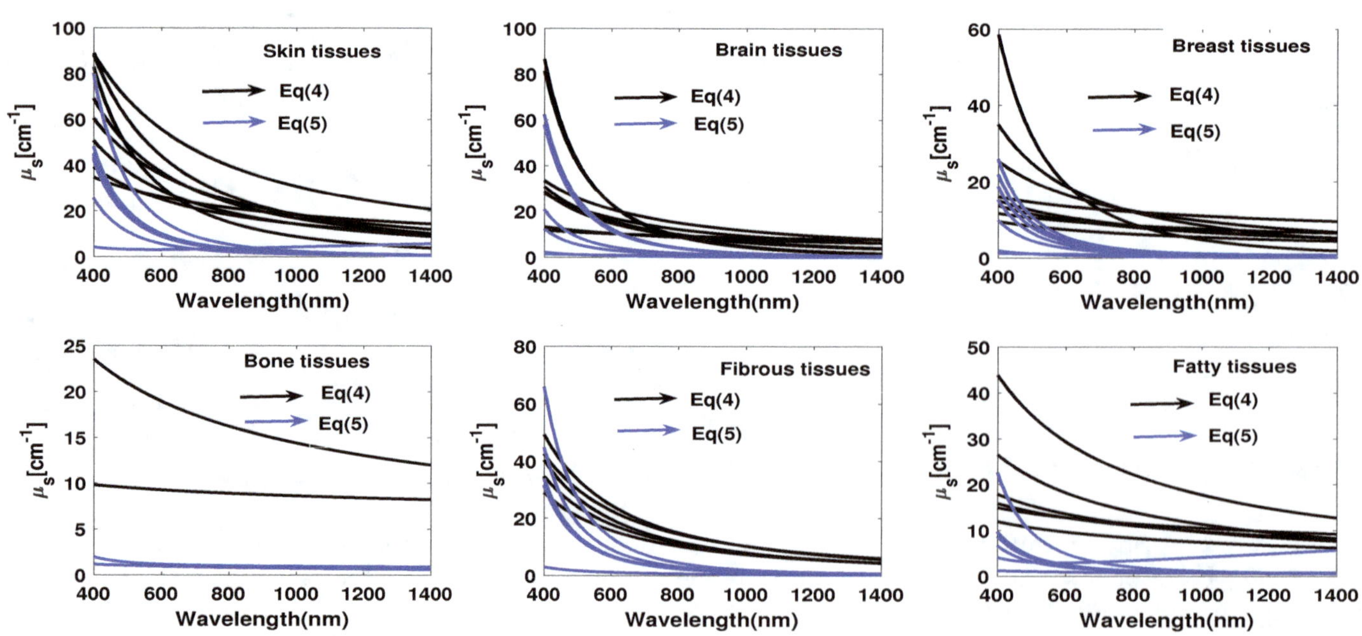

Figure 3. In the review literature, some measurement expressing the optical properties of tissues [27].

Table 1. Represents the different tissues (e.g., skin, brain, breast, bone) description using scattering parameters, where a is the $\mu_s{}'$ value at the reference wavelength and b is the characteristic power dependence and f_{Ray} or f_{Mie} demonstrated the fraction of small and large scatterers, respectively.

#	a	b	a′	f_{Ray}	f_{Mie}	Tissue Description	Ref
					Skin		
1	48.9	1.548	45.6	0.22	1.184	skin	[36]
2	47.8	2.453	42.9	0.76	0.351	skin	[35]
3	37.2	1.39	42.6	0.4	0.919	skin	[37]
4	60.1	1.722	58.3	0.31	0.919	skin	[38]
5	29.7	0.705	36.4	0.48	0.22	skin	[39]
6	45.3	1.292	43.6	0.41	0.562	dermis	[40]
7	68.7	1.161	66.7	0.29	0.689	epidermis	[40]
					Brain		
8	40.8	3.059	40.8	0	3.088	brain	[41]
9	10.9	0.334	13.3	0.36	0	cortex (frontal lobe)	[42]
10	11.6	0.601	15.7	0.53	0	cortex (temporal lobe)	[42]
11	20	1.629	29.1	0.81	0	astrocytoma of optic nerve	[42]
12	25.9	1.156	25.9	0	1.156	normal optic nerve	[42]
13	21.5	1.629	31	0.82	0	cerebellar white matter	[42]
14	41.8	3.254	41.8	0	3.254	medulloblastoma	[42]
15	21.4	1.2	21.4	0	1.2	brain	[25]
					Breast		
16	31.8	2.741	31.8	0	2.741	breast	[41]
17	11.8	0.775	15.2	0.58	0	breast	[41]
18	24.8	1.544	24.8	0	1.544	breast	[41]
19	20.1	1.054	20.2	0.18	0.638	breast	[41]
20	14.6	0.41	18.1	0.41	0	breast	[43]
21	12.5	0.837	17.4	0.6	0.0076	breast	[44]
22	8.3	0.617	11.2	0.54	0.009	breast	[44]
23	10.5	0.464	10.5	0	0.473	breast	[45]
					Bone		
24	9.5	0.141	9.7	0.04	0.116	skull	[42]
25	20.9	0.537	20.9	0	0.537	skull	[46]

Table 2. Represents the different tissues (e.g., fibrous and fatty) description using scattering parameters, where a is the $\mu_s{}'$ value at the reference wavelength and b is the characteristic power dependence and f_{Ray} or f_{Mie} demonstrated the fraction of small and large scatterers, respectivelypectively.

#	a	b	a′	f_{Ray}	f_{Mie}	Tissue Discription	Ref
				Fibrous tissue			
26	33.6	1.712	37.3	0.72	0	tumor	[41]
27	30.1	1.549	30.1	0.02	1.521	prostate	[47]
28	27.2	1.768	29.7	0.61	0.585	glandular breast	[48]
29	24.1	1.618	25.8	0.49	0.7845	fibrocystic breast	[48]
30	20.7	1.487	22.8	0.6	0.327	carcinoma breast	[48]
				Fatty tissues			
31	13.7	o.385	14.7	0.16	0.250	Subcutaneous fat	[37]
32	10.6	0.520	11.2	0.29	0.089	Adipose breast	[48]
33	15.4	0.680	15.4	0.00	0.680	Subcutaneous adipose	[39]
34	35.2	0.988	34.2	0.26	0.567	Subcut. fat	[40]
35	21.6	0.930	21.1	0.17	0.651	Subcut. adipocytes	[40]
36	14.1	0.530	na	na	na	Adipose	[49]

3. Scattering of Light from Nerves, Veins, and Arteries

The polarization of light contributes to the observed appearance of the skin and its relative colour, since the reflection/refraction/diffraction of the light on it depends strictly on the degree of polarization of the light used. Since on some chromatic bands the absorption is very high and on others much less, the observed effects can be either superficial or deep, with light penetrations in the underlying layers either limited to a few microns or extended to several centimeters [50–52].

Based on conventional tissue staining protocols, pathological understanding of arterial diseases is mainly attributable to observations that have been reported in the literature [53]. A new venue for visualizing pathological changes in the extracellular matrix caused by the progression of atherosclerosis is the emerging development of Nonlinear Optical Microscopy (NLOM), especially in second-harmonic generation, two-photon excited fluorescence and, coherent Raman scattering. In general, these techniques can offer rapid three-dimensional imaging in the biomedical sector. In this review, we look at recent progress in applications related to arterial disease imaging using various forms of NLOM [53,54].

During internal propagation, the light undergoes both scattering, due to the strong inhomogeneity of the biological tissue (formed by dispersed micro and nanostructures, filamentous proteins, cells, fibres, successive layers of dermis, fat, veins and capillaries, etc.), and absorption, due to the presence of many chromophores (the main ones being haemoglobin and melanin [39,55,56]. The melanin function is essentially the absorption of light radiation on some spectral bands, for example, the erythemal UV between 290 and 320 nm, which could be harmful to the body). Through the skin, the veins are also visible and with them the blood circulating inside, being able to make remote measurements in a non-invasive and non-bloody way. Focusing attention on it, the absorption spectrum of oxygenated (HbO_2) and deoxygenated haemoglobin (Hb) is shown in Figure 4 [57].

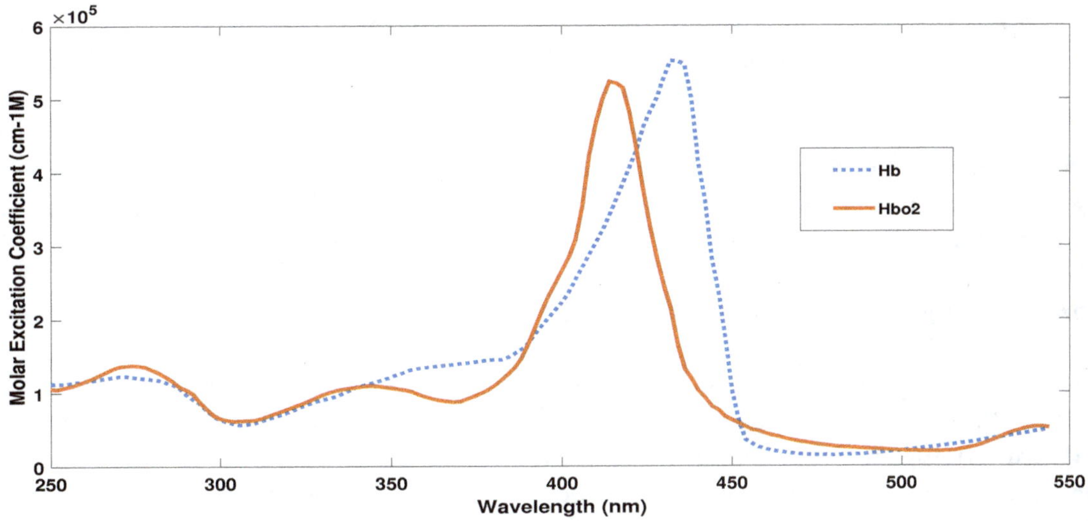

Figure 4. The graph shows the best-estimated spectrum of Hb and HbO_2 from the various sources by Scott Prahl Data [57].

Color	Wavelength Interval	Frequency Interval
Violet	430–380 nm	700–790 THz
Blue	500–430 nm	600–700 THz
Cyan	520–500 nm	580–600 THz
Green	565–520 nm	530–580 THz
Yellow	590–565 nm	510–530 THz
Orange	625–590 nm	480–410 THz
Red	740–625 nm	405–480 THz

Figure 5. White light spectrum with its corresponding wavelength and frequency interval.

3.1. Haemoglobin Absorption

As you can see, the two forms, Hb and HbO_2, have absorption peaks posted with respect to each other. Therefore, by making differential absorption measurements on the different peaks, it is possible to control the level of oxygenation with great precision [58]. This different absorption also influences the observed colour of the blood: oxygenated blood, within arteries, has a cherry red colour while the deoxygenated blood, present in the veins, is dark red (but through the skin it looks blue). The absorption rate of light is higher in the blue band than in the red band, because dark red deoxygenated venous blood has a higher absorption coefficient than cherry red oxygenated arterial blood in the human body [59]. However, the arteries are generally brighter than the veins. This is because they have thick vessel walls as they have to withstand high pressures due to heart beating. The arterial walls are typical of elastic and sometimes muscular tissues, which dilate and contract both to withstand the large pressures induced by heart pulses and to regulate and control the resistance of the flow in the capillary network. The veins, on the other hand, are used only for the transport of low oxygen blood to the organs used for its purification, lungs, and liver. For this reason, venous blood appears very dark to the eye [60,61]. Arteries and veins have different dispositions within the human body too: the arteries travel deep and are difficult to see and not accessible from the outside; the veins, on the other hand, are typically superficial and therefore can be easily monitored with non-invasive imaging techniques. However, it is possible to make non-bloody and non-invasive measurements also on the arteries by monitoring the retinal one: in fact, in the retina, there is a network of arterial capillaries between cones and rods of the retina. The central artery of the retina, through the dural sheath of the optic nerve, reaches the optic papilla, where it divides first into an ascending and descending branch and then, subsequently, into lateral and medial branches. In this way, a dense network of small vessels is formed that never anastomose and that is easily accessible for observation by intraocular retinal imaging techniques. For many medical applications, it is of great importance to measure blood pressure and check for abnormal changes in veins and arteries that could be analyzed in depth using these retinal imaging techniques. In fact, many diseases cause an abnormal ratio between the length, diameter, and cross-linking of arteries and veins. For example, in diabetic patients the veins are abnormally wide, while pancreatic diseases lead to a narrowing of the wall of the vessels which generates an increase in blood pressure [5,62]. Minhaj et al. have shown that by combining together the optical density ratio (ODR) and the tracking of blood vessels (BVT) it is possible to make and characterize the map of the vessels, both arteries and veins. This is often traced starting from the source nodes and uses the curvature and the angle to derive the whole network. This measurement technique, despite being qualitative, has an accuracy of 97.06% in identifying veins and arteries [63]. Furthermore, the different response of oxygenated and deoxygenated hemoglobin to electromagnetic excitation finds application in functional magnetic resonance [64].

3.2. Optical Properties of Human Blood and Its Composition

Normal human blood consists of red blood cells (RBCs or erythrocytes, $\pm 4500 \times 103/\mu L$ blood), white blood cells (leukocytes, $\pm 8 \times 103/\mu L$ blood), platelets (thrombocytes, $\pm 300 \times 103/\mu L$ blood) and blood plasma that mainly contains water, electrolytes, plasma proteins, carbohydrates, lipids and various extracellular vesicles. The major portion of RBCs consists of haemoglobin. In healthy human adults, the haemoglobin concentration in blood is 140 g/L in women and 155 g/L in men on average.

Scattering and absorption of light in the blood is largely conducted by red blood cells for many reasons. Firstly, it should be remembered, that the quantity of red blood cells is about 4000 times greater, than that of white blood cells and therefore, they constitute the largest mass fraction. In humans, red blood cells have the typical shape of flexible biconcave discs, 6–8 μm in diameter, and 2.5 μm thick [58,65,66]. They dominate blood light scattering over any other component of the blood both for their large size and for the contrast index of refraction between the red blood cells and the surrounding blood plasma. In fact, their refractive index has a value of approximately between 1.40 and 1.42 [67], due to the combination of HbO_2 (1.615) and water (1.333) [68], while the refractive index of plasma (and serum) ranges from 1.36 (@400 nm) to 1.34 (@800 nm) [69]. Absorption is instead dominated by hemoglobin, in the two deoxygenated Hb and oxygenated HbO_2 forms (Figure 5). Flow cytometric light scattering measurements are helpful to determine the concentration of RBCs and their volume fraction, the hemoglobin concentration, and to discriminate the health of blood cells, as for example thalassaemic vs normal RBCs [70–73].

4. Computational Techniques in Literature

Many numerical models are used to describe the propagation of light within diffusive environments such as for example liquid suspensions of red blood cells. It is the most used, the Monte Carlo (MC) method is one of the most used statistical methods to describe multivariable dynamic systems. It is based on the dynamic simulation of the propagation of a population of elements which in our case are photons. By imposing the rules of absorption and diffusion of light passing through a suspension of RBCs, the MC method analyses in parallel the propagation of a set of photons statistically independent through the suspension. At each iteration a single photon may (1) not suffer anything and continue straight or (2) be absorbed or (3) be diffused. Statistically reconstructing the evolution of the entire population is initially possible to estimate the behaviour of light when passing through an RBCs suspension. The MC method is accessible to record the transmission and reflection coefficients from the tissues; from a comparison of the numerical results with the experimental data, it is possible to identify the micro topologies developed, the succession of the tissue layers, the properties of the materials, and the efficiencies of absorption and scattering [74,75].

The finite differences in time domain (FDTD) is a method of solving the electromagnetic wave equation using a step integration (finite differences) in the time domain. The method, in principle conceptually simple, is based on the definition of a derivative as a ratio of finite and not infinitesimal increments. This approximation is very delicate and leads to converging results if the rules defined by the Nyquist–Shannon sampling theorem [in the book Advances in FDTD Computational Electrodynamics] are respected [76]. Subsequent versions of the model have been developed over the years to decrease the error resulting from sampling using more complex definitions of the derivative as a ratio of symmetrical increments with respect to the calculation point. The FDTD method is general and flexible in terms of implementation of the full-wave techniques used to solve complex biological scattering problems [77]. It is suitable for the numerical simulation of scattering from non-homogeneous objects of arbitrary forms, as it numerically solves Maxwell's equations and it can calculate the angular dispersion of the scattered light [78,79]. For readers interested in the FDTD method, the book by Taflove [76] is recommended for further information. An effective method of optimizing the scattering results produced by FDTD simulations takes advantage of the Rytov approximation, and is often applied in tomography. Starting from the phase mapping of the scattered light and comparing it with the experimental data, the method exercises an iterative process of convergence to optimize the distribution of the scattering centers [80,81]. The Discrete Dipole Approximation (DDA) is closely related to the method of moments applicable for multiple scattering from RBCs. The working principle of this method is based on the decomposition of the volume into infinitesimal elements, each represented as a dipole. The electromagnetic field is calculated as the superposition of the injected field with the secondary ones emitted by the induced dipole sources [82]. Jiangping et al. performed a comparison of these methods, finding that the Rytov approximation is less accurate than DDA and FDTD methods [80].

5. Theoretical and Experimental Techniques in the Literature

There has been a considerable amount of consequence in applying polarization properties of light to biomedical imaging usage, in the recent years. Optical polarization imaging is examining to be a popular convenient non-invasive technique for the detection of biological structures. The ultimate goal is the detection of millimeter-sized small tissues in the biological texture. A few of the research that used polarization principles for biomedical imaging were expressed in the following section. Demos et al. reported that the techniques regarding polarization principles for non-invasive surface imaging of biological systems [83,84]. Polarization discrimination of the scattered photons were precisely used employing a non-rotating retarder polarimetric configuration to enhance the visualness of the subsurface textures. Jacques et al. [85] used the simple polarization principle for visualizing superficial layers of tissue such as skin, breast, brain, bones, connective tissue and fat. The study gives the detailed information on the transition of linearly polarized light into randomly polarized light using the light propagation through tissues. Results from the study demonstrated that the polarized light imaging of skin yields images based on backscattered photon from apparent epidermal and initial papillary dermis however, the birefringent dermal collagen immediately irregular polarized light.

Sankaran et al. [86] described the light propagates through tissue phantoms with densely packed scatterers show the changes in the properties of polarization. To study the increase and decrease in linear and circular polarization were used polystyrene microspheres suspended in an aqueous solution. This study was playing a vital role in designing and optimizing polarimetric techniques for tissue imaging and diagnostics. Shamaraj et al. [87,88] reported the study of scattered polarized light from highly scattering media are helpful for an analytical model and material characterization techniques. This study might be described in understanding the techniques for imaging tissues and hidden objects, which can be, used for the treatment of malignant diseases and diagnostics. Kari et al. [89] investigated the use of polarized light reflections to image tissues such as wood fibers. The components of the reflected light from the wood fibers contained information regarding the structure of the tissue.

They described the wood-fiber absorption, scattering cross sections, and scattering matrices in the ray-optics approximation. They computed the complicated internal structure of the wood fibers.

5.1. Fundamentals of Polarized Light Scattering

An incident of polarized light on an object can be described as two orthogonal linear polarization components of the incident light field parallel $\mathbf{E_{i||}}$ and perpendicular $\mathbf{E_{i\perp}}$ to the scattering plane shown in Figure 6.

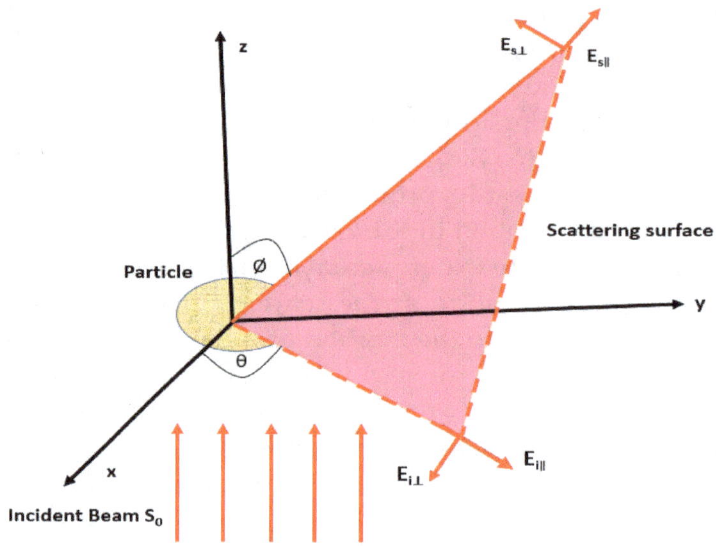

Figure 6. Geometry represents the scattering of light by an object located at the origin.

This figure represents the geometry of the scattering of light by an object (a particle representing the primary components of a biological structure). Here, the incident light beam $\mathbf{S_0}$ is parallel to the $z-axis$, θ and ϕ are the scattering angles in the scattering plane and in the plane perpendicular to the scattering plane, respectively. The detecting plane located at a distance r from the origin along the vector $\mathbf{S_1}$. two orthogonal polarization components, $\mathbf{E_{s\perp}}$ and $\mathbf{E_{s||}}$ of the scattered light formed a specific state of polarization depending on the amplitudes and phase shifts between components. The linear relationship between incident and scattered components can be described by the transformation of an arbitrarily polarized light (linear, circular, or elliptical) [90,91].

$$\begin{bmatrix} \mathbf{E_{s||}} \\ \mathbf{E_{s\perp}} \end{bmatrix} = \frac{e^{-ik(r-z)}}{-ikr} \begin{bmatrix} S_1 & S_2 \\ S_3 & S_4 \end{bmatrix} \begin{bmatrix} \mathbf{E_{i||}} \\ \mathbf{E_{i\perp}} \end{bmatrix} \tag{7}$$

where $k = \frac{2\pi}{\lambda}$ is a wave number, $\iota = \sqrt{-1}$, r represents the distance from the scatterer to the detector, z is the position coordinate of the scatterer. The matrix elements from $\mathbf{S_1}$ to $\mathbf{S_4}$ are described the amplitude of the scattering matrix (S-matrix) or Jones matrix. Each element depends on an elevation and azimuthal angles θ and ϕ, which contain information regarding the scatterer. Both phase and amplitude must be measured to evaluate the amplitude scattering matrix. The Jones matrix elements of transparent optical materials without sign ambiguity can be determined by using polarimetric methods.

5.2. Polarimetric Imaging

Polarimetry is the technique of measuring polarization state and interaction of polarized light with the target object always returns the change in the state of polarization of the interacting light. Weakly scattered light retains its polarization state easily, meanwhile strongly scattered light does not retain its polarization state [92]. Investigating the state of polarization of light interaction with the target results in a better imaging procedure to extract useful information from the target.

5.3. Stokes Parameter

The polarization state of light can be adequately demonstrated by the four Stokes parameters as shown below.

$$I = \mathbf{E}_x^2 + \mathbf{E}_y^2 \tag{8}$$

$$Q = \mathbf{E}_x^2 - \mathbf{E}_y^2 \tag{9}$$

$$U = 2\mathbf{E}_x\mathbf{E}_y \cos\delta \tag{10}$$

$$V = 2\mathbf{E}_x\mathbf{E}_y \sin\delta \tag{11}$$

where $\mathbf{E}_x$ and $\mathbf{E}_y$ describes the maximum amplitudes of the optical components of the field in x and y directions, respectively, and δ describes the phase difference between the optical components of the field.

I expresses the total intensity of light;

Q expresses the amount of linear horizontal or vertical polarization;

U expresses the amount of linear +45° or −45° polarization;

V expresses the amount of right or left circular polarization contained in the light beam. The Stokes matrix may be written as:

$$\mathbf{S} = \begin{bmatrix} I \\ Q \\ U \\ V \end{bmatrix} = \begin{bmatrix} I_H + I_V \\ I_H - I_V \\ I_P - I_M \\ I_R - I_L \end{bmatrix} \tag{12}$$

where I_H and I_V are light intensities measured with horizontally and vertically oriented linear polarizers, I_P and I_M are measured with +45° and −45° oriented linear polarizers, I_R and I_L are measured with right circularly and left circularly oriented linear polarizers in front of a detector, respectively.

5.4. Mueller Matrix

When light comes in contact with the object, the polarization state of the light beam changes with respect to the medium. Eventually, the incident and exciting beam will have a different state of polarized light. The polarization of the scattered light from an object in far field shown in Figure 1. is investigated the Stokes vector S_s associated with the Stokes vector of the incident light S_i connected by the matrix equation S_s = M S_i, where M is the normalized scattering matrix (Mueller matrix) [93,94].

$$\begin{bmatrix} I_s \\ Q_s \\ U_s \\ V_s \end{bmatrix} = \begin{bmatrix} M_{11} & M_{12} & M_{13} & M_{14} \\ M_{21} & M_{22} & M_{23} & M_{24} \\ M_{31} & M_{32} & M_{33} & M_{34} \\ M_{41} & M_{42} & M_{43} & M_{44} \end{bmatrix} \begin{bmatrix} I_i \\ Q_i \\ U_i \\ V_i \end{bmatrix} \tag{13}$$

Elements of the Mueller matrix depends on the scattering angle the wavelength of light, and the optical parameters of the object with the corresponding geometries. Element M_{11} tell us the information of the incident light is unpolarized, and scattered light is a function of the moving angles, it allows long-range structure rather than the other light scattering matrix elements. Element M_{12} is access by measuring the total scattered field intensity for a horizontally linearly polarized incoming light and subtracting the total scattered field intensity for a vertically linearly polarized incoming light. Element M_{22} refers to the ratio of depolarized light to the total scattered light. M_{34} refers to the transformation of the 45° obliquely polarized incident light to circularly polarized scattered light.

The elements M_{33} and M_{44} also displays the accurate measurement of the scattering beam from the object [95–97].

6. Conclusions

In this article, we have reviewed and compiled the optical properties of human tissues and the circulatory system with the main focus on blood. From this literature review, one of the main conclusions is that there are numerous factors of physical and methodological origin that are responsible for the study of the optical properties that anyone should aware of before performing own optical properties measurements. We have pointed out the main factors that influence absorption spectra of whole blood and hence influence optical properties. Revision of available polarimetric techniques can be helpful for the reader in the practice of biomedical optics. From this, we hope that we have provided the reader with a set of optical property spectra for whole blood and different polarimetric techniques that can be used in the practice of biomedical optics.

Author Contributions: The authors S.B. conceived the presented idea. S.B. developed the formulation or evolution of overarching research goals and aims. and performed the computations. Following co-authors (M.N., F.M., F.F., E.F.) encouraged first author to investigate a specific aspect and supervised the findings of this work. All authors provided critical feedback and helped in equal contribution to the formation of the research article. All authors have read and agreed to the published version of the manuscript.

References

1. Tang, J.; Fu, C. Preliminary experimental research on skin reflection, transmission and absorption of light rays. *Chin. J. Lasers* **1987**, *7*, 1-14.
2. Lister, T.; Wright, P.A.; Chappell, P.H. Optical properties of human skin. *J. Biomed. Opt.* **2012**, *17*, 090901. [CrossRef] [PubMed]
3. Cuccia, D.J.; Bevilacqua, F.P.; Durkin, A.J.; Ayers, F.R.; Tromberg, B.J. Quantitation and mapping of tissue optical properties using modulated imaging. *J. Biomed. Opt.* **2009**, *14*, 024012. [CrossRef] [PubMed]
4. Beck, G.C.; Akgun, N.; Ruck, A.; Steiner, R. Design and characterisation of a tissue phantom system for optical diagnostics. *Lasers Med. Sci.* **1998**, *17*, 160–171. [CrossRef]
5. Tuchin, V.V.; Maksimova, I.L.; Zimnyakov, D.A.; Kon, I.L.; Mavlyutov, A.H.; Mishin, A.A. Light propagation in tissues with controlled optical properties. *J. Biomed. Opt.* **1997**, *2*, 401–418. [CrossRef]
6. Kim, M.K. Principles and techniques of digital holographic microscopy. *SPIE Rev.* **2010**, *1*, 018005. [CrossRef]
7. Yodh, A.; Chance, B. Spectroscopy and imaging with diffusing light. *Phys. Today* **1995**, *3*, 34–41. [CrossRef]
8. Hardy, J.D.; Hammel, H.T.; Murgatroyd, D. Spectral transmittance and reflectance of excised human skin. *J. Appl. Physiol.* **1956**, *2*, 257–264. [CrossRef]
9. Papadopoulos, M.G.; Sadlej, A.J.; Leszczynski, J. *Non-Linear Optical Properties of Matter*; Springer: Dordrecht, The Netherlands, 2006.
10. Asahara, A.; Nishiyama, A.; Yoshida, S.; Kondo, K.I.; Nakajima, Y.; Minoshima, K. Dual-comb spectroscopy for rapid characterization of complex optical properties of solids. *Opt. Lett.* **2016**, *41*, 4971–4974. [CrossRef]
11. Lin, S.P.; Wang, L.; Jacques, S.L.; Tittel, F.K. Measurement of tissue optical properties by the use of oblique-incidence optical fiber reflectometry. *Appl. Opt.* **1997**, *1*, 136–143. [CrossRef]
12. Wilson, B.C.; Patterson, M.S.; Flock, S.T. Indirect versus direct techniques for the measurement of the optical properties of tissues. *Photochem. Photobiol.* **1987**, *46*, 601–608. [CrossRef] [PubMed]
13. Schmitt, J.M.; Knuttel, A.; Bonner, R.F. Measurement of optical properties of biological tissues by low-coherence reflectometry. *Appl. Opt.* **1993**, *32*, 6032–6042. [CrossRef] [PubMed]
14. Batool, S.; Nisar, M.; Mangini, F.; Frezza, F.; Fazio, E. Polarization Imaging for Identifying the Microscopical Orientation of Biological Structures. In Proceedings of the URSI GASS Conference, Rome, Italy, 29 August 2020.
15. Frezza, F.; Mangini, F.; Muzi, M.; Stoja, E. In silico validation procedure for cell volume fraction estimation through dielectric spectroscopy. *J. Biol. Phys.* **2015**, *41*, 223–234. [CrossRef] [PubMed]

16. Frezza, F.; Mangini, F.; Tedeschi, N. Introduction to electromagnetic scattering: Tutorial. *JOSA A* **2018**, *35*, 163–173. [CrossRef]
17. Frezza, F.; Mangini, F.; Tedeschi, N. Introduction to electromagnetic scattering, part II. tutorial. *JOSA A* **2020**, *37*, 1300–1315. [CrossRef]
18. Batool, S.; Frezza, F.; Mangini, F.; Xu, Y.L. Scattering from multiple PEC sphere using Translation Addition Theorems for Spherical Vector Wave Function. *J. Quant. Spectrosc. Radiat. Transf.* **2020**, *248*, 106905. [CrossRef]
19. Batool, S.; Naqvi, Q.A.; Fiaz, M.A. Scattering from a cylindrical obstacle deeply buried beneath a planar non-integer dimensional dielectric slab using Kobayashi potential method. *Opt. Int. J. Light Electron Opt.* **2018**, *153*, 95–108. [CrossRef]
20. Prieve, D.C.; Walz, J.Y. Scattering of an evanescent surface wave by a microscopic dielectric sphere. *Appl. Opt.* **1993**, *32*, 1629–1641. [CrossRef]
21. Frezza, F.; Mangini, F. Vectorial spherical-harmonics representation of an inhomogeneous elliptically polarized plane wave. *JOSA A* **2015**, *32*, 1379–1383. [CrossRef]
22. Batool, S.; Benedetti, A.; Frezza, F.; Mangini, F.; Xu, Y.L. Effect of Finite Terms on the Truncation Error of Addition Theorems for Spherical Vector Wave Function, PhotonIcs. In Proceedings of the IEEE Electromagnetics Research Symposium-Spring (PIERS Spring), Rome, Italy, 17–20 June 2019; pp. 2795–2801.
23. Bassan, P.; Kohler, A.; Martens, H.; Lee, J.; Byrne, H.J.; Dumas, P.; Gazi, E.; Brown, M.; Clarke, N.; Gardner, P. Resonant Mie scattering (RMieS) correction of infrared spectra from highly scattering biological samples. *Analyst* **2010**, *135*, 268–277. [CrossRef]
24. Graaff, R.; Aarnoudse, J.G.; Zijp, J.R.; Sloot, P.M.; De Mul, F.F.; Greve, J.; Koelink, M.H. Reduced light-scattering properties for mixtures of spherical particles: A simple approximation derived from Mie calculations. *Appl. Opt.* **1992**, *31*, 1370–1376. [CrossRef]
25. Yi, J.; Backman, V. Imaging a full set of optical scattering properties of biological tissues by inverse spectroscopic optical coherence tomography. *Opt. Lett.* **2012**, *37*, 4443–4445. [CrossRef]
26. Fung, A.K. A note on the Wiener-Khintchine theorem for autocorrelation. *Proc. IEEE* **1967**, *55*, 594–595. [CrossRef]
27. Jacques, S.L. Optical properties of biological tissues: A review. *Phys. Med. Biol.* **2013**, *11*, 37–61. [CrossRef]
28. Jacques, S.L.; Prahl, S.A. *ECE532 Biomedical Optics*; Oregon Graduate Institute: Washington, DC, USA, 1998.
29. Gazdaru, D.; Chilom, C.; Calin, M.A.; Geanta, C.; Popescu, A. Laser radiation propagation and heat transfer into cells and tissues. *Rom. J. Biophys.* **2008**, *18*, 73–85.
30. Schmidt, F.E. Development of a Time-Resolved Optical Tomography System for Neonatal Brain Imaging. Ph.D. Thesis, University of London, London, UK, 2000.
31. Grossweiner, L.I.; Grossweiner, J.B.; Rogers, B.G. *The Science of Phototherapy: An Introduction*; Springer: Dordrecht, The Netherlands, 2005.
32. Johns, M.; Giller, C.A.; German, D.C.; Liu, H. Determination of reduced scattering coefficient of biological tissue from a needle-like probe. *Opt. Express* **2005**, *13*, 4828–4842. [CrossRef]
33. Yariv, I.; Duadi, H.; Fixler, D. Optical method to extract the reduced scattering coefficient from tissue: Theory and experiments. *Opt. Lett.* **2018**, *43*, 5299–5302. [CrossRef]
34. Mourant, J.R.; Fuselier, T.; Boyer, J.; Johnson, T.M.; Bigio, I.J. Predictions and measurements of scattering and absorption over broad wavelength ranges in tissue phantoms. *Appl. Opt.* **1997**, *36*, 949–957. [CrossRef]
35. Jacques, S.L. Origins of tissue optical properties in the UVA, visible, and NIR regions. *OSA TOPS Adv. Opt. Imaging Photon Migr.* **1996**, *1*, 364–371.
36. Anderson, R.R.; Parrish, J.A. *Optical Properties of Human Skin*; Springer: Berlin/Heidelberg, Germany, 1982; pp. 147–194.
37. Simpson, C.R.; Kohl, M.; Essenpreis, M.; Cope, M. Near-infrared optical properties of ex vivo human skin and subcutaneous tissues measured using the Monte Carlo inversion technique. *Phys. Med. Biol.* **1998**, *43*, 2465. [CrossRef]
38. Saidi, I.S.; Jacques, S.L.; Tittel, F.K. Mie and Rayleigh modeling of visible-light scattering in neonatal skin. *Appl. Opt.* **1995**, *34*, 7410–7418. [CrossRef]
39. Bashkatov, A.N.; Genina, E.A.; Tuchin, V.V. Optical properties of skin, subcutaneous, and muscle tissues: A review. *J. Innov. Opt. Health Sci.* **2011**, *4*, 9–38. [CrossRef]
40. Salomatina, E.V.; Jiang, B.; Novak, J.; Yaroslavsky, A.N. Optical properties of normal and cancerous human skin in the visible and near infrared spectral range. *J. Biomed. Opt.* **2006**, *11*, 064026. [CrossRef]

41. Sandell, J.L.; Zhu, T.C. A review of in vivo optical properties of human tissues and its impact on PDT. *J. Biophotonics* **2011**, *4*, 773–787. [CrossRef]
42. Bevilacqua, F.; Berger, A.J.; Cerussi, A.E.; Jakubowski, D.; Tromberg, B.J. Broadband absorption spectroscopy in turbid media by combined frequency-domain and steady-state methods. *Appl. Opt.* **2000**, *39*, 6498–6507. [CrossRef] [PubMed]
43. Spinelli, L.; Torricelli, A.; Pifferi, A.; Taroni, P.; Danesini, G.M.; Cubeddu, R. Bulk optical properties and tissue components in the female breast from multiwavelength time-resolved optical mammography. *J. Biomed. Opt.* **2004**, *9*, 1137–1143. [CrossRef]
44. Cerussi, A.E.; Berger, A.J.; Bevilacqua, F.; Shah, N.; Jakubowski, D.; Butler, J.; Holcombe, R.F.; Tromberg, B.J. Sources of absorption and scattering contrast for near-infrared optical mammography. *Acad. Radiol.* **2001**, *8*, 211–218. [CrossRef]
45. Durduran, T.; Choe, R.; Culver, J.P.; Zubkov, L.; Holboke, M.J.; Giammarco, J.; Chance, B.; Yodh, A.G. Bulk optical properties of healthy female breast tissue. *Phys. Med. Biol.* **2002**, *47*, 2847. [CrossRef]
46. Firbank, H.; Hiraoka, M.; Essenpreis, M.; Delpy, D.T. Measurement of the optical properties of the skull in the wavelength range 650–950 nm. *Phys. Med. Biol.* **1993**, *38*, 503–510. [CrossRef]
47. Newman, C.; Jacques, S.L. Laser penetration into prostate for various wavelengths. *Lasers Surg. Med.* **1991**, *3*, 75.
48. Peters, V.G.; Wyman, D.R.; Patterson, M.S.; Frank, G.L. Optical properties of normal and diseased human breast tissues in the visible and near infrared. *Phys. Med. Biol.* **1990**, *35*, 1317. [CrossRef] [PubMed]
49. Alexandrakis, G.; Rannou, F.R.; Chatziioannou, A.F. Tomographic bioluminescence imaging by use of a combined optical-PET (OPET) system: A computer simulation feasibility study. *Phys. Med. Biol.* **2005**, *50*, 4225. [CrossRef] [PubMed]
50. Brinchmann, H.O.; Heier, H. Theoretical relations between light streak characteristics and optical properties of retinal vessels. *Acta Ophthalmol.* **1986**, *64*, 33–37. [CrossRef]
51. Fitzgerald, A.J.; Berry, E.; Zinovev, N.N.; Homer, V.S.; Miles, R.E.; Chamberlain, J.M.; Smith, M.A. Catalogue of human tissue optical properties at terahertz frequencies. *J. Biol. Phys.* **2003**, *29*, 123–128. [CrossRef]
52. Gerken, M.; Faris, G.W. Frequency-domain immersion technique for accurate optical property measurements of turbid media. *Opt. Lett.* **1999**, *24*, 1726–1728.
53. Ko, A.C.; Ridsdale, A.; Mostaco, G.L.B.; Major, A.; Stolow, A.; Sowa, M.G. Nonlinear optical microscopy in decoding arterial diseases. *Biophys. Rev.* **2012**, *4*, 323–334. [CrossRef]
54. Hu, J.J.; Humphrey, J.D.; Yeh, A.T. Characterization of engineered tissue development under biaxial stretch using nonlinear optical microscopy. *Tissue Eng. Part A* **2009**, *15*, 1553–1564. [CrossRef]
55. Bashkatov, A.N.; Genina, E.A.; Kochubey, V.I.; Tuchin, V.V. Optical properties of human skin, subcutaneous and mucous tissues in the wavelength range from 400 to 2000 nm. *J. Phys. D Appl. Phys.* **2005**, *15*, 2543–2554. [CrossRef]
56. Troy, T.L.; Thennadil, S.N. Optical properties of human skin in the near infrared wavelength range of 1000 to 2200 nm. *J. Biomed. Opt.* **2001**, *2*, 167–177. [CrossRef]
57. Gareau, D.S.; Gratzer, W.B.; Kollias, N. *Personal Communication from Gratzer*; Med. Res. Council Labs: Holly Hill, SC, USA; London, UK; N Kollias, Wellman Laboratories, Harvard Medical School: Boston, MA, USA. Available online: http://omlc.ogi.edu/spectra/hemoglobin/ (accessed on 10 October 2020).
58. Roggan, A.; Friebel, M.; Dorschel, K.; Hahn, A.; Mueller, G.J. Optical properties of circulating human blood in the wavelength range 400–2500 nm. *J. Biomed. Opt.* **1999**, *4*, 36–47. [CrossRef]
59. Kienle, A.; Lilge, L.; Vitkin, I.A.; Patterson, M.S.; Wilson, B.C.; Hibst, R.; Steiner, R. Why do veins appear blue? A new look at an old question. *Appl. Opt.* **1996**, *35*, 1151–1160. [CrossRef]
60. Bosschaart, N.; Edelman, G.J.; Aalders, M.C.; Van Leeuwen, T.G.; Faber, D.J. A literature review and novel theoretical approach on the optical properties of whole blood. *Lasers Med. Sci.* **2014**, *29*, 453–479. [CrossRef] [PubMed]
61. Hammer, M.; Roggan, A.; Schweitzer, D.; Muller, G. Optical properties of ocular fundus tissues-an in vitro study using the double-integrating-sphere technique and inverse Monte Carlo simulation. *Phys. Med. Biol.* **1995**, *40*, 963. [CrossRef] [PubMed]
62. Kondermann, C.; Kondermann, D.; Yan, M. Blood vessel classification into arteries and veins in retinal images. *Int. Soc. Opt. Eng.* **2007**, *12*, 651247.

63. Alam, M.; Son, T.; Toslak, D.; Lim, J.I.; Yao, X. Combining ODR and Blood Vessel Tracking for Artery/Vein Classification and Analysis in Color Fundus Images. *Transl. Vis. Sci. Technol.* **2018**, *2*, 1–23. [CrossRef] [PubMed]
64. Mangini, F.; Dinuzzo, M.; Maugeri, L.; Moraschi, M.; Mascali, D.; Cedola, A.; Frezza, F.; Giove, F.; Fratini, M. Numerical simulation of the blood oxygenation level-dependent functional magnetic resonance signal using finite element method. *Int. J. Numer. Methods Biomed. Eng.* **2020**, *36*, 3290. [CrossRef]
65. Shvalov, A.N.; Soini, J.T.; Chernyshev, A.V.; Tarasov, P.A.; Soini, E.; Maltsev, V.P. Light-scattering properties of individual erythrocytes. *Appl. Opt.* **1998**, *38*, 230–235. [CrossRef]
66. Borovoi, A.G.; Naats, E.I.; Oppel, U.G. Scattering of light by a red blood cell. *J. Biomed. Opt.* **1998**, *3*, 364–372. [CrossRef]
67. Kinnunen, M.; Kauppila, A.; Karmenyan, A.; Myllyla, R. Effect of the size and shape of a red blood cell on elastic light scattering properties at the single-cell level. *Biomed. Opt. Express* **2011**, *2*, 1803–1814. [CrossRef]
68. Mazeron, P.; Muller, S.; El Azouzi, H. Deformation of erythrocytes under shear: A small-angle light scattering study. *Biorheology* **1997**, *34*, 99–110. [CrossRef]
69. Liu, S.; Deng, Z.; Li, J.; Wang, J.; Huang, N.; Cui, R.; Zhang, Q.; Zhou, W.M.; Zhang, C.; Ye, Q.; et al. Measurement of the refractive index of whole blood and its components for a continuous spectral region. *J. Biomed. Opt.* **2019**, *24*, 035003. [CrossRef]
70. Tycko, D.H.; Metz, M.H.; Epstein, E.A.; Grinbaum, A. Flow-cytometric light scattering measurement of red blood cell volume and hemoglobin concentration. *Appl. Opt.* **1985**, *9*, 1355–1365. [CrossRef]
71. Yurkin, M.A.; Semyanov, K.A.; Tarasov, P.A.; Chernyshev, A.V.; Hoekstra, A.G.; Maltsev, V.P. Experimental and theoretical study of light scattering by individual mature red blood cells by use of scanning flow cytometry and a discrete dipole approximation. *Appl. Opt.* **2005**, *25*, 5249–5256. [CrossRef]
72. Amer, J.; Goldfarb, A.; Fibach, E. Flow cytometric measurement of reactive oxygen species production by normal and thalassaemic red blood cells. *Eur. J. Haematol.* **2003**, *2*, 84–90. [CrossRef]
73. Altendorf, E.; Zebert, D.; Holl, M.; Yager, P. Differential blood cell counts obtained using a microchannel based flow cytometer. *Proc. Int. Solid State Sens. Actuators Conf.* **1997**, *1*, 531–534.
74. Sakota, D.; Takatani, S. Quantitative analysis of optical properties of flowing blood using a photon-cell interactive Monte Carlo code: Effects of red blood cells orientation on light scattering. *J. Biomed. Opt.* **2012**, *5*, 1–12. [CrossRef]
75. Friebel, M.; Roggan, A.; Muller, G.J.; Meinke, M.C. Determination of optical properties of human blood in the spectral range 250 to 1100 nm using Monte Carlo simulations with hematocrit-dependent effective scattering phase functions. *J. Biomed. Opt.* **2006**, *3*, 21–34. [CrossRef]
76. Taflove, A. *Computational Electrodynamics: The Finite Difference Time-Domain Method*; Artech House: Norwood, MA, USA, 1995.
77. Lu, J.Q.; Yang, P.; Hu, X.H. Simulations of light scattering from a biconcave red blood cell using the finite-difference time-domain method. *J. Biomed. Opt.* **2005**, *10*, 024022. [CrossRef]
78. Brock, R.S.; Hu, X.H.; Yang, P.; Lu, J.Q. Evaluation of a parallel FDTD code and application to modeling of light scattering by deformed red blood cells. *Opt. Express* **2005**, *14*, 5279–5292. [CrossRef]
79. Brock, R.S.; Hu, X.H.; Weidner, D.A.; Mourant, J.R.; Lu, J.Q. Effect of detailed cell structure on light scattering distribution: FDTD study of a B-cell with 3D structure constructed from confocal images. *J. Quant. Spectrosc. Radiat. Transf.* **2006**, *1*, 25–36. [CrossRef]
80. He, J.; Karlsson, A.; Swartling, J.; Andersson-Engels, S. Light scattering by multiple red blood cells. *JOSA A* **2004**, *10*, 1953–1961. [CrossRef] [PubMed]
81. Karlsson, A.; He, J.; Swartling, J.; Andersson-Engels, S. Numerical simulations of light scattering by red blood cells. *IEEE Trans. Biomed. Eng.* **2005**, *1*, 13–18. [CrossRef] [PubMed]
82. Wriedt, T.; Hellmers, J.; Eremina, E.; Schuh, R. Light scattering by single erythrocyte: Comparison of different methods. *J. Quant. Spectrosc. Radiat. Transf.* **2006**, *1*, 444–456. [CrossRef]
83. Demos, S.G.; Alfano, R.R. Optical polarization imaging. *Appl. Opt.* **1997**, *36*, 150–155. [CrossRef] [PubMed]
84. Demos, S.G.; Radousky, H.B.; Alfano, R.R. Deep subsurface imaging in tissues using spectral and polarization filtering. *Opt. Express* **2000**, *7*, 23–28. [CrossRef]
85. Jacques, S.L.; Roman, J.R.; Lee, K. *Imaging Superficial Tissues with Polarized Light*; Wiley Interscience: New York, NY, USA, 1999.

86. Sankaran, V.; Walsh, J.T.; Maitland, D.J. Polarized light propagation through tissue phantoms containing densely packed scatterers. *Opt. Lett.* **2000**, *25*, 239–241. [CrossRef]
87. Firdous, S.; Ikram, M. Polarized Laser Beam Scattering through Turbid Medium for Application in Tissue Imaging. *Sci. Asia* **2005**, *31*, 167–172. [CrossRef]
88. Anderson, R.R. Polarized light examination and photography of the skin. *Arch. Dermatol.* **1991**, *127*, 1000–1005. [CrossRef]
89. Saarinen, K.; Muinonen, K. Light scattering by wood fibers. *Appl. Opt.* **2001**, *40*, 06477. [CrossRef]
90. Mischenko, M.I.; Hovenier, J.W.; Travis, L.D. *Light Scattering by Nonspherical Particles Theory Measurement and Applications*; Academic Press: Cambridge, MA, USA, 2000.
91. Mishchenko, M.I.; Travis, L.D.; Lacis, A.A. *Scattering Absorption and Emission of Light by Small Particles*; Cambridge University Press: Cambridge, UK, 2002.
92. Giakos, G.C. Multispectral, multifusion laser polarimetric imaging principles. *IEEE Int. Workshop Imaging Syst. Tech.* **2004**, *4*, 54–59.
93. Khos, O.T.; Munkhbaatar, P.; Yang, B.K.; Kim, H.W.; Kim, J.S.; Kim, M.W. Polarimetric measurement of Jones matrix of a twisted nematic liquid crystal spatial light modulator. *J. Opt. Soc. Korea* **2012**, *16*, 443–448. [CrossRef]
94. Jiao, S.; Wang, L.V. Jones-matrix imaging of biological tissues with quadruple-channel optical coherence tomography. *J. Biomed. Opt.* **2002**, *7*, 1083–3668. [CrossRef]
95. Layden, D.; Ghosh, N.; Vitkin, A. Quantitative polarimetry for tissue characterization and diagnosis. *Adv. Biophotonics Tissue Opt. Sect.* **2013**, *5*, 73–108.
96. Arteaga, O.; Freudenthal, J.; Wang, B.; Kahr, B. Mueller matrix polarimetry with four photoelastic modulators theory and calibration. *Appl. Opt.* **2012**, *28*, 6805–6817. [CrossRef]
97. Pezzaniti, J.L.; Chipman, R.A. Mueller matrix imaging polarimetry. *Opt. Eng.* **1995**, *34*, 1558–1569. [CrossRef]

16

Visible and Extended Near-Infrared Multispectral Imaging for Skin Cancer Diagnosis

Laura Rey-Barroso [1,*], Francisco J. Burgos-Fernández [1], Xana Delpueyo [1], Miguel Ares [1], Santiago Royo [1], Josep Malvehy [2], Susana Puig [2] and Meritxell Vilaseca [1]

1 Centre for Sensors, Instruments and Systems Development, Technical University of Catalonia, Terrassa 08222, Spain; francisco.javier.burgos@upc.edu (F.J.B.-F.); xana.delpueyo@upc.edu (X.D.); miguel.ares@oo.upc.edu (M.A.); santiago.royo@upc.edu (S.R.); meritxell.vilaseca@upc.edu (M.V.)

2 Dermatology Department of the Hospital Clinic of Barcelona, IDIBAPS; Barcelona 08036, Spain; jmalvehy@gmail.com (J.M.); susipuig@gmail.com (S.P.)

* Correspondence: laura.rey.barroso@upc.edu

Abstract: With the goal of diagnosing skin cancer in an early and noninvasive way, an extended near infrared multispectral imaging system based on an InGaAs sensor with sensitivity from 995 nm to 1613 nm was built to evaluate deeper skin layers thanks to the higher penetration of photons at these wavelengths. The outcomes of this device were combined with those of a previously developed multispectral system that works in the visible and near infrared range (414 nm–995 nm). Both provide spectral and spatial information from skin lesions. A classification method to discriminate between melanomas and nevi was developed based on the analysis of first-order statistics descriptors, principal component analysis, and support vector machine tools. The system provided a sensitivity of 78.6% and a specificity of 84.6%, the latter one being improved with respect to that offered by silicon sensors.

Keywords: InGaAs camera; multispectral imaging; infrared; skin cancer; melanoma

1. Introduction

Due to the uncontrolled growth of abnormal cells in skin cancer, chromophores such as melanin, hemoglobin, and water might differ among tumors of different etiologies; thus, skin cancer lesions can be identified clinically when a lesion changes its color, increases its size or thickness, and gets an unusual texture or its outline becomes irregular [1,2]. In this context, multispectral imaging systems, which provide precise quantification of spectral, colorimetric, and spatial features, have been employed over the last few years to analyze spectral and colorimetric properties of the skin reliably and non-invasively [3,4]. Specifically, they have also been used to improve the detection of skin cancer, especially melanoma, which is the most aggressive and lethal form.

In 2005, Tomatis et al. [5] developed an automated multispectral imaging system for the diagnosis of pigmented lesions. The device consisted of a spectrophotometer with a light source, a monochromator, and a bundle of optical fibers coupled to a probe head. The spectral range from 483 nm to 950 nm was covered with 15 spectral bands. A region-growing algorithm segmented the lesions and extracted descriptors to be used as input for setting and testing a neural network classifier.

Some years later, Kuzmina et al. [6] used a multispectral system that incorporated halogen lamps and filters from 450 nm to 950 nm with a spectral bandwidth of 15 nm. They observed that wavelengths closer to the infrared (IR) range penetrate deeper into the skin, resulting in decreased contrast due to higher light scattering. However, in the case of melanomas the contrast at 950 nm was found to be much higher, indicating considerably deeper structural damage.

In 2012, Bekina et al. [7] analyzed lesions under a multispectral system with four different spectral bands, each one to obtain information from specific structures of the skin: 450 nm for superficial layers, 545 nm for blood distribution, 660 nm for melanin detection, and 940 nm for the evaluation of deeper skin layers. Then, a ratio was calculated between the intensities of green light (545 nm), where the hemoglobin absorption is high, and red light (660 nm), where it is low. It was proven that pathological tissues showed higher values of this index than the surrounding skin as a consequence of having higher blood content. The same authors developed a similar system [8] that consisted of a multispectral imaging system with a CCD imaging sensor and a liquid crystal tunable filter (LCTF) (with spectral bands from 450 nm to 950 nm in steps of 10 nm) (Nuance EX), a spectral optimized lens, and internal optics. The illumination system was a ring of halogen lamps with a polarizer orthogonal to the camera in order to remove the artifacts caused by light reflection. In order to differentiate between melanoma and nevi, a new parameter was suggested based on skin optical density differences at three wavelengths: 540 nm, 650 nm, and 950 nm.

Additionally, Jakovels et al. [9] used principal component analysis (PCA) of multispectral imaging data in the wavelength range from 450 nm to 950 nm for distant skin melanoma recognition, which resulted in clear separation between malignant melanomas and pigmented nevi.

Delpueyo et al. [10] also proposed a light-emitting diodes (LEDs)-based multispectral imaging system with eight different wavelengths (414–995 nm) but using the analysis of the spatial distribution of color and spectral features through descriptors based on the first-order statistics of the histogram to improve the detection of skin cancer lesions, specifically melanomas and basal cell carcinomas.

Recently, Kim et al. [11] have investigated the potential of mobile smartphone-based multispectral imaging for the quantitative diagnosis and management of skin lesions. The authors miniaturized a spectral imaging system so that it could be attached to a smartphone, allowing users to obtain ten images sequentially within a range of wavelengths from 440 nm to 690 nm, with one white-light image. The results suggested that smartphone-based multispectral imaging and analysis had great potential as a healthcare tool for quantitative mobile skin diagnosis.

Despite the fact that sensitivity and specificity obtained with the former multispectral imaging systems based on silicon imaging sensors have reached similar values to those obtained by experienced dermatologists through dermoscopy [10,12], they have not yet superseded histological examination. In fact, this continues to be the clinical gold standard, providing diagnostic confirmation after surgical excision of the tumor.

Digital cameras based on silicon have a spectral response in the visible (VIS) up to the near-infrared (NIR) (900 nm–1000 nm). However, multispectral, extended, near-infrared (exNIR) optical imaging is nowadays available thanks to new indium gallium arsenide (InGaAs) cameras with high quantum efficiency within 900 nm–1600 nm. This has sparked interest among biologists in this relatively unexplored spectral region also known as "the second near-infrared window" (900 nm–1400 nm) [13].

Going further than 900 nm into the exNIR enables deeper in vivo optical imaging as photons at these wavelengths penetrate deeper into living tissue [14]; this could be a hint to explore further this spectral region as a means of improving skin cancer diagnosis and prognosis, as it may release information about how tissues are damaged due to ultraviolet radiation, water content, and other factors that might be different in benign and malignant lesions. For instance, due to the increased absorption of water in this spectral range, spectral images in the exNIR can provide information about the presence of angiogenesis, a tumorous growth of blood vessels around the malignant lesion.

In fact, the near-infrared region has been widely utilized in the past decade, and a number of clinical imaging applications have already been developed [15].

In this study, we investigate the possibilities of a multispectral imaging system based on an InGaAs camera and light-emitting diodes (LEDs) for the detection of skin cancer, especially melanomas, in the exNIR range, specifically from 995 nm to 1613 nm. Although InGaAs sensors tend to be noisier than CMOS or CCD sensors and the deeper scattering at exNIR wavelengths can reduce image contrast, we consider that the study of this unexplored spectral range can bring very interesting results to the scientific community.

2. Experimental Setup and Clinical Measurements

The device developed to perform exNIR multispectral imaging of skin cancer is depicted in Figure 1b,c. It integrates a 16-bit depth InGaAs camera (Hamamatsu C10633-23, Hamamatsu Photonics, Shizuoka, Japan) with spectral sensitivity from 900 nm to 1600 nm, readout speed of 50 fps, and 320 × 256 pixels together with a Kowa LM12HC-SW 1.4/12.5 mm short-wave infrared (SWIR) lens with high transmission from 800 nm to 2000 nm (Kowa Company, Ltd., Aichi, Japan). Additionally, a LED-based light source was built on a cylinder of polyvinyl chloride (PVC) including high power Surface Mounted Displays (SMD) LEDs with peak wavelengths at 995 nm, 1081 nm, 1214 nm, 1340 nm, 1486 nm, and 1613 nm (Figure 2b); they were selected in accordance with the absorption curves of the principal chromophores of the skin, such as bilirubin, hemoglobin, and water, especially taking into account their most representative minimums and maximums, and the spectral bands with considerable differences among them allowing characterization of the tissue constituents [10]. The tip of the cylinder is a cone with an opening of 20 mm × 20 mm and a diffuser. Four LEDs per spectral band were included in the light source with a separation of 90° among them to ensure a uniform illumination over the skin; a total amount of 24 LEDs was finally placed on the ring. All parts were assembled in a handheld configuration with a trigger to start the acquisition. A base was also designed and constructed to hold the multispectral system when it was not being used. It incorporated a calibrated reference at the bottom that consisted of the Neutral 5 gray color of an X-Rite ColorChecker® (Grand Rapids, MI, USA) with level of reflectance similar to that of the skin in the exNIR range. The degradation of the reference over time was controlled by visual inspection and spectrally by means of a spectrometer. If the reference showed dirty areas or scratches or its reflectance spectrum presented variations up to 5% with respect to the spectrum when it was brand new, it was replaced.

The exNIR system was used together with another multispectral imaging system previously built [10] for capturing reflectance and color features in the VIS and NIR ranges (Figure 1a). In this case, the camera integrated in the multispectral head is a 12-bit depth DMK 23U445 with a 1/3" CCD sensor of Sony ICX445ALA with 1280 × 960 pixels of resolution and readout speed of 30 fps; it represented an advantage over the spatial resolution of the exNIR camera, which limited the performance of the analysis in this spectral range. The lens coupled was a Schneider-Kreuznack Cinegon with spectral sensitivity from 400 nm to 1000 nm and a working distance from infinite to 20 mm, which allowed focusing the skin lesions at a distance of 40 mm with a field of view of 15 mm × 20 mm. As in the previous case, sequential multiplexed illumination is used by means of a ring of 32 LEDs (four per wavelength) with the following peak wavelengths: 414 nm, 447 nm, 477 nm, 524 nm, 671 nm, 735 nm, 890 nm, and 995 nm (Figure 2a). For each wavelength, the forward current of the LEDs was tuned to obtain a constant temporal behavior in terms of radiance. The final currents used for each wavelength were selected, taking into account a compromise between emission stability and the exposure time needed to make use of the whole dynamic range of the cameras: from 0 to 4095 digital levels in the case of the VIS-NIR system and from 0 to 65,533 in the case of the exNIR system. In general, measurements of radiance over time showed that LEDs needed at least two seconds to stabilize, and therefore this delay was added when any LED was switched on (Figure 3). Infrared LEDs used in the exNIR device showed a much more stable behavior than those in the VIS-NIR range; for this reason, the two-second delay was not implemented in this system. Despite that, the spectral assessment in the exNIR was less accurate than in the VIS-NIR, because exNIR LEDs presented a wider Full Width at Half Maximum (FWHM). In consequence, the information captured at each spectral band and then associated with the wavelength peak of each LED includes a broader range of data coming from more wavelengths.

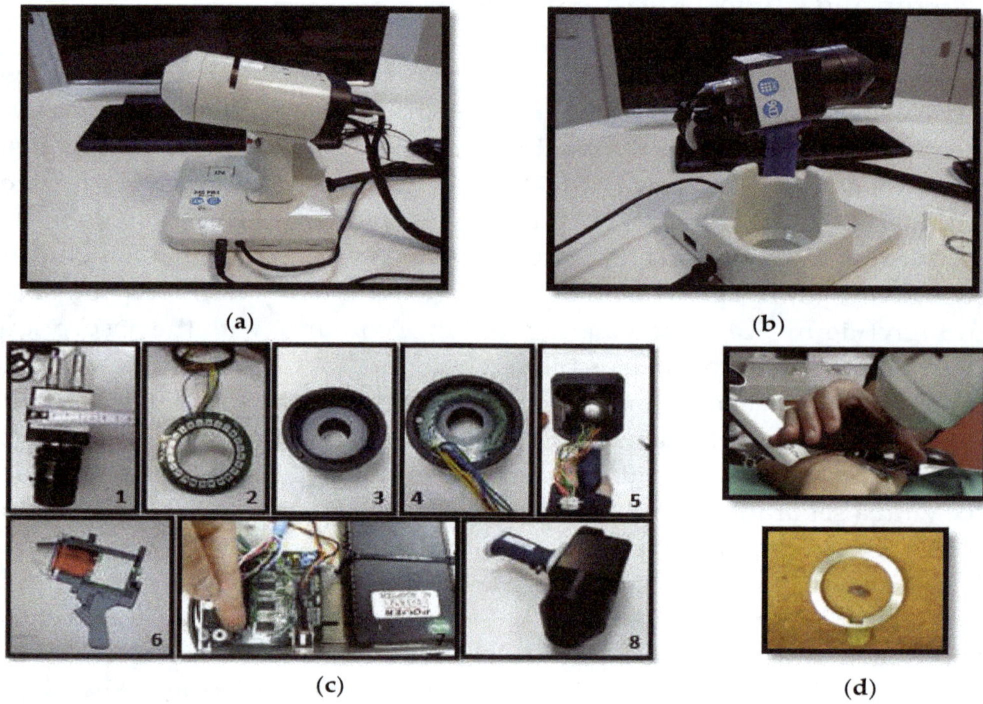

Figure 1. (**a**) General view of the previously developed handheld VIS-NIR multispectral device. (**b**) General view of the handheld exNIR multispectral device. (**c**) Components of the exNIR imaging system: 1—InGaAs camera, 2—Ring of LEDs, 3—Tip of PVC cone, 4—Ring of LEDs placed at the tip. 5—Handheld case, 6—AutoCad design, 7—Electronic control, and 8—Handheld case with camera inside. (**d**) Clinical measurement and metallic ring, which is glued to the patient's skin for the tip of both systems to place them in the same position and parallel to the skin, without making any contact.

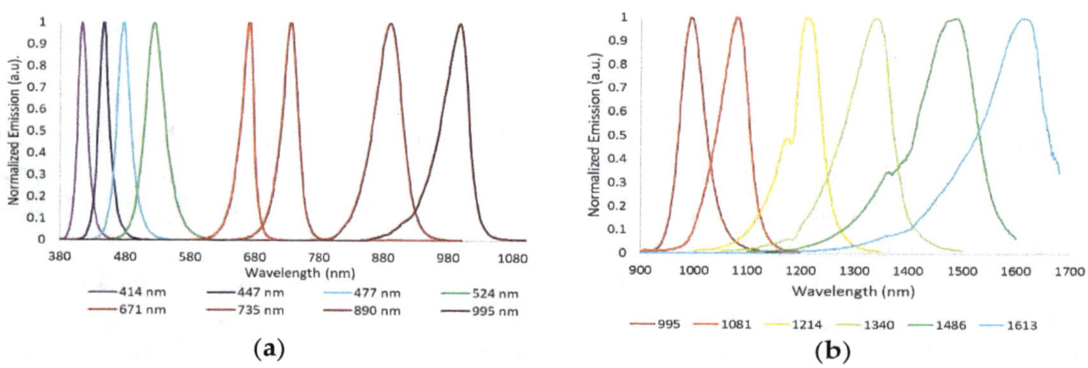

Figure 2. Normalized spectral emission of the LEDs in (**a**) the VIS-NIR and (**b**) exNIR ranges.

A user-friendly acquisition software was built based on Borland Builder C++ to be used for physicians in a clinical environment. The software controls individually and synchronously the emission of the LEDs and the acquisition of spectral images. The software interface asks for a daily calibration to guarantee accurate measurements at all wavelengths along LEDs lifecycle. It involves the acquisition of images of the neutral reference (Neutral 5) at each spectral band and at ten different exposure times to adapt the dynamic range of the system to every skin phenotype, thus avoiding saturated or noisy areas. This set of calibration images is used later for calculating the reflectance images from the raw spectral images (see next section). Then, a measurement over the actual skin lesion can be taken, and the system will make a sequence of acquisitions at every spectral band. In the case of the multispectral system with LEDs in the VIS and NIR ranges, eight images are obtained, while for the one in the exNIR, six images of a lesion are taken. Each one is acquired with a given exposure time, chosen from a learning table among the ten exposure times previously used to take images of the reference. The exposure times are chosen by an algorithm with a target averaged digital level (DL) for each image that is about half of the dynamic range of the camera; in this way, saturated images are avoided. This active exposure time selection also contributes to compensating variations of LEDs' power output due to their lifecycle. Another advantage of this algorithm is that it allows the evaluation of all kinds of skin, from brighter to darker ones. A set of dark current images also needs to be acquired by just making another calibration in a room in dark conditions, to take into account the straylight caused by internal reflections and noise sensed by the camera at the time of calculating the reflectance curve of a pixel area; the same ten exposure times previously used are applied. The straylight was measured sequentially switching on the LEDs, as during the calibration with the reference, in order to remove from the image the reflections caused by the inner surface of the PVC painted cone. Environmental illumination barely affects the measurement, because the tip of the devices is fully covered by the metallic ring and the patient's skin. One lesion is fully analyzed when sequentially measured with the VIS-NIR and the exNIR multispectral imaging systems. Apart from the additional spectral information from 414 nm to 995 nm, the use of the VIS-NIR system allows to locate with higher accuracy some lesions that present blurry boundaries in the IR.

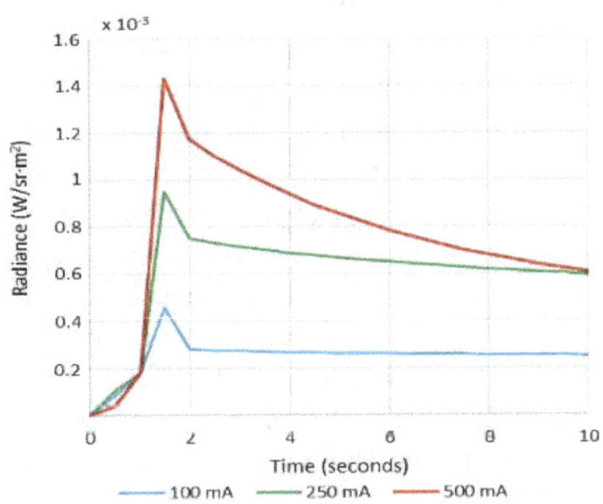

Figure 3. Radiance (W/sr·m^2) of the 414 nm LEDs at different forward currents measured every second over 10 s.

As a pilot study, the VIS-NIR and exNIR multispectral systems were used to analyze 39 nevi and 14 melanomas from Caucasian patients at the Hospital Clínic *i* Provincial de Barcelona (Barcelona, Spain). Patients could be seated or lying down on the hospital bed while capturing.

All of them provided written informed consent before any examination and ethical committee approval (Spanish Agency of Drugs and Clinical Products, document number 7576) was obtained. The study complied with the tenets of the 1975 Declaration of Helsinki (Tokyo revision, 2004). The lesions were diagnosed by dermatologists (SP and JM) using a commercial dermoscope and the confocal laser scanning microscope VivaScope® 1500 from MAVIG GmbH (Munich, Germany). When malignancy was suspected, the lesion was excised and a histological analysis was carried out.

3. Data Processing

The images from the multispectral systems were processed through a graphical user interface (GUI) built in Matlab R2015a (The MathWorks Inc., Natick, MA, USA). It has different functions to make internal calibration algorithms and also to compute reflectance spectra that can be used to compare subtle differences between benign and malignant lesions. In order to calculate the reflectance images, the corresponding calibration images from the reference and dark current images are selected by the program. Then, for a given exposure time and wavelength, being different the exposure time for each wavelength, the reflectance at each pixel (i, j) is calculated as follows:

$$R_{Lesion}(i,j) = k\frac{I(i,j) - I_D(i,j)}{I_N(i,j) - I_D(i,j)}, \tag{1}$$

where $R_{Lesion}(i,j)$ is the spectral reflectance image; $I(i,j)$, $I_N(i,j)$, and $I_D(i,j)$ contain the DLs of the raw, neutral gray reference and dark current images, respectively; and k is the calibrated reflectance of the neutral gray reference, given by the manufacturer.

Since the purpose was to obtain information about the lesions themselves and not from the whole reflectance images, which also contain spectral information about the surrounding healthy skin, every lesion was segmented. The segmentation of lesions from the IR images was a challenge, because in many cases they were hardly distinguishable from the surrounding skin because of the decreased contrast due to higher scattering at these wavelengths. In order to overcome this, two different algorithms of segmentation were used for each multispectral system.

For the images of the lesion in the exNIR range, manual segmentation coupled with previous image registration was used. In this case, the corresponding images of the lesion taken in the VIS range were correlated to those captured by the exNIR multispectral system in order to overcome the constraint of the second device. This could be easily done by means of a mathematical transformation of the images matrices, since skin lesions were measured by both systems at the same position and in the same orientation thanks to a metallic ring were the tip of both systems could be attached to the patient's skin (Figure 1d). The metallic ring was glued to the patient's skin by means of a medical adhesive ring that was different for every patient; this combination prevents the systems from touching the skin. Afterwards, when the corresponding images were shown together, one on top of the other, manual segmentation was performed over the images in the exNIR range (Figure 4a).

The algorithm used for the images in the VIS-NIR range consisted of searching the DL threshold to establish those pixels belonging to the patient's lesion (foreground) and those to the surrounding healthy skin (background). The DL threshold was calculated with the Otsu's method, which maximizes the between-class variance of the lesion and the skin pixel values based on the intensity of the histogram [16]. A binary image is created according to the threshold, and pixels below are transformed into zeros and above into ones. This binary image can be used as a mask to be applied to all the spectral images and obtain the DLs corresponding to the pixels of the lesion. However, Otsu's method is based on a global threshold that can only be used in lesions that are clearly different from the skin. In order to solve skin inhomogeneity, reflectance images were divided into four subimages, allowing different thresholds adapted to the local characteristics to be calculated (Figure 4b). The image used for performing VIS-NIR segmentation was taken at 414 nm, since this spectral band enhanced the detection of melanin, and therefore it extended the contour of the lesion to its real size.

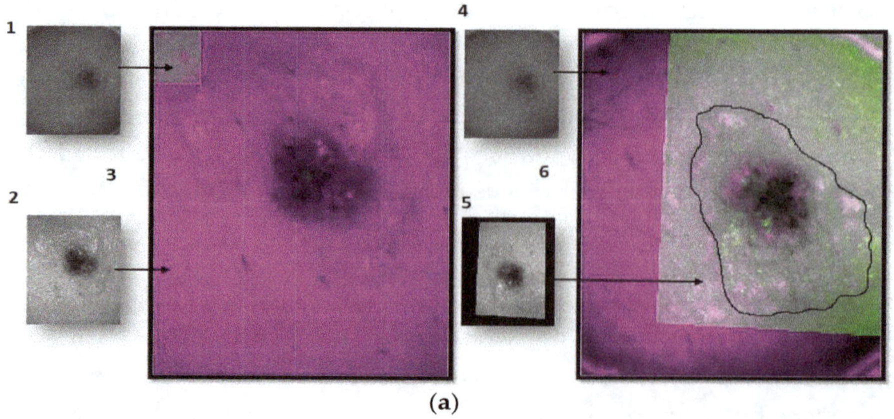

(a)

Figure 4. *Cont.*

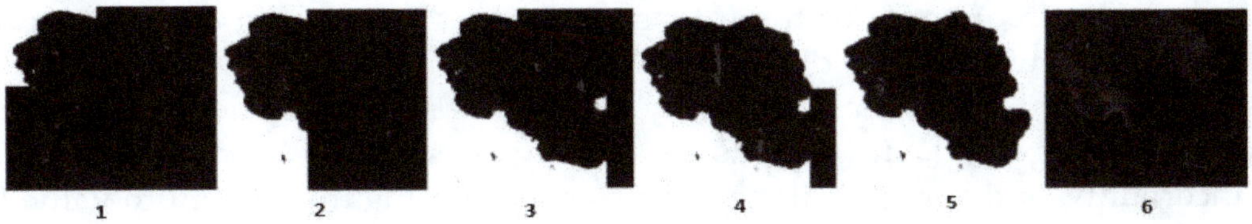

(**b**)

Figure 4. Steps of the segmentation algorithm for both multispectral imaging systems. (**a**) Example of how the segmentation is done for a lesion taken with the exNIR system: (1) Reflectance image taken with the exNIR device. (2) Reflectance image taken with the VIS-NIR camera. (3) Reflectance images from both cameras superimposed. Here, it can be seen how both systems take images at different resolutions, rotated with respect to each other a certain angle. (4) Reflectance image of the exNIR imaging system. (5) Reflectance image from the VIS-NIR system, to which a mathematical operation for correlation has been applied. (6) These last images were superimposed. (**b**) Example of how the segmentation is done for a lesion taken with the VIS-NIR imaging system: images correspond to the implementation of the Otsu method for each subimage. A mask for each of them is calculated in (1–4), and they are put together to form the (5) final mask for segmentation. (6) is the result of segmenting the lesion.

Different parameters to discriminate between benign and malignant lesions were also calculated based on spectral features additionally to the reflectance images (Equation (1)). To avoid the influence of the patient's healthy skin, another set of reflectance images were calculated by subtraction of the mean reflectance value of the patient's skin from the reflectance images of the segmented lesion (Equation (2)). This was proposed as an empirical approach to improve the results, if possible, due to the different penetration depths of wavelengths owing to the different absorption of structures inside the tissue; however, in multispectral technology, images contain a mixture of light coming from not only a specific depth inside the tissue but also from the preceding layers due to backscattering.

Another two set of images were also computed by taking the logarithm of the latter ones, in order to obtain information in terms of absorbance, too.

$$R_{Lesion-Skin}(i,j) = k\frac{I_{lesion}(i,j) - I_D(i,j)}{I_N(i,j) - I_D(i,j)} - mean\left(k\frac{I_{skin}(i,j) - I_D(i,j)}{I_N(i,j) - I_D(i,j)}\right), \quad (2)$$

At a second stage, a statistical analysis over the former images was carried out as a first approach to characterize the spatial features based on the histogram of the lesions and obtain further information for the classification algorithm. This analysis was envisaged to provide information about the distribution of digital levels at each spectral band and all over the sample rather than only taking into account the traditional statistical descriptors: mean (μ), maximum (max), minimum (min), and standard deviation (σ). Accordingly, first order statistics descriptors such as the energy (En), the entropy (Ep), and the third central moment (μ_3) were obtained from the histogram of the segmented lesion in terms of the spectral reflectance and absorbance; these parameters have been shown to provide useful information about human features such as the iris pattern [17]. They are defined as follows:

$$E_n = \sum_{i=0}^{N-1} P(i)^2, \quad (3)$$

$$E_p = -\sum_{i=0}^{N-1} P(i)^2 \log\left[P(i)^2\right], \quad (4)$$

$$\mu_3 = \sum_{i=0}^{N-1} (i-\mu)^3 P(i)^2, \quad (5)$$

where $P(i)$ is the value (frequency) of the intensity element i (bin) of the histogram and N is the number of levels that the histogram is divided into.

Energy is a numerical descriptor of uniformity that ranges between 0 and 1, reaching the maximum value for a constant image [18]. In regards to entropy, it is a well-known statistical measure of randomness, uncertainty, or disorder in image values, with 0 being the minimum value for a constant image and $\log^2(N)$ the maximum [18]. The third central moment or skewness, μ_3, refers to the skewness of the histogram about its mean; it has a range of values between -1 and 1, positive for histograms skewed to the right, negative for the ones skewed to the left, and 0 for symmetric ones [18]. According to all this, these descriptors can be used to account for reflectance distribution features of skin lesions besides the more classical averaged spectral information obtained from traditional multispectral imaging systems.

4. Classification Algorithm

In order to determine which of the former statistical descriptors related with reflectance and absorbance values were useful to discriminate between malignant and benign tumors, as well as reflectance/absorbance minus the average of the healthy skin, scatter plots with the values for every lesion analyzed were evaluated. In total, there were 392 scatter plots, 224 from the VIS-NIR system and 168 from the exNIR. A Matlab-based classification algorithm was then used to find the best ones. The algorithm included the definition of upper and lower thresholds on the scatterplots that were experimentally set to delimit the area where benign lesions were prone to lay down. The lesions that fell outside the thresholds for at least one parameter were considered to be malignant (i.e., melanomas).

The classification algorithm worked as follows: after setting the thresholds of all parameters, they were ordered according to the number of malignant lesions that they allowed to classify. Accordingly, the first parameter on the list was such allowing the greatest number of malignant lesions to be classified, the second one was such allowing the second greatest number, and so forth. The algorithm then started from the first of the list alone and calculated the corresponding sensitivity, i.e., the percentage of malignant lesions classified as such. The second parameter of the list was then chosen to perform the classification together with the first one, and the sensitivity was computed again. If the second parameter did not allow for the improvement of the classification with at least one more malignant lesion detected, it was discarded as it was considered to be redundant. Otherwise, it was included. Next, the third parameter on the list was added to the first two, and the sensitivity was calculated again, repeating the described process until the addition of more parameters did not improve the sensitivity of malignant lesions.

Thresholds were not set to include all nevi or all melanomas, because preliminary tests showed large values of false positives and false negatives, which would considerably increase the complexity of the algorithm.

After choosing the best statistical descriptors as those allowing more melanomas to be classified as melanomas, a Principal Component Analysis (PCA) [19] was carried out to automatize and enhance the performance of the classification algorithm by avoiding the use of experimental thresholds manually selected.

At first, the matrix of data was standardized. This was done by subtracting the mean and dividing by the standard deviation of every descriptor as follows:

$$Descriptor_{norm} = \frac{Descriptor_{Lesion} - mean(Descriptor)}{stdv(Descriptor)}, \tag{6}$$

Then, Singular Value Decomposition (SVD) [19] was performed over the matrix containing the d best descriptors to detect melanomas for every of the 53 lesions (Y_{dx53}). SVD represents an expansion of the original data in a coordinate system in which the covariance matrix is diagonal. This operation is performed with the *svd* Matlab function obtaining the matrices U_{dxd}, whose columns correspond to nonzero singular values form a set of orthonormal basis vectors for the range of

Y; D_{dx53}, whose diagonal values are the square roots of the eigenvalues; and V_{53x53}, where the columns are the eigenvectors of the standardized data matrix. V therefore contains the principal directions to form a base in which the variance between classes is maximized and D the coefficients by which these eigenvectors are multiplied, to obtain the data coordinates transformed into the base of principal directions.

The initial data could be reproduced from the following matrices as follows:

$$\hat{Y}(i,j) = U(i,j) \cdot D(i,j) \cdot V^t(i,j), \tag{7}$$

The first principal components (PCs) can then be calculated as follows:

$$PC_1(i,j) = D(1,1) \cdot V(i,1), \tag{8}$$

$$PC_2(i,j) = D(2,2) \cdot V(i,2), \tag{9}$$

$$PC_3(i,j) = D(3,3) \cdot V(i,3), \tag{10}$$

Many PCs as descriptors originally available are obtained, although the first three PCs are those that are known to contain the higher variability among data (in descendent order).

PCs were represented one against the others, as it is shown in the next section with the aim of transforming the actual descriptors to another coordinate axes where the different classes, nevi, and melanomas are thought to be represented as separate as possible. Additionally, a decision boundary using a Support Vector Machine (SVM) training algorithm was implemented to classify nevi and melanomas [19]. It looks for a hyperplane that separates the space of descriptors into two classes with the maximum margin. This maximum margin is the distance from the decision surface to the closest data point and determines the margin of the classifier. This method of construction necessarily means that the decision function for an SVM is fully specified by a (usually small) subset of the data that defines the position of the separator. These points are referred to as the support vectors; in a vector space, a point can be thought of as a vector between the origin and that point. In the end, the different positions of the separator form the decision boundary from which sensitivity and specificity values can be established. Sensitivity corresponds to the true positive rate defined as the proportion of melanomas that lay inside the boundaries, correctly identified as such; specificity relates to the true negative rate defined as the proportion of nevi that lay outside the boundaries.

5. Results and Discussion

Figure 5 shows the mean reflectance ($\pm\sigma$) of the whole set of melanomas and nevi measured, separately. The mean reflectance of melanomas in the VIS-NIR and exNIR ranges is lower than that of nevi, being that of nevi, which is especially higher from 995 nm to 1350 nm than for melanomas. This wavelength range, often called second near-infrared window, corresponds to that in which radiation can penetrate deeper into the tissue (longer wavelengths are highly absorbed by water) and thus can inform about deeper structures, which could be notably different between nevi and melanomas.

This behavior agreed with a previous study in which the average reflectance of the nevi was found to be higher with respect to the melanoma population in the VIS range [10], although the standard deviation of the data that was analyzed made it quite entangled.

Figure 6 depicts representative reflectance images of a nevus and a melanoma for all the spectral range evaluated (414 nm–1613 nm). It can be seen that nevi are usually more homogeneous at all wavelengths, while melanomas grow deeper in the skin as it was found in IR images. Our results correlate with those found by Zhang et al. [20], who identified a strong absorption between 1400 nm and 1450 nm, and also beyond this range, due to the presence of water in tissue, causing a contrast decrease of spectral images. They also evaluated the spectral behavior of tissues for different thicknesses but ex-vivo samples were used; therefore, an accurate comparison with our findings cannot be performed, since we carried out in-vivo measurements.

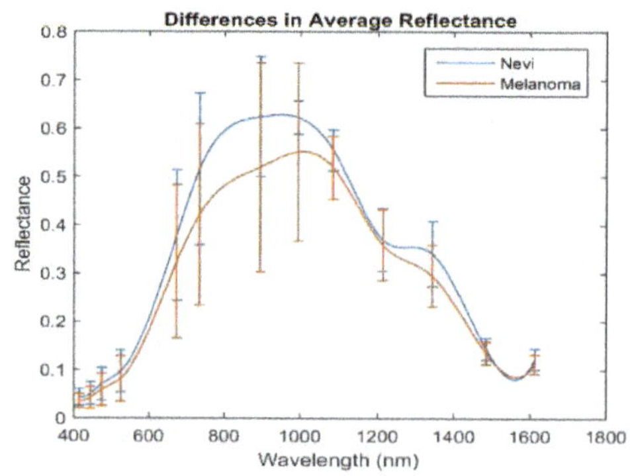

Figure 5. Averaged spectral reflectance curves ($\pm\sigma$) of nevi and melanomas in the VIS-NIR and exNIR ranges.

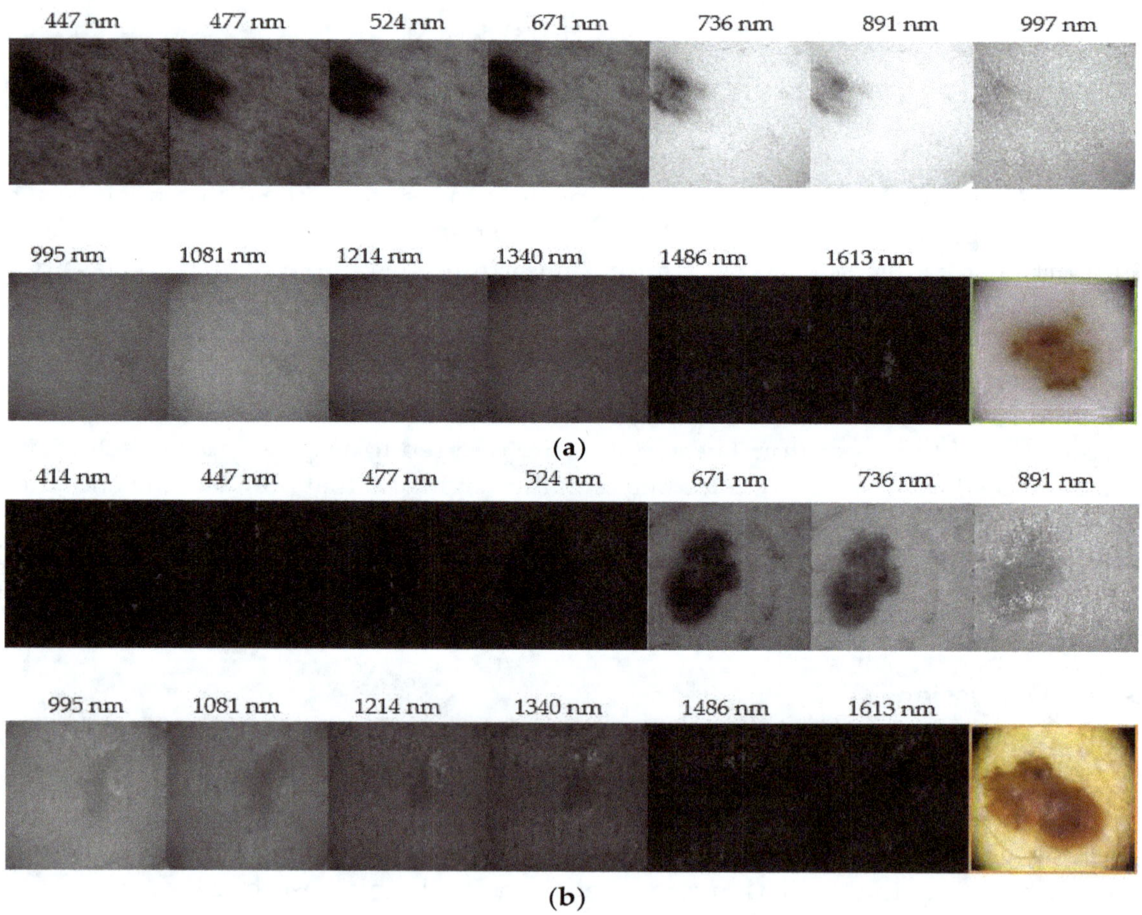

Figure 6. Reflectance images obtained with the systems in the VIS-NIR and exNIR ranges: (**a**) nevus and (**b**) melanoma. (**a**) shows that nevi are usually more homogeneous at all wavelengths. Furthermore, the IR light, which penetrates deeper in the skin, shows that melanomas generally grow deeper in (**b**). Color images were taken with a dermoscope.

In the end, the number *d* of best statistical descriptors exhibiting a more accurate classification of lesions that the Matlab algorithm retrieved was eight, corresponding to seven different spectral bands:

- Minimum of the spectral reflectance (minus the average of the healthy skin) at 414 nm.
- Spectral absorbance in terms of the standard deviation at 477 nm.
- Spectral absorbance in terms of the energy at 477 nm.

- Spectral reflectance in terms of energy at 524 nm.
- Spectral reflectance in terms of the skewness at 671 nm.
- Spectral reflectance in terms of the mean at 995 nm.
- Spectral absorbance (minus the average of the healthy skin) in terms of standard deviation at 1214 nm.
- Minimum of the spectral absorbance at 1613 nm.

Table 1 shows these parameters, how the total sensitivity is increased when a new selected parameter is added to the set in the iterative algorithm, and where the experimental thresholds were set in order to obtain the highest possible values of sensitivity.

Table 1. Best statistical descriptors, corresponding experimental upper and lower thresholds, and total cumulative sensitivity.

Parameter	Upper Threshold	Lower Threshold	Cummulative Sensitivity
Min. of the reflectance at 414 nm (minus skin)	0.8	−0.33	36%
Absorbance in terms of σ at 477 nm	0.082	0.039	43%
Absorbance in terms of the energy at 477 nm	0.125	0.046	50%
Reflectance in terms of energy at 524 nm	0.28	0.03	64%
Reflectance in terms of the skewness at 721 nm	1.8×10^{-3}	−2	71.5%
Reflectance in terms of the mean at 995 nm	0.55	0.4	83%
Absorbance (minus skin) in terms of σ at 1214 nm	0.082	0.04	91%
Minimum of the absorbance at 1613 nm	1.95	1.18	100%

Combinations of more parameters did not produce better discrimination between nevi and melanomas, taking into account the manual experimental thresholding defined in the scatterplots.

Figure 7a shows two representative histograms of a nevus (left) and a melanoma (right) from which the statistical descriptors were computed; they correspond to reflectance images at 1214 nm. The averaged spectral reflectance (μ); the standard deviation (σ); and corresponding Ep, En, and μ_3 are also shown. It can be seen that the En is lower, and the Ep and μ_3 are higher for the melanoma. It means that they are characterized by less uniform images, with a higher disorder in terms of reflectance and a histogram more skewed than that of the nevus. However, it can be appreciated that the μ of the melanoma is higher than that of the nevus. Figure 7b depicts a scatter plot of the spectral absorbance minus the average of the healthy skin in terms of standard deviation at 1214 nm. It can be observed that the experimental thresholding was not accurate enough to separate melanomas and nevus.

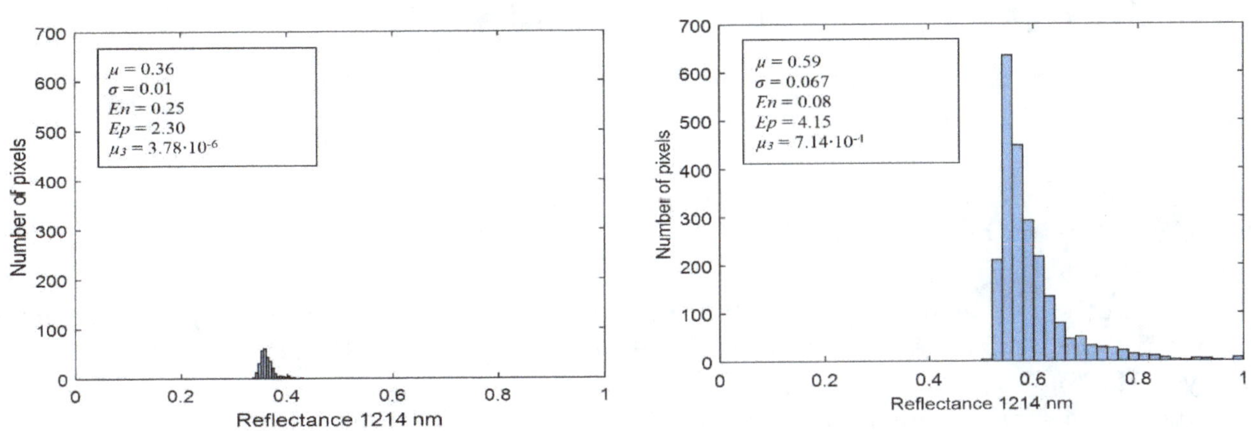

(a)

Figure 7. *Cont.*

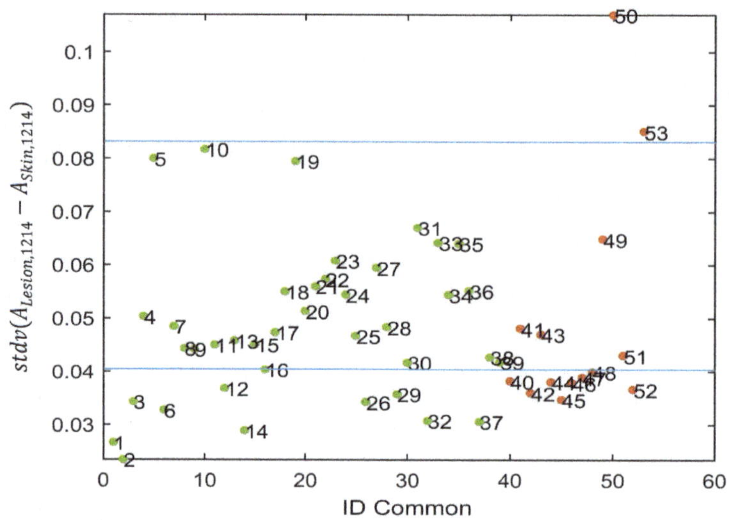

(b)

Figure 7. (**a**) Reflectance histogram at 1214 nm including the mean (μ), standard deviation (σ), energy (En), entropy (Ep), and skewness or third central moment (μ_3) values of a nevus (left) and a melanoma lesion (right). (**b**) Scatter plot of the spectral absorbance minus the average of the healthy skin in terms of standard deviation at 1214 nm in which manual thresholds have been identified.

In this preliminary study, the first three PCs were found to contain most of the variability among data (98.3%); PC1 explained 73.3%, while PC1 and PC2 explained 83.3% of the variability. Figure 8 shows the PCs plotted against each other to obtain the best descriptor's space to separate the two types of lesions, as well as the decision boundaries established using a SVM. As it can be seen, the standardization of the descriptors used and the posterior PCA showed to be useful for separating away benign and malignant lesions.

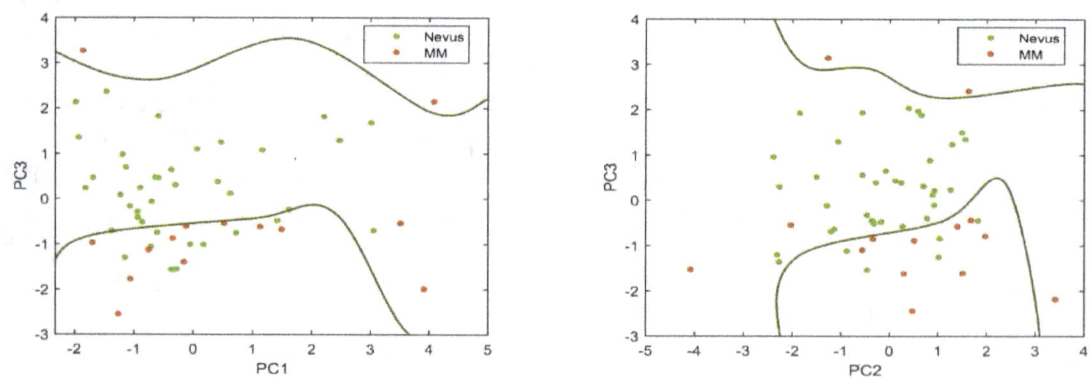

(**a**) (**b**)

Figure 8. (**a**) PC3 vs. PC1 and (**b**) PC3 vs. PC2 descriptors for nevi (green markers) and melanoma (orange markers) are represented.

Among all the PCs evaluated, those that produced more precise classifications were the PC3 vs. PC1 (sensitivity = 85.7% and specificity = 76.9%) and the PC3 vs. PC2 (sensitivity = 78.6% and specificity = 84.6%).

Delpueyo et al. found sensitivity and specificity values of 87.2% and 54.5%, respectively, when using only the VIS-NIR device for the analysis of 290 nevi and 95 melanomas [10]. Even though the sensitivity values were similar or slightly lower than when using only the VIS-NIR device [10], the specificity was clearly increased so that exNIR information seems to be relevant for the classification between benign and malignant lesions.

In fact, the detection of malignant lesions at early stages, when they can still be controlled and successfully excised, is crucial when dealing with skin cancer, and this is the reason why dermatologists are more concerned with increasing sensitivity than specificity. However, many of the multispectral systems used for detection of skin cancer in the VIS range generate a large number of false positives and, consequently, a large number of unnecessary biopsies [21,22]. Therefore, the inclusion of longer wavelengths seems to be helpful in order to improve the specificity values reached at the time of the study.

6. Conclusions

In this pilot study, a novel exNIR multispectral imaging system for skin cancer diagnosis has been presented. The preliminary analysis of melanomas and nevi from 995 nm to 1613 nm considering spectral and spatial descriptors showed the potential of this technique, particularly for the information obtained from deeper layers of the skin by the use of IR light. In order to improve its performance, the data collected was combined with that provided by a VIS-NIR multispectral imaging system developed in a previous study. The evaluation of lesions from 414 nm to 1613 nm offered an exhaustive spectral assessment of skin lesions.

In addition, the combination of the selected as best parameters for classification, the experimental thresholding, and the use of PCA and SVM enhanced the accuracy of the initial discrimination methodology, leading to similar values of sensitivity but increased ones for specificity. Therefore, exNIR spectral information seems to be relevant for the diagnosis of skin cancer, particularly when nevi and melanomas are taken into account.

The developed methodology was limited by some factors that should be considered for future improvements of the system. Firstly, the resolution of the InGaAs sensor was rather low, limiting the performance of this device. Secondly, the selection of exNIR LEDs was a challenge due to the current state of the art of solid-state technology within this spectral range and the limited availability of wavelengths; their wider FWHMs also contributed to a less accurate spectral reconstruction. Thirdly, the need of the VIS-NIR images for the segmentation of the lesions captured with the exNIR system was also a restriction of this system. Finally, the field of view (FOV) of both systems was another limitation, since only image lesions smaller than 20 mm could be acquired.

The set of lesions was large enough to train the SVM with accurate results but was not to check with other lesions how good the decision boundaries were to separate nevi from melanoma. Future work will be focused on increasing the sample set. Also, combining spectral and 3D data available from a former study [10,23] will increase noticeably the morphological and textural information of lesions and hopefully improve the sensitivity and specificity values. Moreover, usage of the proposed methodology may benefit from conjoint use with the VIS-NIR and exNIR modality to maximize specificity. However, a solution to address the course of action in case of conflict between categorization within the two ranges would be needed. Alternative algorithms considering not only the detection of melanomas but the rate of true positives and true negatives should also be investigated.

Author Contributions: L.R.-B. and X.D. performed the experiment and analyzed the data; F.J.B.-F. contributed to technical aspects of the experiment; J.M. and S.P. coordinated the clinical assessments; M.V. conceived the experiment; F.J.B.-F., M.V., M.A., and S.R. carried out the experiments; and L.R.-B., F.J.B.-F., and M.V. wrote the paper.

References

1. Guy, G.P.; Ekwueme, D.U. Melanoma Treatment Costs: A systematic review of the literature, 1990–2011. *Am. J. Prev. Med.* **2012**, *43*, 537–545. [CrossRef] [PubMed]
2. Stern, R.S. Prevalence of a History of Skin Cancer in 2007: Results of an incidence-based model. *Arch. Dermatol.* **2010**, *146*, 279–282. [CrossRef] [PubMed]
3. Pladellorens, J.; Pintó, A.; Segura, J.; Cadevall, C.; Antó, J.; Pujol, J.; Vilaseca, M.; Coll, J. A Device for the Color Measurement and Detection of Spots on the Skin. *Skin Res. Technol.* **2008**, *14*, 65–70. [CrossRef] [PubMed]
4. Jolivot, R.; Benezeth, Y.; Marzani, F. Skin Parameter Map Retrieval from a dedicated Multispectral Imaging System Applied to Dermatology/Cosmetology. *J. Biomed. Imaging* **2013**, *2013*, 1–15. [CrossRef] [PubMed]
5. Tomatis, S.; Carrara, M.; Bono, A.; Bartoli, C.; Lualdi, M.; Tragni, G. Automated Melanoma Detection with a Novel Multispectral Imaging System: Results of a prospective study. *Phys. Med. Biol.* **2005**, *50*, 1675–1687. [CrossRef] [PubMed]
6. Kuzmina, I.; Diabele, I.; Jakovels, D.; Spigullis, J.; Valeine, L.; Kapsotinsh, J.; Berzina, A. Towards Non-Contact Skin Melanoma Selection by Multispectral Analysis. *J. Biomed. Opt.* **2011**, *16*, 060502. [CrossRef] [PubMed]
7. Bekina, A.; Diebele, I.; Rubins, U.; Zaharans, J.; Dejarbo, A.; Sigulis, J. Multispectral assessment of skin malformations using a modified video-microscope. *Latv. J. Phys. Tech. Sci.* **2012**, *49*, 4–8. [CrossRef]
8. Diebele, I.; Kuzmina, I.; Lihachev, A.; Kapsotinsh, J.; Dejarbo, A.; Valiene, L.; Spigulis, J. Clinical evaluation of melanomas and common nevi by spectral imaging. *Biomed. Opt. Express* **2012**, *3*, 467–472. [CrossRef] [PubMed]
9. Jakovels, D.; Lihacova, I.; Kuzmina, I.; Sigulis, J. Evaluation of Skin Melanoma in Spectral Range 450–950 nm Using Principal Component Analysis. In Proceedings of the European Conference on Biomedical Optics, Munich, Germany, 24 June 2013; Volume 8803. [CrossRef]
10. Delpueyo, X.; Vilaseca, M.; Royo, S.; Ares, M.; Rey-Barroso, L.; Sanabria, F.; Puig, S.; Malvehy, J.; Pellacani, J.; Noguero, F.; et al. Multispectral imaging system based on light-emitting diodes for the detection of melanomas and basal cell carcinomas: A pilot study. *J. Biomed. Opt.* **2017**, *22*, 065006. [CrossRef] [PubMed]
11. Kim, S.; Cho, D.; Kim, J.; Kim, M.; Youn, S.; Jang, J.E.; Je, M.; Lee, D.H.; Lee, B.; Farkas, D.L.; et al. Smartphone-based multiespectral imaging: System development and potential for mobile skin diagnosis. *Biomed. Opt. Express* **2016**, *7*, 005294. [CrossRef] [PubMed]
12. Langley, R.G.; Walsh, N.; Sutherland, A.E.; Propperova, I.; Delaney, L.; Morris, S.F.; Gallant, C. The diagnostic accuracy of in vivo confocal scanning laser microscopy compared to dermoscopy of bening and malignant melanocytic lesions: A prospective study. *Arch. Dermatol.* **2007**, *215*, 365–372. [CrossRef]
13. Salo, D.; Kim, D.; Cao, Q.; Berezin, M.Y. Multispectral imaging/deep tissue imaging: Extended near-infrared: A new window on in vivo bioimaging. *BioOpt. World* **2014**, *7*, 22–25.
14. Mourant, J.R.; Fuselier, T.; Boyer, J.; Johnson, T.M.; Bigio, I.J. Predicrions and measurements of scattering and absorption over broad wavelength ranges in tissue phantoms. *Arch. Dermatol.* **2007**, *215*, 365–372. [CrossRef]
15. Godoy, S.E.; Ramirez, D.A.; Myers, S.A.; von Winckel, G.; Krishna, S.; Berwick, M.; Padilla, S.; Sen, P.; Krishna, S. Dynamic infrared imaging for skin cancer screening. *Infrared Phys. Technol.* **2015**, *70*, 147–152. [CrossRef]
16. El-Baz, A.; Jiang, X.; Suri, J.S. *Biomedical Image Segmentation*, 1st ed.; CRC Press: Boca Raton, FL, USA, 2017; pp. 249–271. ISBN 9781482258554.
17. Herrera, J.A.; Vilaseca, M.; Düll, J.; Arjona, M.; Torrecilla, E.; Pujol, J. Iris color and texture: A comparative analysis of real irises, ocular prostheses, and colored contact lenses. *Color Res. Appl.* **2011**, *36*, 373–382. [CrossRef]
18. Martinez, W.L.; Martinez, A.R.; Solka, J.L. *Exploratory Data Analysis with Matlab*, 3rd ed.; Chapman and Hall CRC Press: New York, NY, USA, 2017; Part II; ISBN 9781498776066.
19. Ritter, G.; Wilson, J. Image Features and Descriptors. In *Handbook of Computer Vision Algorithms in Image Algebra*, 2nd ed.; CRC Press: Boca Raton, FL, USA, 2000; pp. 299–305. ISBN 0849300754.

20. Zhang, H.; Salo, D.; Kim, D.M.; Komarov, S.; Tai, Y.C.; Berezin, M.Y. Penetration depth of photons in biological tissues from hyperspectral imaging in shortwave infrared in transmission and reflection geometries. *J. Biomed. Opt.* **2016**, *21*, 126006. [CrossRef] [PubMed]
21. Monheit, G.; Cognetta, A.B.; Rabinovitz, H.; Gross, K.; Martini, M.; Grichnik, J.M.; Mihm, M.; Prieto, V.G.; Googe, P.; King, R.; et al. The performance of MelaFind: A prospective study. *Arch. Dermatol.* **2011**, *147*, 188–194. [CrossRef] [PubMed]
22. Burroni, M.; Sbano, P.; Cevenini, G.; Risulo, M.; Dell'Eva, G.; Barbini, P.; Miracco, C.; Fimiani, M.; Adreassi, L.; Rubegni, P. Dysplastic naevus vs. in situ melanoma: Digital dermoscopy analysis. *Br. J. Dermatol.* **2005**, *152*, 679–684. [CrossRef] [PubMed]
23. Ares, M.; Royo, S.; Vilaseca, M.; Herrera, J.A.; Delpueyo, X.; Sanabria, F. Handheld 3D Scanning System for In-Vivo Imaging of Skin Cancer. In Proceedings of the 5th International Conference on 3D Body Scanning Technologies, Lugano, Switzerland, 21–22 October 2014. [CrossRef]

17

Diagnostic Accuracy of Cross-Polarization OCT and OCT-Elastography for Differentiation of Breast Cancer Subtypes

Ekaterina V. Gubarkova [1,*], Elena B. Kiseleva [1], Marina A. Sirotkina [1], Dmitry A. Vorontsov [2], Ksenia A. Achkasova [1], Sergey S. Kuznetsov [3], Konstantin S. Yashin [4], Aleksander L. Matveyev [5], Aleksander A. Sovetsky [6], Lev A. Matveev [6], Anton A. Plekhanov [1], Alexey Y. Vorontsov [2], Vladimir Y. Zaitsev [6] and Natalia D. Gladkova [1]

1 Institute of Experimental Oncology and Biomedical Technologies, Privolzhsky Research Medical University, 603950 Nizhny Novgorod, Russia; kiseleva84@gmail.com (E.B.K.); sirotkina_m@mail.ru (M.A.S.); achkasova.k@bk.ru (K.A.A.); strike_gor@mail.ru (A.A.P.); natalia.gladkova@gmail.com (N.D.G.)

2 Department of Oncology, Nizhny Novgorod Regional Oncologic Hospital, 603126 Nizhny Novgorod, Russia; dr.vorontsovdmitriy@rambler.ru (D.A.V.); doctorvorontsov@mail.ru (A.Y.V.)

3 Department of Pathology, Privolzhsky Research Medical University, 603950 Nizhny Novgorod, Russia; zunek@mail.ru

4 University Clinic, Privolzhsky Research Medical University, 603950 Nizhny Novgorod, Russia; jashinmed@gmail.com

5 Laboratory of Multidimensional Signal Processing, Institute of Applied Physics of the Russian Academy of Sciences, 603950 Nizhny Novgorod, Russia; matveyev@appl.sci-nnov.ru

6 Laboratory of Wave Methods for Studying Structurally Inhomogeneous Media, Institute of Applied Physics of the Russian Academy of Sciences, 603950 Nizhny Novgorod, Russia; alex.sovetsky@mail.ru (A.A.S.); lionnn52rus@mail.ru (L.A.M.); vyuzai@ipfran.ru (V.Y.Z.)

* Correspondence: kgybarkova@mail.ru

Abstract: The possibility to assess molecular-biological and morphological features of particular breast cancer types can improve the precision of resection margin detection and enable accurate determining of the tumor aggressiveness, which is important for treatment selection. To enable reliable differentiation of breast-cancer subtypes and evaluation of resection margin, without performing conventional histological procedures, here we apply cross-polarization optical coherence tomography (CP-OCT) and compare it with a novel variant of compressional optical coherence elastography (C-OCE) in terms of the diagnostic accuracy (Ac) with histological verification. The study used 70 excised breast cancer specimens with different morphological structure and molecular status (Luminal A, Luminal B, Her2/Neo+, non-luminal and triple-negative cancer). Our first aim was to formulate convenient criteria of visual assessment of CP-OCT and C-OCE images intended (i) to differentiate tumorous and non-tumorous tissues and (ii) to enable more precise differentiation among different malignant states. We identified such criteria based on the presence of heterogeneities and characteristics of signal attenuation in CP-OCT images, as well as the presence of inclusions/mosaic structures combined with visually feasible assessment of several stiffness grades in C-OCE images. Secondly, we performed a blinded reader study of the Ac of C-OCE versus CP-OCT, for delineation of tumorous versus non-tumorous tissues followed by identification of breast cancer subtypes. For tumor detection, C-OCE showed higher specificity than CP-OCT (97.5% versus 93.3%) and higher Ac (96.0 versus 92.4%). For the first time, the Ac of C-OCE and CP-OCT were evaluated for differentiation between non-invasive and invasive breast cancer (90.4% and 82.5%, respectively). Furthermore, for invasive cancers, the difference between invasive but low-aggressive and highly-aggressive subtypes can be detected. For differentiation between non-tumorous tissue and low-aggressive breast-cancer subtypes, Ac was 95.7% for C-OCE and 88.1% for CP-OCT. For differentiation between non-tumorous tissue and highly-aggressive breast cancers, Ac was found to be 98.3% for C-OCE and

97.2% for CP-OCT. In all cases C-OCE showed better diagnostic parameters independently of the tumor type. These findings confirm the high potential of OCT-based examinations for rapid and accurate diagnostics during breast conservation surgery.

Keywords: breast cancer; cross-polarization optical coherence tomography (CP-OCT); compressional optical coherence elastography (C-OCE); image assessment

1. Introduction

Intraoperative detection of breast malignancy margins would allow minimization of the risk of tumor recurrence in patients undergoing breast conservation surgery (BCS). Intraoperative pathological estimation can be performed through frozen section analysis and imprint cytology [1]; however, these techniques are characterized by several restrictions such as resource intensity, sampling only a small percentage of the surgical margins and limited efficacy, especially for ductal carcinoma in situ (DCIS) [2]. Consequently, these methods have not been widely adopted [3]. Fluorescent techniques that utilize molecular contrast, potentially affording surgeons to visualize tumor in the cavity, are currently in the development [4,5]. Ultrasound elastography has been developed for a number of applications, and specifically for preoperative diagnosis of breast lesions [6–8]. However, its relatively low spatial resolution makes it inappropriate to use this method for intraoperative tumor margin assessment.

Optical coherence tomography (OCT) presents a very promising method for surgical tasks solving due to the clear benefits of this method such as: safety (using a near infrared light source does not risk tissue damage); accuracy (high resolution ~10–15 micron); there being no need for contrast agents; and the short duration of image attainment. OCT can be used both in the resected specimen of tumor and in the surgical cavity. OCT can be added to biopsy needle probes and can be used to guide correct sampling of tumor biopsies [9–11]. OCT is a promising method for intraoperative guidance during the resection of breast cancer and for identifying positive margins in specimens from BCS [12–15]. Recently, OCT has been proposed for intraoperative use in distinguishing tumorous and non-tumorous tissues using handheld probes [16,17]. To overcome the limited imaging depth ~2 mm typical for OCT (which usually requires sufficiently close approaching of the OCT probe towards the studied tissue), utilization of endoscopic and/or needle OCT probes are considered [11]. Moreover, it is known that structural OCT scans exhibit low contrast between tumor and uninvolved dense stromal tissue, which makes it challenging to accurately assess margin status [18]. In view of this, improvements in several aspects of OCT attract much attention, in particular, the development of functional OCT extensions based on polarization effects and stiffness analysis as considered below.

Based on the birefringence of the tissue structure, polarization-sensitive (PS) OCT provides advanced imaging of collagen fibers in the breast tissue and enhances intraoperative differentiation of breast cancer [19–21]. Stroma state assessment is fundamentally important, because tumor collagen matrix plays a crucial role in breast cancer invasion and metastatic spreading [22]. Several studies have developed quantitative diagnosis algorithms for intraoperative assessing breast cancer margins and validated them against OCT, both alone and in combination with other modalities [23]. Cross-polarization OCT (CP-OCT) is a variant of PS OCT that allows imaging of the initial polarization state changes due to both birefringence and cross-scattering in biological tissues [24]. Only orthogonally polarized backscattered light, which is mutually coherent with the incident wave, contributes to the cross-polarized (CP) OCT image. CP-OCT is a promising method for differentiating tumorous from non-tumorous tissues in human breast tissues [25], human brain tissues [26,27], as well as for diagnosis of bladder cancer [28–31]. OCT can also measure attenuation, which can be helpful for improving contrast of breast imaging research [32,33].

Attention to the problem of determining tissue stiffness (elastographic mapping) by optical coherence elastography (OCE) methods has been increasing in recent years [34–37]. Sufficiently high resolution of quantitative stiffness maps enabled by compressional OCE opened the possibility to perform morphological segmentations of tumor tissue constituents very similar to morphological segmentation of conventional histological images [25,38,39]. In these studies of experimental tumor models on animals, this technique allowed in vivo monitoring of morphological variation in tumor tissue during tumor growth and response to therapies. In studies [25,40–42], application of compressional OCE (C-OCE) for characterization of mechanical properties of excised human breast cancer specimens was demonstrated. New possibilities for intraoperative assessment of the breast cancer borders by means of optical coherence micro-elastography (OCME) were reported in a recent study [43,44]. It has been demonstrated that OCME provides additional contrast of tumor compared to OCT alone. Additionally, the potential of OCME images for evaluation of tumor margins in specimens excised during BCS was demonstrated in [41,43]. In our previous paper it was shown that CP-OCT and C-OCE can be helpful in breast cancer margin identification, as well as for grading breast cancer subtypes [25].

For more accurate evaluation of the resection margin, it is advantageous to take into account the genetic heterogeneity of breast cancer, as well as the variety of molecular-biological and morphological features influencing prognosis of the disease course (degree of aggressiveness) and treatment selection [45,46]. Indeed, it was demonstrated that probability of tumor recurrence mainly depends on molecular-biological characteristic of the tumor [47,48], while an increase in the size of the removed tissue, free of cancer cells, is not associated with a decrease in the recurrence rate [49].

Various molecular-biological and morphological features of breast cancer are anticipated to differently influence the polarizing and elastic tumor and peritumoral tissue qualities. This stimulates interest in evaluation of the clinical potential of polarization-sensitive and elastographic OCT techniques for determining breast cancer subtypes (malignancy grade) and improving tumor boundary detection based on the ability of these methods to identify different tumor subtypes. In this way, surgeons are expected to be provided with essential information that can improve reliability of the positive resection margin detection during BCS, at least for some breast cancer subtypes.

The goals of this research are (1) to define the visual assessment criteria required for the CP-OCT and C-OCE images in order to enable differentiation among various breast cancer subtypes; (2) to determine the diagnostic accuracy (sensitivity and specificity) of C-OCE in comparison with CP-OCT, for delineation of tumorous and non-tumorous breast tissues and subsequent identification of breast cancer subtypes in a blinded reader study.

2. Materials and Methods

2.1. Human Breast Specimens

This study was approved by the institutional review board of the Privolzhsky Research Medical University (Protocol #10 from 28 September 2018). All of the patients included in the study provided written informed consent. A total of 70 breast tumor tissue specimens were taken from 50 patients post partial (n = 35) or complete (n = 15) mastectomy with different diagnosis (Table 1). To minimize the effect tissue degrading, the excised specimens were immediately placed in gauze saturated with phosphate buffer and closed to prevent dehydration. CP-OCT and C-OCE images of the fresh, un-fixed breast tissue were acquired within 2 h after surgical excision. The studies were done on specimens with sizes from 0.5 × 1 cm to 1 × 2 cm. Specimens were taken from central zone of tumors for diagnostics of breast cancer subtypes and in the peritumoral area for visualization of normal (non-tumorous) breast tissue. A special motorized table for convenient positioning the specimen under the OCT probe was used. The entire CP-OCT and C-OCE study of each specimen was no longer than 20 min (including preliminary sample preparation and orientation).

Table 1. Clinical specimens' characteristics and number of imaged specimens.

Diagnosis	Number of Specimens	Age of Patients (Range)	Tumor Size
	Benign breast conditions		
Non-tumorous breast tissue	20	43–68	-
Fibroadenoma/fibroadenomatosis	4	35–48	≤1 cm
	Malignant breast lesions		
Ductal carcinoma in situ (DCIS)	5	44–63	≤1 cm
Invasive ductal carcinoma (IDC) of scirrhous structure	24	41–82	≤2 cm
Invasive ductal carcinoma (IDC) of solid structure	10	41–82	≤2 cm
Invasive lobular carcinoma (ILC) of solid structure	7	48–72	≤2 cm

2.2. Multimodal OCT Device

This study used a common path spectral domain multimodal OCT system with a central wavelength of 1310 nm and spectral width of 100 nm, with an axial resolution of 10 μm, lateral resolution is 15 μm, a scanning depth of 2 mm in air, a scanning speed of 20,000 A-scans per second. The OCT-system acquired 3D blocks of OCT data, 2 mm in depth (in air) over 2.4 × 2.4 mm^2 area and 2D lateral scanning with a similar field of view were acquired in 26 s. The CP-OCT and C-OCE images were generated in real time during the acquisition process. For living tissues, real-time angiographic imaging was also possible by processing the same data [50]. For the described OCT studies, the total scanning time along a 1–2 cm trajectory on a biopsy sample was 3–5 min depending on the number of stitched images.

Structural 2D (cross-sectional images) CP-OCT images were constructed in two virtual channels, one of which was co-polarized with the incident polarization (co-polarization channel) and the other one was orthogonal (cross-polarization channel) to the incident polarization, respectively [24]. CP-OCT aims to obtain the information contained in the cross-polarization channel, which allows one to form cross-polarization images caused by birefringence of the tissue from optically anisotropic structures (evaluate the state of connective tissue component), as well as due to contribution of coherent cross-polarization backscattering on non-spherical particles and particles with dimensions much larger than the wavelength. In view of low informativity of the co-polarization images (as found in previous studies [25]), only cross-polarization images were used for diagnostic conclusions in this study.

An advanced variant of phase-sensitive compression OCE [37,39,51–55] was used to visualize inter-frame strains in the tissue and subsequently map the Young modulus. The probe was slightly pressed onto the studied sample surface, and strain distribution in the probe vicinity was reconstructed. Strain mapping was based on estimation of axial gradients of interframe phase variations of the OCT signal using the "vector" method [51,53]. The name "vector" is due to the fact that, without explicitly singling out amplitude and phase, the complex-valued OCT signals in this method are considered as vectors in the complex plane, and the phase is singled out at the very last step of the processing. Such vector representation allows one to perform flexibly-tuned amplitude-weighted averaging over the processing-window area. As a result, noisy contributions of small-amplitude pixels and, at the same time, especially strong phase errors (by ~π rad.) are very efficiently suppressed. This allows obtaining strain maps with fairly high quality even without periodic averaging (which is very important for the one-directional single-step loading of the tissue used in the described studies). In addition to the exceptionally high tolerance to various measurement noises, the vector method is very efficient computationally, so that the elastographic processing of the acquired sequence of several hundreds of OCT scans requires ~5–10 s using a "typical" PC without the necessity of GPU computations.

Another important point is that the estimated interframe phase-variation gradient is averaged over a processing window, the dimensions of which being the main factor determining the resolution of the resultant OCE scans. For a rectangular processing window with comparable axial and lateral sizes, the resolution in strain maps is also comparable in these directions and corresponds to $\sim\frac{1}{2}$ of the window size. For the described system, the window size was ~90–100 μm, which defined the strain-mapping resolution ~45–50 μm. Such a window size was chosen empirically as a compromise between worse quality of the OCE-images for smaller windows (because of insufficiently averaged noise) and too-strong smoothing of spatial inhomogeneities for larger windows.

The next important point is quantification of the tissue Young's modulus, to enable which a reference silicone layer with preliminary calibrated stiffness (with the Young's modulus in the range 50–100 kPa) was used as described in [42,54–56]. Of key importance in the used variant of C-OCE technique is that all OCE images are formed using a pre-selected pressure level (4 kPa in the described study) standardized over the entire image area, despite the fact that for real OCE scans, the local pressure over the lateral coordinate usually varies several times because of the non-ideally planar boundary of the sample, its mechanical inhomogeneity, etc. The pressure standardization technique is based on the usage of the reference silicone layer as a sensor of local pressure as described in detail in [55]. To synthesize such a single "standardized OCE image", a series of initial structural OCT-scans acquired during monotonic compression of the sample was first processed to obtain a series of cumulative-strain maps as described in [54,57,58]. Then vertical A-scans corresponding to the selected pressure were picked up from the initial series of cumulative-strain maps and reassembled to synthesize a single cumulative-strain image in which all A-scans now correspond to the same preselected pressure onto the tissue [55]. To be sure that the strain in silicone can be considered linearly proportional to stress (pressure), high linearity of silicone was specially verified as described in [42,54,55]. Real biological tissues usually demonstrate a pronouncedly nonlinear stress–strain law. The described C-OCE method allows one to determine this law by plotting the strain in the linear precalibrated silicone against strain in any region of interest in the tissue beneath the silicone. The elasticity of the tissue can then be estimated as the tangent Young's modulus (the slope of the stress-strain curve) corresponding to the desired pre-selected pressure. It was empirically found that for breast-cancer tissue the sought tangent modulus could be conveniently estimated as the slope of the chorde corresponding to the pressure range 4 ± 1 kPa. At lower pressures, very small strain of stiffer regions was difficult to estimate, whereas at higher pressures, the elasticity contrast among various tumor components became worse because of strong nonlinearity-induced stiffening of the initially softer components of the tumor (see examples in [55]). Without such standardization the intrinsic elastic nonlinearity of breast-cancer tissues may result in uncontrollable variability of the estimated elastic modulus in different measurements and even different parts of the same image. This unpredictable variability may be rather significant (several times and greater) even for apparently moderate strains within a few percent [42,55]. Thus, the developed pressure-standardization procedures were critically important for enabling meaningful quantitative comparisons of elastographic data obtained from different measurements.

The so-obtained OCE-images were represented in the color-coded form, such that stiffer areas (those with weaker strain) are shown in blue, and soft areas, where deformation is greater, are shown in red.

2.3. *Histological Study*

After CP-OCT and C-OCE imaging of the freshly-excised sample with yet non-modified optical and biomechanical properties, the scanned area was marked on the specimen with histological ink. Then the specimen was fixed in 10% formalin for 48 h and resectioned through the marked area, so that the plane of the histological sections coincided to the cross-sectional CP-OCT and C-OCE images. For the histological evaluation, haematoxylin and eosin (H&E) staining was used. Two independent histopathologists interpreted the histological slices photographed in transmitted light with a Leica DM2500 DFC (Leica Microsystems, Wetzlar, Germany) microscope, equipped with a digital camera. Based on histopathological analysis, all samples were classified into tumorous and non-tumorous breast tissues. The revealed histological types of breast tissue include: adipose tissue with streaks of connective tissue (number of specimens $n = 20$); fibroadenomatosis/fibroadenoma ($n = 4$); DCIS ($n = 5$); invasive lobular carcinoma (ILC) ($n = 7$); invasive ductal carcinoma (IDC) of scirrhous ($n = 24$) and solid ($n = 10$) structure (Table 1). In addition, to assess tumor aggressiveness (prognosis of the disease course) immunohistochemistry (for $n = 46$ samples) was performed, identifying five molecular subtypes of the tumors: Luminal A, Luminal B (Her2/Neo-), Her2/Neo+, Non-luminal, Triple-negative cancer (TNC). Luminal A and Luminal B (Her2/Neo-) are reported to be low-aggressive tumors characterized by predominantly favorable prognosis of disease course and treatment in comparison with Her2/Neo+, Non-luminal and TNC [24]. Furthermore, it should be noted that Luminal A and Luminal B subtypes were characterized by scirrhous architectonics, while Her2/Neo+, Non-luminal, TNC had solid structure.

The results of histopathology were compared with the corresponding CP-OCT-based and C-OCE-based findings. For the blinded reader study, all images were divided into 4 groups: adipose and normal stromal breast tissue, benign breast tissue (fibroadenoma/fibroadenomatosis), non-invasive DCIS, and images portraying cancerous features of invasive low and highly-aggressive breast cancer.

2.4. *Reader Analysis of CP-OCT and C-OCE Images*

A blinded reader study was performed to evaluate the statistical performance of assessing tumorous and non-tumorous breast tissues based on the CP-OCT imaging (first test) and C-OCE visualization (second test). In the study, 115 CP-OCT and 115 C-OCE images from 50 patients were interpreted by 6 readers specially trained for this OCT-based assessment (2 biologists experienced in optical imaging, but unskilled in recognizing breast cancer pathology; 2 post-graduate students of the Medical University unexperienced both in optical imaging and in recognizing breast cancer pathology; 2 surgeons skilled in detecting breast cancer pathology, but without work experience in optical imaging) who were unaware whether the image contained cancer or not. The readers were given a training set of sample CP-OCT and C-OCE images (3 images of each histological type of breast tissue).

The criteria evaluated by the readers are summarized in Tables 2 and 3. Each image group had its own set of visual criteria. The reader's goal was to distinguish between tumorous and non-tumorous breast tissues. If an image was considered to represent non-tumorous breast tissue, the reader indicated a score of "0" whether it was normal breast tissue or fibroadenoma. If the reader identified malignant lesion marks, a score from "1" to "3" was assigned to the sample depending on the estimated tumor aggressiveness. The score of "1" means that the reader thinks that the image represents non-invasive DCIS; a score of "2" means that the reader considers the cancer to be invasive, but less aggressive; a score of "3" means that the reader thinks that invasive cancer is more aggressive.

The first test was based on assessment of signal architecture in cross- polarization images (Table 2). The cross-polarization channel enables more contrast visualization of the presence and state of connective tissue in comparison with the co-polarization OCT images.

Structural features in the CP-OCT images were distinguished by the following features of the scattering intensity and lateral uniformity of the signal attenuation (Table 2):

(i) the average level of the CP-OCT signal throughout the image is visually estimated as "low" like in Figure 1(b5) or "high" for the used 0–50 dB signal range, where "low" corresponded to intensities below 25 dB, i.e., the noise range in the used scale, and "high" related to the level above 25 dB on the used scale like in Figure 1(b2);

(ii) the presence of structures with a sharp boundary between contrasting-in-brightness regions with well-circumscribed boundary architecture like in Figure 1(b3) (which was graded as "yes"/"no");

(iii) the attenuation rate as estimated by the penetration depth of the probing radiation ("high" attenuation like in Figure 1(b5) and "low" like in Figure 1(b2));

(iv) the uniformity of attenuation along the interior border of the structural CP-OCT image ("uniform" like in Figure 1(b2)/"non-uniform" like in Figure 1(b4)).

Table 2. Visual assessment criteria of cross-polarization optical coherence tomography (CP-OCT) images for distinguishing between non-tumorous and tumorous breast tissue.

	Normal (Non-Tumorous) Breast Tissue ($n = 20$)	Fibroadenoma/ Fibroadenomatosis ($n = 13$)	DCIS ($n = 10$)	Low-Aggressive Invasive Breast Cancer ($n = 47$)	Highly-Aggressive Invasive Breast Cancer ($n = 25$)
			Main criterion:		
Typical architecture	honeycomb structure, areas of high intensity signal	predominance of areas with high signal intensity	alternating signal of high, medium and low intensity; the presence of structures with no signal with clear boundaries (ducts)	alternating signal of medium and low intensity	homogenous low intensity signal
			Additional criteria:		
Signal penetration depth	high	high	high	high	low
Structures with clear (contrasting) boundaries	no	no	yes	no	no
Uniformity of the OCT signal attenuation along the inferior border of the image	uniform	uniform	highly uneven	non-uniform	uniform
Final score	0	0	1	2	3

n—number of images.

Table 3. Visual assessment criteria of compressional optical coherence elastography (C-OCE) images for distinguishing between non-tumorous and tumorous breast tissue.

	Normal (Non-Tumorous) Breast Tissue ($n = 20$)	Fibroadenoma/ Fibroadenomatosis ($n = 13$)	DCIS ($n = 10$)	Low-Aggressive Invasive Breast Cancer ($n = 47$)	Highly-Aggressive Invasive Breast Cancer ($n = 25$)
			Main criterion:		
Typical stiffness pattern	uniform low stiffness level over the C-OCE image		low stiffness level of the stiffness throughout the image with high-contrast zones with strongly increased stiffness	non-uniform high stiffness level over the C-OCE image	
			Additional criteria:		
Predominance of uniform distribution of high stiffness values (>500 kPa)	no	no	no	no	yes
Presence of multiple moderately contrast inclusions of high stiffness (Mosaic structure)	no	no	no	yes	no
Final score	0	0	1	2	3

n—number of images.

The second test was based on the analysis of stiffness values distributions on C-OCE images. Stiffness maps are presented in a color palette, where hard areas (blue—above 500 kPa) indicate the presence of tumor cells, and soft regions (red—below 100 kPa) represent adipose and connective tissues. At the same time, tissues with intermediate stiffness (the predominance of orange and yellow colors corresponding to ~200–400 kPa) correspond to the presence of such degenerative changes of breast-tissue stroma as fibrosis or hyalinosis of collagen fibers. The threshold values for stiffness (Table 3) of the main types of breast-tissue components were identified as described in detail in our previous work [25], in which accurate comparison of histological and OCE images was performed.

Main and additional criteria of subsuming the images to one or another group were formulated for cross-polarization and C-OCE images, the additional criteria of visual assessment being needed for more precise differentiation among different malignant states (Tables 2 and 3).

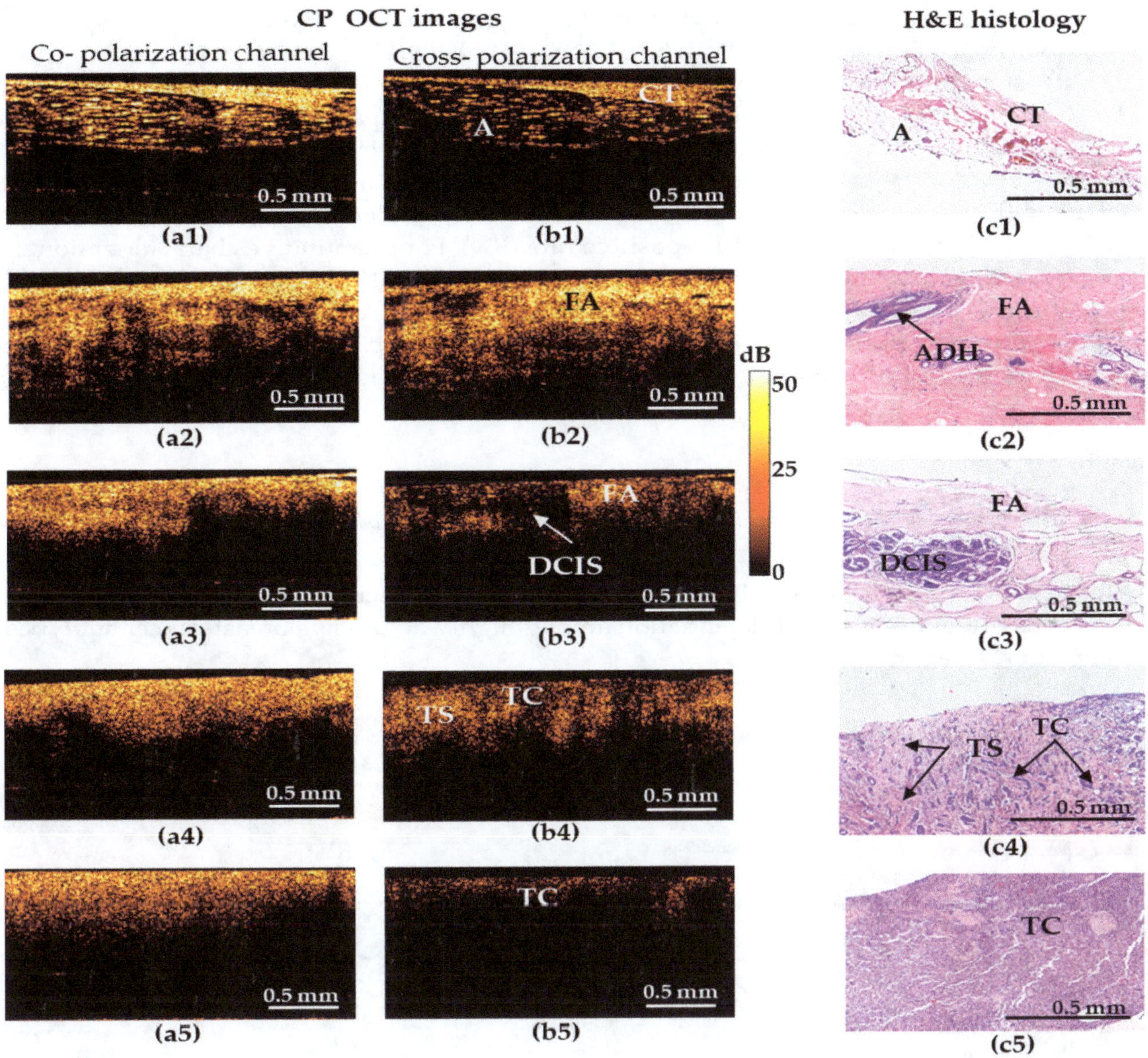

Figure 1. Representative depth-wise co- and cross-polarization OCT images (**a**,**b**) of non-tumorous and tumorous breast tissue with the corresponding histology (**c**). (**a1**–**c1**) Adipose tissue with streaks of connective tissue; (**a2**–**c2**) fibroadenomatosis/fibroadenoma; (**a3**–**c3**) DCIS; (**a4**–**c4**) invasive ductal carcinoma (IDC) of scirrhous structure (low-aggressive breast cancer subtype); (**a5**–**c5**) IDC of solid structure (highly-aggressive breast cancer subtype). (**a1**–**a5**) OCT images in co-polarization channel; (**b1**–**b5**) OCT images in cross-polarization channel; (**c1**–**c5**) histological images, haematoxylin and eosin (H&E) staining. Abbreviations: A—adipose, CT—connective tissue, FA—fibroadenomatosis, ADH—atypical ductal hyperplasia, DCIS—ductal carcinoma in situ, TS—tumor stroma, TC—cluster of tumor cells.

2.5. Statistical Analysis

The results of the blinded reader study of CP-OCT and C-OCE images analysis were collected for determining the diagnostic accuracy for distinguishing: (1) non-tumorous breast tissues (n = 33) from tumor (n = 82); (2) non-invasive DCIS (n = 10)) from invasive breast cancer (n = 72); (3) low-aggressive invasive tumors (Luminal A, Luminal B (Her2/Neo-)) (n = 47) with favorable prognosis from highly aggressive invasive tumors (Her2/Neo+, Non-luminal, TNC) (n = 25) with unfavorable prognosis;

(4) non-tumorous breast tissues (n = 33) from low-aggressive invasive tumors (n = 47), and (5) non-tumorous breast tissues (n = 33) from highly-aggressive invasive tumors (n = 25).

The statistical analysis was performed using Statistica 10.0 and IBM SPSS Statistics software.

The assessment of the informative value and diagnostic capabilities of the studied methods (CP-OCT and C-OCE) was carried out with an estimation of their sensitivity (Se), specificity (Sp), and diagnostic accuracy (Ac). Based on the sensitivity and specificity values, Receiver operating characteristic (ROC) curves were constructed, which show the dependence of the number of true positive rate (TP) on the number of false positive rate (FN). For quantitative characterization of the ROC curves, we evaluated the area under the ROC curve (AUC), i.e., the area bounded by the ROC curve and the axis of the false positive rate [59]. The higher the AUC, the better the classifier is.

The inter-reader agreement was calculated using Cohen's kappa coefficient (k): k ≥ 0.81—perfect agreement; 0.61 ≤ k < 0.80—substantial agreement; k < 0.6—poor agreement [60].

3. Results

3.1. Visual Assessment of the CP-OCT and C-OCE Images for Distinguishing between Non-Tumorous and Tumorous Breast Tissue

The results based on the CP-OCT and C-OCE images for representative cases of the non-tumorous and tumorous breast tissue and differentiation among highly-aggressive breast-cancer subtypes are shown in Figures 1 and 2.

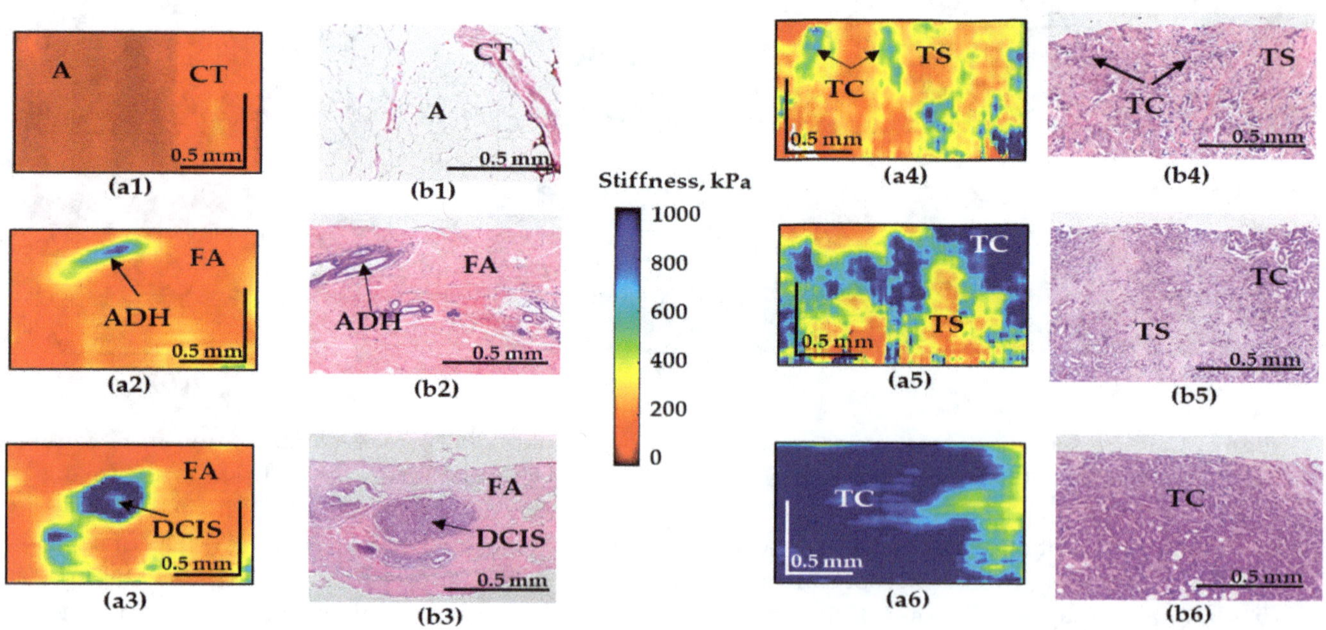

Figure 2. Representative depth-wise C-OCE images (**a1**–**a6**) of non-tumorous and tumorous breast tissue with corresponding histological images (**b1**–**b6**). (**a1**–**b1**) Adipose tissue with streaks of connective tissue; (**a2**–**b2**) fibroadenomatosis/fibroadenoma; (**a3**–**b3**) DCIS; (**a4**,**a5**–**b4**,**b5**) IDC of scirrhous structure (low-aggressive breast cancer subtypes); (**a6**–**b6**) IDC of solid structure (highly-aggressive breast cancer subtype). Abbreviations: A—adipose, CT—connective tissue, ADH—atypical ductal hyperplasia, FA—fibroadenomatosis, DCIS—ductal carcinoma in situ, TS—tumor stroma, TC—cluster of tumor cells.

Figure 1 shows five types of representative CP-OCT and histological images: "adipose tissue with streaks of connective tissue" (a1–c1)/"fibroadenomatosis/fibroadenoma" (a2–c2)/"DCIS" (a3–c3)/invasive low-aggressive breast cancer of scirrhous structure (a4–c4)/invasive highly-aggressive breast cancer of solid structure (a5–c5).

Benign breast tissue states are characterized by high signal-penetration depth and uniformity of the signal attenuation along the inferior border in co- and cross-polarized structural OCT images (Figure 1). The hallmark of normal adipose (fatty) tissue is a "honeycomb" structure with low sparse scattering, while fibrous structures are characterized by high uniform scattering in co- and cross-polarized structural OCT images (Figure 1(a1–c1)). Fibroadenoma is characterized by a predominance of high-intensity OCT signal in co- and cross-polarization channels (Figure 1(a2–c2)) in comparison with normal breast tissue that has a dense structure due to the presence of large fibrous collagen fibers (Figure 1(c2)).

Cases suspicious for malignancy are characterized by general reduction in signal intensity and its penetration depth, irregular inferior border. All these features cause heterogeneity of the image. In particular, DCIS (Figure 1(c3)) is characterized by the presence of localized structures with low signal intensity and clear boundaries in the surrounding fibrous stroma with a high signal intensity in the cross-polarization channel (Figure 1(b3)). In co-polarization channels DCIS is not detectable (Figure 1(a3)).

In case of invasive breast cancer, the OCT signal in the cross-polarization channel for highly-aggressive (Figure 1(b5)) and less-aggressive (Figure 1(b4)) cancer subtypes is greatly different. IDC of solid structure (highly-aggressive) demonstrates a uniform low-level OCT signal, which is associated with an increased density of tumor cells and an almost total absence of anisotropic (fibrous) structures in this tumor subtype (Figure 1(b5)). For IDC of scirrhous structure (less-aggressive subtype), the heterogeneity of the OCT signal was observed: an alternating signal of medium and low intensity was revealed (Figure 1(b4)). On the corresponding histological images, there were clusters of tumor cells surrounded by connective tissue in a state of fibrosis and hyalinosis (Figure 1(c4)), which clearly leads to an increase in the level of OCT signal in these areas. It should be noted that in these cases, there is no pronounced contrast between low-aggressive (Figure 1(a4)) and highly-aggressive (Figure 1(a5)) breast cancer subtypes in the co-polarization channel.

Thus, in the structural OCT images, the most informative is the cross- polarization channel showing both regions with fairly high cross-polarization backscattering and (corresponding to the presence of connective tissue) and regions with a reduced cross-polarization signal (corresponding to the clusters of tumor cells), see Figure 1(b1–b5)). Therefore, in view of low informativity of the co-polarization images, only cross- polarization images were used for diagnostic accuracy analysis in this study.

The C-OCE image of the normal mammary gland (normal connective tissue and adipose tissue) is characterized by the lowest stiffness (Figure 2(a1)). However, fibroadenomatosis/fibroadenoma is characterized by a slight overall increase in stiffness (Figure 2(a2)) and the presence of well-localized areas with an increased elastic modulus in the regions of atypical ductal hyperplasia (ADH).

C-OCE images of malignancy demonstrate the appearance of regions with pronouncedly increased stiffness. Moreover, for IDC of solid structure (highly-aggressive), these areas occupy up to 90% of the entire image, which sharply distinguishes this breast cancer subtype (Figure 2(a6)). The ducts filled with tumor cells for DCIS are visualized as high-contrast zones with strongly increased stiffness (Figure 2(a3)) which coincide well with the histological image. The surrounding fibrous tissue is characterized by fairly low stiffness values (Figure 2(a3)). The OCE images of IDC of scirrhous structure demonstrate an increased stiffness in the regions of the clusters of tumor cells and significantly lower stiffness in the regions of the tumor stroma, causing multiple moderately contrast inclusions with elevated stiffness, which represents a feature of low-aggressive tumor subtype (Figure 2(a4–a5)).

In addition, it is necessary to mention that images of IDC of scirrhous structure and fibroadenoma may have similar patterns that may be challenging to differentiate for the reader. To solve this problem an additional criteria (Table 3) of "presence the numerous and less contrasting inclusions of increased stiffness" was included in cases of IDC (Figure 2(a4)) in contrast to single inclusions in cases of fibroadenoma (Figure 2(a2)) and DCIS (Figure 2(a3)).

3.2. Diagnostic Accuracy of CP-OCT and C-OCE Based on Visual Assessment of Images

The results of the two tests, using the identified main and additional criteria, separately in CP-OCT images and C-OCE images demonstrate their great agreement among the readers. The concordance coefficient in the determination of tumorous or non-tumorous breast tissue in the analysis of CP-OCT images between two researchers was k = 0.68, between two post-graduate students k = 0.93, between the two surgeons k = 0.80. The concordance coefficient in the detection of tissue type in the analysis of C-OCE images between two researchers was k = 0.86, between two post-graduate students k = 0.93, between the two surgeons k = 0.82.

To demonstrate the variability of the test results, ROC-curves were presented for each reader (Figures 3 and 4). ROC-curves analysis confirmed that visual assessment of CP-OCT and C-OCE images has a high diagnostic value for differentiating non-tumorous and tumorous breast tissue (AUC values for all readers were 0.90–0.97 and 0.93–0.99, respectively) and also for distinguishing between low- and highly-aggressive invasive breast-cancer subtypes (AUC values for all readers were 0.84–0.90 and 0.80–1.00, respectively) (Figure 3c, Figure 4c). Slightly lower values were obtained for differentiation between non-invasive breast lesion and invasive breast cancer (AUC values for all readers were 0.74–0.93 and 0.86–0.95, respectively) (Figure 3b, Figure 4b). The ROC-curves show that the best results were demonstrated by the researches experienced in optical imaging.

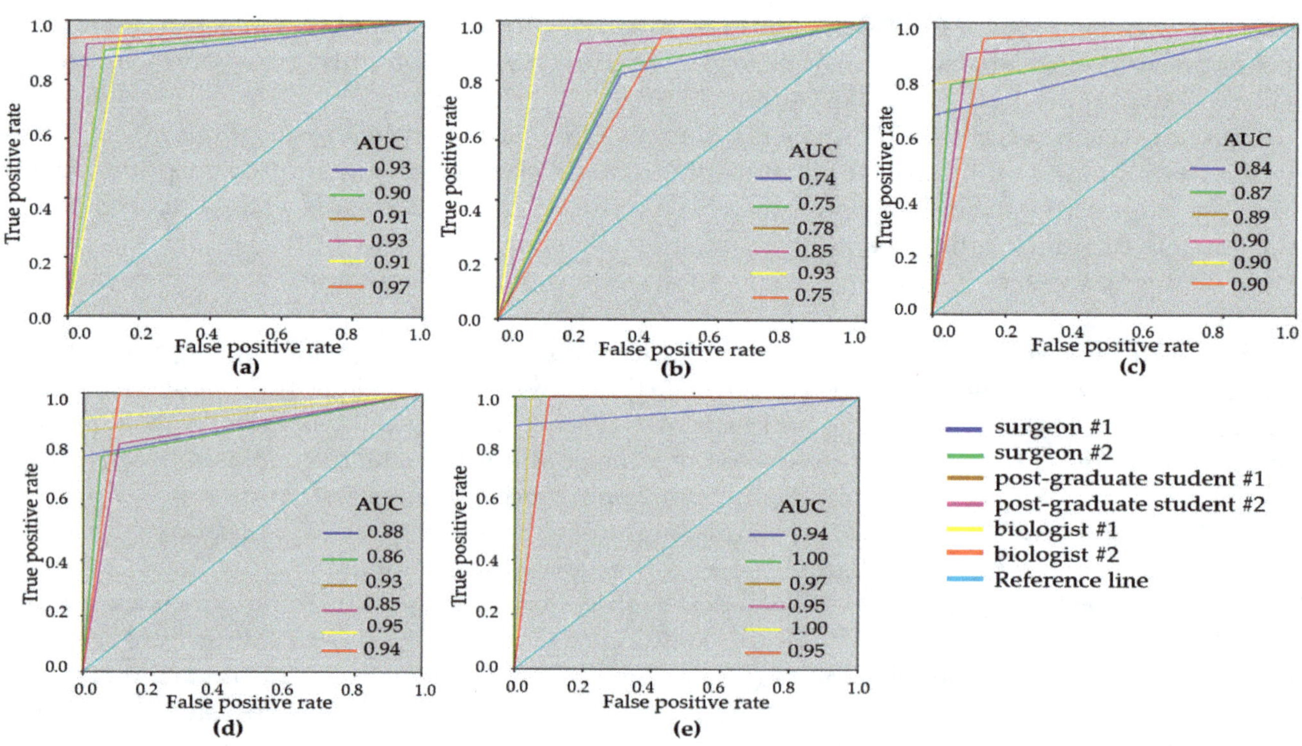

Figure 3. Receiver operating characteristic (ROC)-curves showing the results of visual assessment CP-OCT images for distinguishing non-tumorous breast tissue from tumor (**a**), DCIS from invasive breast cancer (**b**), low-aggressive invasive breast cancer from highly aggressive (**c**), non-tumorous breast tissue from low-aggressive breast cancer (**d**), non-tumorous breast tissue from highly aggressive breast cancer (**e**) for six "blinded" readers.

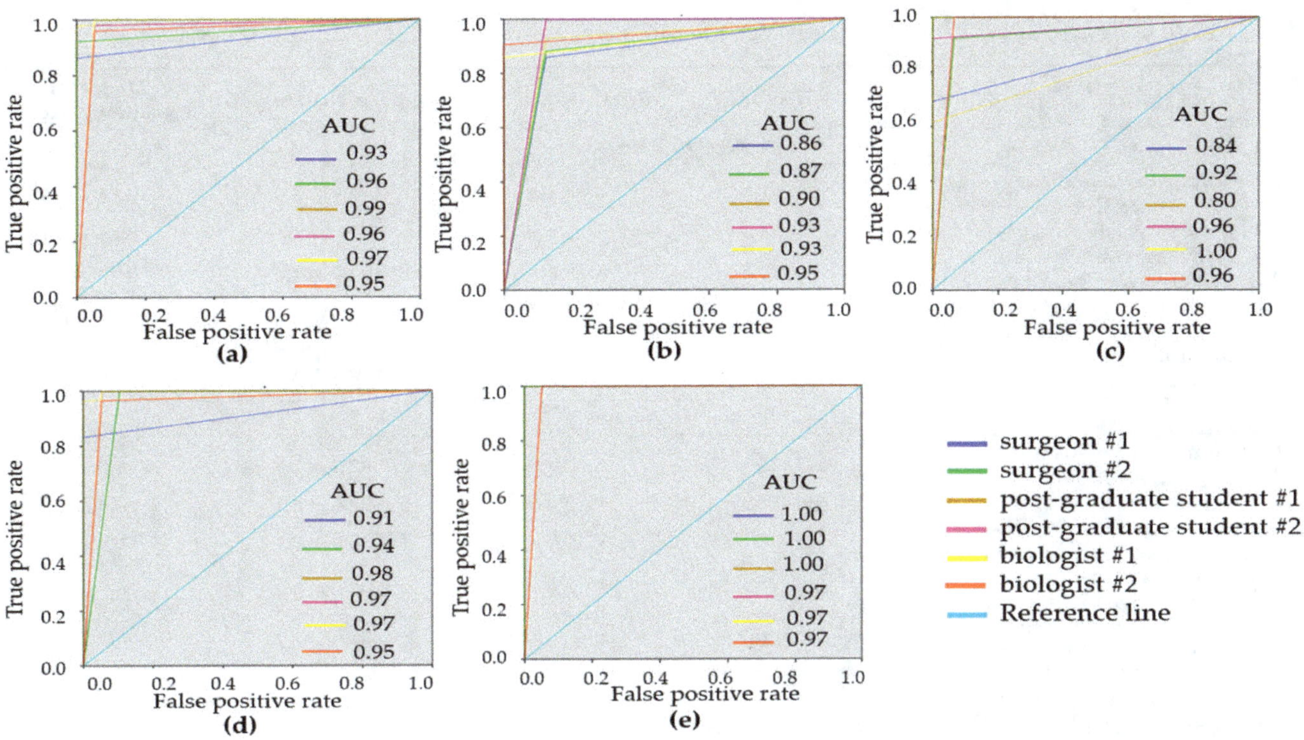

Figure 4. ROC-curves showing the results of visual assessment of C-OCE images for distinguishing non-tumorous from tumorous breast tissue (**a**), DCIS from invasive breast cancer (**b**), low-aggressive invasive breast cancer from highly-aggressive (**c**), non-tumorous breast tissue from low-aggressive breast cancer (**d**), non-tumorous breast tissue from highly-aggressive breast cancer (**e**) for six "blinded" readers.

The results of the blinded reader analysis are summarized in Table 4, showing the sensitivity, specificity and diagnostic accuracy. Each diagnostic index was averaged among all six readers. High diagnostic values were obtained for the differential diagnosis of all analyzed groups. The diagnostic accuracy of distinguishing non-tumorous tissue from tumor was 92.4 ± 2.3% for CP-OCT and 96.0 ± 3.3% for OCE, which determines the OCE method as more specific for detecting tumorous tissue.

For the first time, the diagnostic efficiency of CP-OCT and C-OCE methods for the differential diagnosis of non-invasive from invasive breast cancer was established (Se = 90.1 ± 5.7%, Sp = 70.6 ± 11.3%, Ac = 82.5 ± 7.1% and Se = 90.5 ± 5.3%, Sp = 92.0 ± 6.1%, Ac = 90.4 ± 2.7%, respectively). Furthermore, we demonstrated the possibility to differentiate invasive low-aggressive breast cancer subtypez with a favorable prognosis from highly-aggressive breast cancer subtypes with a poor prognosis for treatment and the course of the disease (Se-83.5 ± 10.5%, Sp-93.5 ± 6.0%, Ac-87.8 ± 6.5% and Se-87.3 ± 13.8 ± 6.5%, Sp-98.0 ± 3.1%, Ac-89.5 ± 10.0%, respectively). In both cases, it was demonstrated that C-OCE showed the best diagnostic indicators (Table 4).

Additionally, we performed a diagnostic analysis of the possibility to distinguish non-tumorous breast tissue from low- and highly-aggressive breast cancer subtypes. It has been shown that the diagnostic accuracy of the difference between non-tumorous breast tissue and a low-aggressive subtype of cancer is 88.1 ± 6.0% for CP-OCT and 95.7 ± 4.1% for C-OCE. The diagnostic accuracy of the difference between non-tumorous breast tissue and highly-aggressive cancer is 97.2 ± 2.8% for CP-OCT and for C-OCE—98.3 ± 2.2%.

Thus, we demonstrated the possibility to use CP-OCT and C-OCE methods for detecting different breast cancer subtypes on the resection margin which would minimize the risk of recurrence and reoperations.

Table 4. The results of diagnostic test for visual assessment of the CP-OCT and C-OCE images.

	AUC (Range)	Sensitivity (Se), %	Specificity (Sp), %	Diagnostic Accuracy (Ac), %
CP-OCT imaging				
Non-tumorous versus tumorous breast tissue	0.90–0.97	92.0 ± 4.0	93.3 ± 6.0	92.4 ± 2.3
DCIS versus invasive breast cancer	0.74–0.93	90.1 ± 5.7	70.6 ± 11.3	82.5 ± 7.1
Low-aggressive versus highly-aggressive breast cancer	0.84–0.90	83.5 ± 10.5	93.5 ± 6.0	87.8 ± 6.5
Non-tumorous breast tissue versus low-aggressive breast cancer	0.85–0.95	85.1 ± 8.8	95.8 ± 4.9	88.1 ± 6.0
Non-tumorous breast tissue versus highly-aggressive breast cancer	0.94–1.00	98.1 ± 4.4	95.8 ± 4.9	97.2 ± 2.8
C-OCE imaging				
Non-tumorous versus tumorous breast tissue	0.93–0.99	95.0 ± 5.1	97.5 ± 2.7	96.0 ± 3.3
DCIS versus invasive breast cancer	0.86–0.95	90.5 ± 5.3	92.0 ± 6.1	90.4 ± 2.7
Low-aggressive versus highly-aggressive breast cancer	0.80–1.00	87.3 ± 13.8	98.0 ± 3.1	89.5 ± 10.0
Non-tumorous breast tissue versus low-aggressive breast cancer	0.91–0.98	95.8 ± 6.5	95.8 ± 3.7	95.7 ± 4.1
Non-tumorous breast tissue versus highly-aggressive breast cancer	0.97–1.00	98.6 ± 3.2	97.5 ± 2.7	98.3 ± 2.2

3.3. Assessment of Human Breast Cancer Margins

The tests performed in this study demonstrated that, in distinguishing the norm from low-aggressive cancers (and, moreover, highly aggressive ones), the analysis of both CP-OCT and C-OCE images the both methods enable high diagnostic accuracy. However, when searching for the transition between IDC of scirrhous structure and non-cancerous tissue, the C-OCE-based stiffness mapping (Figure 5c) visualizes the tumor margin much more clearly in comparison with the cross-polarization images (Figure 5b).

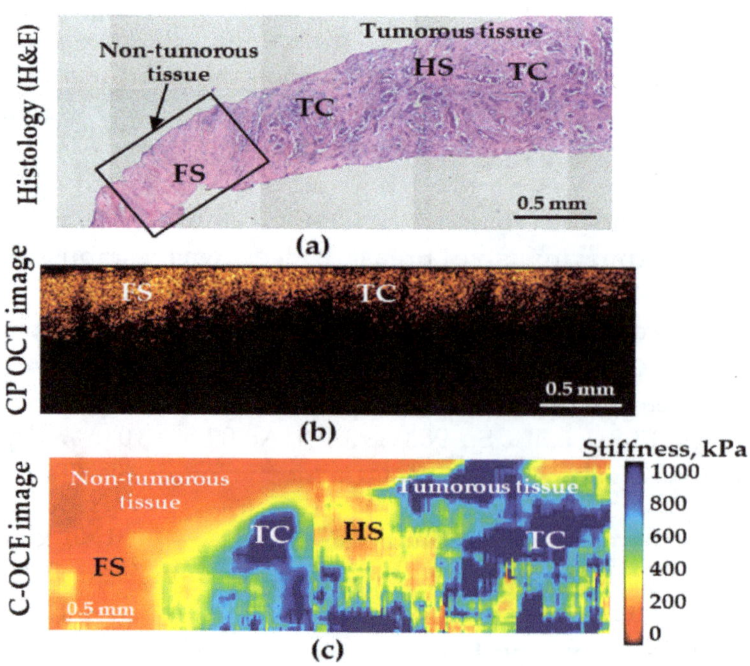

Figure 5. Histological image (**a**) demonstrating transition between non-tumorous (fibrous stroma—FS) and tumorous breast tissues (low-aggressive IDC of scirrhous structure); (**b**) is the corresponding CP-OCT image in the cross-polarization channel and (**c**) is the C-OCE images of the same area. HS denotes hyalinized stroma, and TC—clusters of tumor cells.

4. Discussion

The results presented here show the high diagnostic value and efficiency of CP-OCT and C-OCE methods for differential diagnosis of non-tumorous and tumorous breast tissue, with the further prospect of intraoperative determination of the "positive" margin of tumor resection during breast-conserving surgery in real time. In addition, the diagnostic efficiency of CP-OCT and C-OCE methods for differentiation between non-invasive and invasive breast cancers, as well as between invasive low-aggressive breast cancer subtype with a favorable prognosis (Luminal A, Luminal B (Her2/Neo-)) and highly aggressive breast cancer subtypes with a poor prognosis for course of the disease (Her2/Neo+, Non-luminal, TNC).

In previous studies, only standard visual imaging criteria, such as signal intensity and high/low stiffness, were used for differentiation between tumorous and non-tumorous breast tissues. In this study, additional analysis criteria were proposed, which made it possible to increase the diagnostic sensitivity and specificity, significantly reducing the number of erroneous diagnoses. We identified such additional analysis criteria as the presence of structures and the characteristics of signal attenuation in depth on cross-polarization images, as well as the presence of inclusions and mosaic structure on C-OCE images with visually feasible assessment of several stiffness grades.

Previous works have demonstrated that conventional, intensity-based OCT can provide differentiation between tumorous and non-tumorous breast tissues through both quantitative [18,61–63] and qualitative [32,61,63] assessment of the OCT signal. Several studies demonstrated that OCE has the high potential to delineate tumor in breast tissue based on elevated elasticity on a microscale [33,40,41,44]. A recent study [16] demonstrated the ability of structural OCT to identify positive margins in specimens from BCS. The qualitative assessment of OCT images showed the high diagnostic accuracy of structural OCT for distinguishing normal and cancerous tissue within the resection bed following wide local excision of the human breast: sensitivity of 91.7% and specificity of 92.1% [16]. Additionally, visual assessment of C-OCE images for evaluation of tumor margins in specimens excised during breast-conserving surgery also provides high sensitivity of (92.9%) and specificity (96.4%) [43].

Breast cancer is a highly heterogeneous disease, both morphologically and genetically. The surgical approach and the amount of resection depend on the subtype of breast cancer, which, as this study has shown, can be determined in rapid OCT-based tests, including the possibility of intraoperative use. The C-OCE and CP-OCT images provide additional contrast between tumor and normal tissue in comparison with structural OCT. C-OCE and CP-OCT analysis of excised tissue specimens can distinguish between normal and cancerous tissues by identifying the heterogeneous and disorganized connective tissue structures indicative for malignancy. We have demonstrated that differences in the microstructural features of cross-polarization and stiffness images enable differentiation between highly and low-aggressive breast cancer subtypes confirmed by histopathology. For this purpose, the main and additional criteria for assigning an image to a particular group were formulated, which are necessary for a more accurate differentiation of malignant conditions among themselves. For example, a uniform low-intensity in CP-OCT images and a uniform high level of stiffness in C-OCE images characterize tumor of a solid structure, while tumor tissue of a scirrhous structure in the immediate vicinity of non-tumorous breast tissue can also retain homogeneity, or it can lose it and may be represented by different levels of signal intensity and stiffness.

ROC curves were constructed as a measure of overall accuracy for each reader when non-cancerous tissue was distinguished from tumor by CP-OCT and C-OCE methods (Figure 3). In this case, C-OCE showed higher specificity (97.5 ± 2.7% vs. 93.3 ± 6.0%) and diagnostic accuracy (96.0 ± 3.3% vs. 92.4 ± 2.3%) compared to cross-polarized images. This fact may be caused by the difficulty in interpreting qualitative OCT criteria based on signal intensity by readers, in comparison with the criteria for interpreting quantitative OCE images that usually have more contrast and visually easier assessable differences. Overall, for differentiation between tumorous and non-tumorous tissues, the C-OCE method has proved to be more efficient.

Additionally, for more specific differentiation between non-invasive breast cancer and invasive breast cancer, the following diagnostic parameters were determined for CP-OCT and C-OCE methods: Se = 90.1 ± 5.7%, Sp = 70.6 ± 11.3%, Ac = 82.5 ± 7.1% and Se = 90.5 ± 5.3%, Sp = 92.0 ± 6.1%, Ac = 90.4 ± 2.7%, respectively. For distinguishing between invasive low-aggressive and highly-aggressive breast cancer subtypes, the CP-OCT and C-OCE gave the following results: Se = 83.5 ± 10.5%, Sp = 93.5 ± 6.0%, Ac = 87.8 ± 6.5% and Se = 87.3 ± 13.8 ± 6.5%, Sp = 98.0 ± 3.1%, Ac = 89.5 ± 10.0%, respectively. Therefore, in both cases, C-OCE showed better diagnostic indicators (Table 4).

The diagnostic accuracy of the difference between non-tumorous breast tissue and low-aggressive breast cancer for CP-OCT and C-OCE was found to be fairly high, 88.1 ± 6.0% and 95.7 ± 4.1%, respectively. Even higher was the Ac of CP-OCT and C-OCE for the difference between non-tumorous breast tissue and highly-aggressive breast cancer (97.2 ± 2.8% and 98.3 ± 2.2%, respectively).

Accurate determining of the boundaries of tumor resection is more feasible for tumors of a solid structure in comparison with tumors of scirrhous structure that may resemble fibroadenomas in OCT-based images. However, the performed targeted histological examination has given a clue for better understanding of the causes of stiffness increase or decrease and made it possible to define additional criteria that improved the diagnostic accuracy of C-OCE for various breast cancer subtypes detection, including non-invasive and low-aggressive tumors.

Thus, the formulated additional (clarifying) criteria for visual assessment of CP-OCT and C-OCE images provided a higher diagnostic accuracy in differentiation between tumorous and non-tumorous breast tissues with various grades of aggressiveness. In the future, this will increase the value of these OCT-based methods in detecting the boundaries of tumor resection during BCS.

5. Conclusions

Both CP-OCT and C-OCE data may be helpful to a surgeon–oncologist for more accurate detection of a "clean" resection margin during breast-conserving surgery. The test based on assessment of C-OCE images has shown higher diagnostic accuracy (96%) and sensitivity (95%) in comparison with CP-OCT images (Se—92%, Ac—92.4%) for breast cancer detection. Furthermore, the preformed study demonstrated high potential of CP-OCT and C-OCE for differentiating particular molecular-biological and morphological subtypes of breast cancer with assessment of the tumor aggressiveness, which is important for subsequent treatment selection.

Author Contributions: Conceptualization, N.D.G. and M.A.S.; images analysis, M.A.S., E.B.K., K.A.A., A.A.P., K.S.Y. and D.A.V.; C-OCE methodology and software, A.L.M., L.A.M., A.A.S. and V.Y.Z.; histological analysis, S.S.K., D.A.V.; data curation, E.V.G., E.B.K.; writing—original draft preparation, E.V.G.; writing—review and editing, N.D.G., A.Y.V. and V.Y.Z.; visualization, E.V.G.; supervision, N.D.G. All authors have read and agreed to the published version of the manuscript.

References

1. Esbona, K.; Li, Z.; Wilke, L.G. Intraoperative imprint cytology and frozen section pathology for margin assessment in breast conservation surgery: A systematic review. *Ann. Surg. Oncol.* **2012**, *19*, 3236–3245. [CrossRef] [PubMed]
2. Decker, M.R.; Trentham-Dietz, A.; Loconte, N.K.; Neuman, H.B.; Smith, M.A.; Punglia, R.S.; Greenberg, C.C.; Wilke, L.G. The Role of Intraoperative Pathologic Assessment in the Surgical Management of Ductal Carcinoma In Situ. *Ann. Surg. Oncol.* **2016**, *23*, 2788–2794. [CrossRef] [PubMed]
3. Harness, J.K.; Giuliano, A.E.; Pockaj, B.A.; Downs-Kelly, E. Margins: A status report from the Annual Meeting of the American Society of Breast Surgeons. *Ann Surg Oncol Ann. Surg. Oncol.* **2014**, *21*, 3192–3197. [CrossRef] [PubMed]

4. Lamberts, L.E.; Koch, M.; de Jong, J.S.; Adams, A.L.L.; Glatz, J.; Kranendonk, M.E.G.; van Scheltinga, A.G.T.T.; Jansen, L.; de Vries, J.; Lub-de Hooge, M.N.; et al. Tumor-Specific Uptake of Fluorescent Bevacizumab-IRDye800CW Microdosing in Patients with Primary Breast Cancer: A Phase I Feasibility Study. *Clin. Cancer Res.* **2017**, *23*, 2730–2741. [CrossRef]
5. Tummers, Q.R.; Verbeek, F.P.; Schaafsma, B.E.; Boonstra, M.C.; van der Vorst, J.R.; Liefers, G.J.; van de Velde, C.J.; Frangioni, J.V.; Vahrmeijer, A.L. Real-time intraoperative detection of breast cancer using near-infrared fluorescence imaging and Methylene Blue. *Eur. J. Surg. Oncol.* **2014**, *40*, 850–858. [CrossRef]
6. Wojcinski, S.; Farrokh, A.; Weber, S.; Thomas, A.; Fischer, T.; Slowinski, T.; Schmidt, W.; Degenhardt, F. Multicenter study of ultrasound real-time tissue elastography in 779 cases for the assessment of breast lesions: Improved diagnostic performance by combining the BI-RADS®-US classification system with sonoelastography. *Ultraschall. Med.* **2010**, *31*, 484–491. [CrossRef]
7. Dua, S.M.; Gray, R.J.; Keshtgar, M. Strategies for localisation of impalpable breast lesions. *Breast* **2011**, *20*, 246–253. [CrossRef]
8. Xu, H.; Varghese, T.; Jiang, J.; Zagzebski, J.A. In vivo classification of breast masses using features derived from axial-strain and axial-shear images. *Ultrason. Imaging* **2012**, *4*, 222–236. [CrossRef]
9. Wang, J.; Xu, Y.; Boppart, S.A. Review of optical coherence tomography in oncology. *J. Biomed. Opt.* **2017**, *22*, 1–23. [CrossRef]
10. Curatolo, A.; McLaughlin, R.A.; Quirk, B.C.; Kirk, R.W.; Bourke, A.G.; Wood, B.A.; Robbins, P.D.; Saunders, C.M.; Sampson, D.D. Ultrasound-guided optical coherence tomography needle probe for the assessment of breast cancer tumor margins. *AJR Am. J. Roentgenol.* **2012**, *199*, W520–W522. [CrossRef]
11. Kennedy, K.M.; McLaughlin, R.A.; Kennedy, B.F.; Tien, A.; Latham, B.; Saunders, C.M.; Sampson, D.D. Needle optical coherence elastography for the measurement of microscale mechanical contrast deep within human breast tissues. *J. Biomed. Opt.* **2013**, *18*, 121510. [CrossRef] [PubMed]
12. Nguyen, F.T.; Zysk, A.M.; Chaney, E.J.; Kotynek, J.G.; Oliphant, U.J.; Bellafiore, F.J.; Rowland, K.M.; Johnson, P.A.; Boppart, S.A. Intraoperative evaluation of breast tumor margins with optical coherence tomography. *Cancer Res.* **2009**, *69*, 8790–8796. [CrossRef] [PubMed]
13. Ha, R.; Friedlander, L.C.; Hibshoosh, H.; Hendon, C.; Feldman, S.; Ahn, S.; Schmidt, H.; Akens, M.K.; Fitzmaurice, M.; Wilson, B.C.; et al. Optical Coherence Tomography: A Novel Imaging Method for Post-lumpectomy Breast Margin Assessment-A Multi-reader Study. *Acad. Radiol.* **2018**, *25*, 279–287. [CrossRef] [PubMed]
14. Schmidt, H.; Connolly, C.; Jaffer, S.; Oza, T.; Weltz, C.R.; Port, E.R.; Corben, A. Evaluation of surgically excised breast tissue microstructure using wide-field optical coherence tomography. *Breast J.* **2020**, *26*, 917–923. [CrossRef] [PubMed]
15. Savastru, D.; Chang, E.W.; Miclos, S.; Pitman, M.B.; Patel, A.; Iftimia, N. Detection of breast surgical margins with optical coherence tomography imaging: A concept evaluation study. *J. Biomed. Opt.* **2014**, *19*, 056001. [CrossRef]
16. Erickson-Bhatt, S.J.; Nolan, R.M.; Shemonski, N.D.; Adie, S.G.; Putney, J.; Darga, D.; McCormick, D.T.; Cittadine, A.J.; Zysk, A.M.; Marjanovic, M.; et al. Real-time Imaging of the Resection Bed Using a Handheld Probe to Reduce Incidence of Microscopic Positive Margins in Cancer Surgery. *Cancer Res.* **2015**, *75*, 3706–3712. [CrossRef]
17. Zysk, A.M.; Chen, K.; Gabrielson, E.; Tafra, L.; May Gonzalez, E.A.; Canner, J.K.; Schneider, E.B.; Cittadine, A.J.; Scott Carney, P.; Boppart, S.A.; et al. Intraoperative Assessment of Final Margins with a Handheld Optical Imaging Probe During Breast-Conserving Surgery May Reduce the Reoperation Rate: Results of a Multicenter Study. *Ann. Surg. Oncol.* **2015**, *22*, 3356–3362. [CrossRef]
18. Zhou, C.; Cohen, D.W.; Wang, Y.; Lee, H.C.; Mondelblatt, A.E.; Tsai, T.H.; Aguirre, A.D.; Fujimoto, J.G.; Connolly, J.L. Integrated optical coherence tomography and microscopy for ex vivo multiscale evaluation of human breast tissues. *Cancer Res.* **2010**, *70*, 10071–10079. [CrossRef]
19. de Boer, J.F.; Hitzenberger, C.K.; Yasuno, Y. Polarization sensitive optical coherence tomography—A review [Invited]. *Biomed. Opt. Express* **2017**, *8*, 1838–1873. [CrossRef]
20. Wang, J.; Xu, Y.; Mesa, K.J.; South, F.A.; Chaney, E.J.; Spillman, D.R.; Barkalifa, R., Jr.; Marjanovic, M.; Carney, P.S.; Higham, A.M.; et al. Complementary use of polarization-sensitive and standard OCT metrics for enhanced intraoperative differentiation of breast cancer. *Biomed. Opt. Express* **2018**, *9*, 6519–6528. [CrossRef]

21. South, F.A.; Chaney, E.J.; Marjanovic, M.; Adie, S.G.; Boppart, S.A. Differentiation of ex vivo human breast tissue using polarization-sensitive optical coherence tomography. *Biomed. Opt. Express* **2014**, *5*, 3417–3426. [CrossRef]

22. Provenzano, P.P.; Eliceiri, K.W.; Campbell, J.M.; Inman, D.R.; White, J.G.; Keely, P.J. Collagen reorganization at the tumor-stromal interface facilitates local invasion. *BMC Med.* **2006**, *4*, 1741–7015. [CrossRef]

23. Patel, R.; Khan, A.; Quinlan, R.; Yaroslavsky, A.N. Polarization-sensitive multimodal imaging for detecting breast cancer. *Cancer Res.* **2014**, *74*, 4685–4693. [CrossRef] [PubMed]

24. Gelikonov, V.M.; Romashov, V.N.; Shabanov, D.V.; Ksenofontov, S.Y.; Terpelov, D.A.; Shilyagin, P.A.; Gelikonov, G.V.; Vitkin, I.A. Cross-polarization optical coherence tomography with active maintenance of the circular polarization of a sounding wave in a common path system. *Radiophys. Quantum Electron.* **2018**, *60*, 897–911. [CrossRef]

25. Gubarkova, E.V.; Sovetsky, A.A.; Zaitsev, V.Y.; Matveyev, A.L.; Vorontsov, D.A.; Sirotkina, M.A.; Matveev, L.A.; Plekhanov, A.A.; Pavlova, N.P.; Kuznetsov, S.S.; et al. OCT-elastography-based optical biopsy for breast cancer delineation and express assessment of morphological/molecular subtypes. *Biomed. Opt. Express* **2019**, *10*, 2244–2263. [CrossRef] [PubMed]

26. Yashin, K.S.; Kiseleva, E.B.; Gubarkova, E.V.; Moiseev, A.A.; Kuznetsov, S.S.; Shilyagin, P.A.; Gelikonov, G.V.; Medyanik, I.A.; Kravets, L.Y.; Potapov, A.A.; et al. Cross-Polarization Optical Coherence Tomography for Brain Tumor Imaging. *Front. Oncol.* **2019**, *9*, 201. [CrossRef] [PubMed]

27. Yashin, K.S.; Kiseleva, E.B.; Moiseev, A.A.; Kuznetsov, S.S.; Timofeeva, L.B.; Pavlova, N.P.; Gelikonov, G.V.; Medyanik, I.A.; Kravets, L.Y.; Zagaynova, E.V.; et al. Quantitative nontumorous and tumorous human brain tissue assessment using microstructural co- and cross-polarized optical coherence tomography. *Sci. Rep.* **2019**, *9*, 2024. [CrossRef] [PubMed]

28. Kiseleva, E.; Kirillin, M.; Feldchtein, F.; Vitkin, A.; Sergeeva, E.; Zagaynova, E.; Streltzova, O.; Shakhov, B.; Gubarkova, E.; Gladkova, N. Differential diagnosis of human bladder mucosa pathologies in vivo with cross-polarization optical coherence tomography. *Biomed. Opt. Express* **2015**, *6*, 1464–1476. [CrossRef]

29. Gladkova, N.; Kiseleva, E.; Streltsova, O.; Prodanets, N.; Snopova, L.; Karabut, M.; Gubarkova, E.; Zagaynova, E. Combined use of fluorescence cystoscopy and cross-polarization OCT for diagnosis of bladder cancer and correlation with immunohistochemical markers. *J. Biophotonics* **2013**, *6*, 687–698. [CrossRef]

30. Gladkova, N.; Streltsova, O.; Zagaynova, E.; Kiseleva, E.; Gelikonov, V.; Gelikonov, G.; Karabut, M.; Yunusova, K.; Evdokimova, O. Cross-polarization optical coherence tomography for early bladder-cancer detection: Statistical study. *J. Biophotonics* **2011**, *4*, 519–532. [CrossRef]

31. Gladkova, N.; Kiseleva, E.; Robakidze, N.; Balalaeva, I.; Karabut, M.; Gubarkova, E.; Feldchtein, F. Evaluation of oral mucosa collagen condition with cross-polarization optical coherence tomography. *J. Biophotonics* **2013**, *6*, 321–329. [CrossRef] [PubMed]

32. Foo, K.Y.; Chin, L.; Zilkens, R.; Lakhiani, D.D.; Fang, Q.; Sanderson, R.; Dessauvagie, B.F.; Latham, B.; McLaren, S.; Saunders, C.M.; et al. Three-dimensional mapping of the attenuation coefficient in optical coherence tomography to enhance breast tissue microarchitecture contrast. *J. Biophotonics* **2020**, *13*, e201960201. [CrossRef]

33. Gubarkova, E.V.; Moiseev, A.A.; Kiseleva, E.B.; Vorontsov, D.A.; Kuznetsov, S.S.; Vorontsov, A.Y.; Gelikonov, G.V.; Sirotkina, M.A.; Gladkova, N.D. Tissue optical properties estimation from cross-polarization OCT data for breast cancer margin assessment. *Laser Phys. Lett.* **2020**, *17*, 075602. [CrossRef]

34. Kennedy, K.M.; Chin, L.; McLaughlin, R.A.; Latham, B.; Saunders, C.M.; Sampson, D.D.; Kennedy, B.F. Quantitative micro-elastography: Imaging of tissue elasticity using compression optical coherence elastography. *Sci. Rep.* **2015**, *5*, 15538. [CrossRef] [PubMed]

35. Kennedy, B.F.; Wijesinghe, P.; Sampson, D.D. The emergence of optical elastography in biomedicine. *Nat. Photonics* **2017**, *11*, 215–221. [CrossRef]

36. Larin, K.V.; Sampson, D.D. Optical coherence elastography—OCT at work in tissue biomechanics [Invited]. *Biomed. Opt. Express* **2017**, *8*, 1172–1202. [CrossRef]

37. Zaitsev, V.Y.; Matveyev, A.L.; Matveev, L.A.; Sovetsky, A.A.; Hepburn, M.S.; Mowla, A.; Kennedy, B.F. Strain and elasticity imaging in compression optical coherence elastography: The two-decade perspective and recent advances. *J. Biophotonics* **2020**, e202000257. [CrossRef] [PubMed]

38. Sirotkina, M.A.; Gubarkova, E.V.; Plekhanov, A.A.; Sovetsky, A.A.; Elagin, V.V.; Matveyev, A.L.; Matveev, L.A.; Kuznetsov, S.S.; Zagaynova, E.V.; Gladkova, N.D.; et al. In vivo assessment of functional and morphological alterations in tumors under treatment using OCT-angiography combined with OCT-elastography. *Biomed. Opt. Express* **2020**, *11*, 1365–1382. [CrossRef]
39. Plekhanov, A.A.; Sirotkina, M.A.; Sovetsky, A.A.; Gubarkova, E.V.; Kuznetsov, S.S.; Matveyev, A.L.; Matveev, L.A.; Zagaynova, E.V.; Gladkova, N.D.; Zaitsev, V.Y. Histological validation of in vivo assessment of cancer tissue inhomogeneity and automated morphological segmentation enabled by Optical Coherence Elastography. *Sci. Rep.* **2020**, *10*, 11781. [CrossRef]
40. Kennedy, B.F.; McLaughlin, R.A.; Kennedy, K.M.; Chin, L.; Wijesinghe, P.; Curatolo, A.; Tien, A.; Ronald, M.; Latham, B.; Saunders, C.M.; et al. Investigation of Optical Coherence Microelastography as a Method to Visualize Cancers in Human Breast Tissue. *Cancer Res.* **2015**, *75*, 3236–3245. [CrossRef]
41. Allen, W.M.; Foo, K.Y.; Zilkens, R.; Kennedy, K.M.; Fang, Q.; Chin, L.; Dessauvagie, B.F.; Latham, B.; Saunders, C.M.; Kennedy, B.F. Clinical feasibility of optical coherence micro-elastography for imaging tumor margins in breast-conserving surgery. *Biomed. Opt. Express* **2018**, *9*, 6331–6349. [CrossRef] [PubMed]
42. Zaitsev, V.Y.; Matveyev, A.L.; Matveev, L.A.; Gubarkova, E.V.; Sovetsky, A.A.; Sirotkina, M.A.; Gelikonov, G.V.; Zagaynova, E.V.; Gladkova, N.D.; Vitkin, A. Practical obstacles and their mitigation strategies in compressional optical coherence elastography of biological tissues *J. Innovative Opt. Health Sci.* **2017**, *10*, 1742006. [CrossRef]
43. Kennedy, K.M.; Zilkens, R.; Allen, W.M.; Foo, K.Y.; Fang, Q.; Chin, L.; Sanderson, R.W.; Anstie, J.; Wijesinghe, P.; Curatolo, A.; et al. Diagnostic Accuracy of Quantitative Micro-Elastography for Margin Assessment in Breast-Conserving Surgery. *Cancer Res.* **2020**, *80*, 1773–1783. [CrossRef] [PubMed]
44. Allen, W.M.; Kennedy, K.M.; Fang, Q.; Chin, L.; Curatolo, A.; Watts, L.; Zilkens, R.; Chin, S.L.; Dessauvagie, B.F.; Latham, B.; et al. Wide-field quantitative micro-elastography of human breast tissue. *Biomed. Opt. Express.* **2018**, *9*, 1082–1096. [CrossRef]
45. Aleskandarany, M.A.; Vandenberghe, M.E.; Marchiò, C.; Ellis, I.O.; Sapino, A.; Rakha, E.A. Tumour Heterogeneity of Breast Cancer: From Morphology to Personalised Medicine. *Pathobiology* **2018**, *85*, 23–34. [CrossRef]
46. Iwao, K.; Matoba, R.; Ueno, N.; Ando, A.; Miyoshi, Y.; Matsubara, K.; Noguchi, S.; Kato, K. Molecular classification of primary breast tumors possessing distinct prognostic properties. *Hum. Mol. Genet.* **2002**, *11*, 199–206. [CrossRef]
47. Lowery, A.J.; Kell, M.R.; Glynn, R.W.; Kerin, M.J.; Sweeney, K.J. Locoregional recurrence after breast cancer surgery: A systematic review by receptor phenotype. *Breast Cancer Res. Treat.* **2012**, *133*, 831–841. [CrossRef]
48. Cancello, G.; Maisonneuve, P.; Rotmensz, N.; Viale, G.; Mastropasqua, M.G.; Pruneri, G.; Montagna, E.; Dellapasqua, S.; Iorfida, M.; Cardillo, A.; et al. Prognosis in women with small (T1mic,T1a,T1b) node-negative operable breast cancer by immunohistochemically selected subtypes. *Breast Cancer Res. Treat.* **2011**, *127*, 713–720. [CrossRef]
49. Houssami, N.; Macaskill, P.; Marinovich, M.L.; Morrow, M. The association of surgical margins and local recurrence in women with early-stage invasive breast cancer treated with breast-conserving therapy: A meta-analysis. *Ann. Surg. Oncol.* **2014**, *21*, 717–730. [CrossRef]
50. Moiseev, A.; Ksenofontov, S.; Sirotkina, M.; Kiseleva, E.; Gorozhantseva, M.; Shakhova, N.; Matveev, L.; Zaitsev, V.; Matveyev, A.; Zagaynova, E.; et al. Optical coherence tomography-based angiography device with real-time angiography B-scans visualization and hand-held probe for everyday clinical use. *J. Biophotonics* **2018**, *11*, e201700292. [CrossRef]
51. Zaitsev, V.Y.; Matveyev, A.L.; Matveev, L.A.; Gelikonov, G.V.; Sovetsky, A.A.; Vitkin, A. Optimized phase gradient measurements and phase-amplitude interplay in optical coherence elastography. *J. Biomed. Opt.* **2016**, *21*, 116005. [CrossRef] [PubMed]
52. Zaitsev, V.Y.; Matveyev, A.L.; Matveev, L.A.; Gelikonov, G.V.; Gubarkova, E.V.; Gladkova, N.D.; Vitkin, A. Hybrid method of strain estimation in optical coherence elastography using combined sub-wavelength phase measurements and supra-pixel displacement tracking. *J. Biophotonics* **2016**, *9*, 499–509. [CrossRef] [PubMed]
53. Matveyev, A.L.; Matveev, L.A.; Sovetsky, A.A.; Gelikonov, G.V.; Moiseev, A.A.; Zaitsev, V.Y. Vector method for strain estimation in phase-sensitive optical coherence elastography. *Laser Phys. Lett.* **2018**, *15*, 065603. [CrossRef]

54. Sovetsky, A.A.; Matveyev, A.L.; Matveev, L.A.; Shabanov, D.V.; Zaitsev, V.Y. Manually-operated compressional optical coherence elastography with effective aperiodic averaging: Demonstrations for corneal and cartilaginous tissues. *Laser Phys. Lett.* **2018**, *15*, 85602. [CrossRef]
55. Sovetsky, A.A.; Matveyev, A.L.; Matveev, L.A.; Gubarkova, E.V.; Plekhanov, A.A.; Sirotkina, M.A.; Gladkova, N.D.; Zaitsev, V.Y. Full-optical method of local stress standardization to exclude nonlinearity-related ambiguity of elasticity estimation in compressional optical coherence elastography. *Laser Phys. Lett.* **2020**, *17*, 065601. [CrossRef]
56. Sovetsky, A.A.; Matveev, L.A.; Gubarkova, E.V.; Matveyev, A.L.; Gladkova, N.D.; Zaitsev, V.Y. Characterization of elastic nonlinear properties of the tissues using compressional optical coherence elastography. *Proc. SPIE* **2020**, *11359*, 113590H. [CrossRef]
57. Zaitsev, V.Y.; Matveyev, A.L.; Matveev, L.A.; Gelikonov, G.V.; Omelchenko, A.I.; Shabanov, D.V.; Baum, O.I.; Svistushkin, V.M.; Sobol, E.N. Optical coherence tomography for visualizing transient strains and measuring large deformations in laser-induced tissue reshaping. *Laser Phys. Lett.* **2016**, *13*, 115603. [CrossRef]
58. Zaitsev, V.Y.; Matveyev, A.L.; Matveev, L.A.; Gelikonov, G.V.; Omelchenko, A.I.; Baum, O.I.; Avetisov, S.E.; Bolshunov, A.V.; Siplivy, V.I.; Shabanov, D.V.; et al. Optical coherence elastography for strain dynamics measurements in laser correction of cornea shape. *J. Biophotonics* **2017**, *10*, 1450–1463. [CrossRef]
59. Feuerman, M.; Miller, A.R. Relationships between statistical measures of agreement: Sensitivity, specificity and kappa. *J. Eval. Clin. Pract.* **2008**, *14*, 930–933. [CrossRef]
60. Viera, A.J.; Garrett, J.M. Understanding interobserver agreement: The kappa statistic. *Fam. Med.* **2005**, *37*, 360–363.
61. Yao, X.; Gan, Y.; Chang, E.; Hibshoosh, H.; Feldman, S.; Hendon, C. Visualization and tissue classification of human breast cancer images using ultrahigh-resolution OCT. *Lasers Surg. Med.* **2017**, *49*, 258–269. [CrossRef] [PubMed]
62. Assayag, O.; Antoine, M.; Sigal-Zafrani, B.; Riben, M.; Harms, F.; Burcheri, A.; Grieve, K.; Dalimier, E.; Le Conte de Poly, B.; Boccara, C. Large field, high resolution full-field optical coherence tomography: A pre-clinical study of human breast tissue and cancer assessment. *Technol. Cancer Res. Treat.* **2014**, *13*, 455–468. [CrossRef] [PubMed]
63. Zysk, A.M.; Boppart, S.A. Computational methods for analysis of human breast tumor tissue in optical coherence tomography images. *J. Biomed. Opt.* **2006**, *11*, 054015. [CrossRef] [PubMed]

18

Bio-Photonic Detection and Quantitative Evaluation Method for the Progression of Dental Caries Using Optical Frequency-Domain Imaging Method

Ruchire Eranga Wijesinghe [1,†], Nam Hyun Cho [2,3,†], Kibeom Park [1], Mansik Jeon [1,*] and Jeehyun Kim [1]

1 School of Electronics Engineering, College of IT Engineering, Kyungpook National University, 80, Daehak-ro, Buk-gu, Daegu 41566, Korea; eranga@knu.ac.kr (R.E.W.); pepl10@knu.ac.kr (K.P.); jeehk@knu.ac.kr (J.K.)
2 Eaton-Peabody Laboratories, Massachusetts Eye and Ear Infirmary(MEEI), 243, Charles Street, Boston, MA 02114, USA; namhyun_cho@meei.harvard.edu
3 Department of Otology and Laryngology, Harvard Medical School, 243, Charles Street, Boston, MA 02114, USA
* Correspondence: msjeon@knu.ac.kr
† These authors contributed equally to this work.

Academic Editors: Dragan Indjin, Željka Cvejić and Małgorzata Jędrzejewska-Szczerska

Abstract: The initial detection of dental caries is an essential biomedical requirement to barricade the progression of caries and tooth demineralization. The objective of this study is to introduce an optical frequency-domain imaging technique based quantitative evaluation method to calculate the volume and thickness of enamel residual, and a quantification method was developed to evaluate the total intensity fluctuation in depth direction owing to carious lesions, which can be favorable to identify the progression of dental caries in advance. The cross-sectional images of the *ex vivo* tooth samples were acquired using 1.3 μm spectral domain optical coherence tomography system (SD-OCT). Moreover, the advantages of the proposed method over the conventional dental inspection methods were compared to highlight the potential capability of OCT. As a consequence, the threshold parameters obtained through the developed method can be used as an efficient investigating technique for the initial detection of demineralization.

Keywords: optical frequency domain imaging (OFDI); optical coherence tomography; dental caries; demineralization; Bio-photonic detection

1. Introduction

Precise structural imaging and quantitative evaluation are critical for the diagnosis of dental caries and research to prevent the formation of initial demineralized regions [1,2]. The depth imaging of enamel, dentin, cavities, pits, and fissures with a high-resolution is particularly important for the study of anatomical and pathological changes of the dental structure [3]. Optical coherence tomography (OCT) is a rapidly advancing optical frequency-domain imaging modality, which can provide non-invasive high-resolution cross-sectional images of dental tissues and various biological tissues [4]. This near-infrared (NIR) biomedical imaging method provides images with high axial and lateral resolutions (i.e., below 8 μm and 15 μm, respectively) [5,6], and, furthermore, OCT has been widely used in different medical applications such as ophthalmology [7,8], dermatology [9], and otolaryngology [10,11]. The methods currently in use for the detection of dental caries such as radiography, microradiography, and X-rays do not provide sufficient resolution, sensitivity, and contrast compared to OCT. Radiography is the most frequently applied inspection method in dentistry with a resolution of 50 μm, which is comparatively lower than the resolution of OCT. Furthermore, radiography is not quantitative, and it is relatively difficult to apply for the initial detection of dental caries [12,13]. Microradiography is another method that can be used to analyze caries quantitatively, but it is hard to apply this method for clinical applications [14]. Other conventional diagnostic methods such as infrared (IR) imaging, dental explorer, and visual inspection are unable to provide more accurate cross-sectional images [15]. Several research groups have determined the mineral loss and the depth of enamel caries using a histology analysis method called transversal microradiography (TMR). However, due to the requirement of a thin sectioning process, applications of the method in dentistry have been scarce [16]. The main drawback of this method is that caries can be detected only at a relatively advanced stage when remineralization is no longer possible, and due to the incapability of obtaining precise quantitative measurements, it is hard to barricade the progression of caries. Thus, owing to the non-invasive and non-destructive imaging capability, and the capability of acquiring precise quantifications such as accurate thickness and volumetric measurements, OCT has gained a significant demand in the medical field as an early diagnosis method. Although OCT has been extensively used as a powerful dental imaging technique, quantitative evaluation of enamel thickness variation, depth dependent intensity fluctuation, and volumetric analysis of enamel residual has not been broadly studied for the initial diagnosis of demineralization.

Especially in dentistry, OCT has been used to produce longitudinal images of dental tissues and caries of an orientation similar to that of the B-scan ultrasound images [17,18]. In these studies, a reduction in enamel reflectivity was observed in areas of dental caries [19]. It is considered that the decrease in reflectivity during demineralization is related to the amount of mineral loss. Few studies have demonstrated that there is two to threefold increase in the scattering coefficient at a wavelength of 1.3 μm [20]. Furthermore, a polarization sensitive OCT (PS-OCT) endoscopic system using a swept source has been implemented as a compact system for dentistry application [21]. Similarly, surface demineralization can be detected using linearly polarized light and measured backscattered signal in two orthogonal axes [22]. Some other OCT techniques have been applied to diagnose dental caries as a result of changes in the optical properties of enamel after undergoing demineralization [23]. The obtained images were quantitatively evaluated by the identification of structures, dimensions, and properties [24]. Moreover, in several review reports and research studies, OCT based dental experiments were demonstrated to verify the stronger optical backscattering signals acquired from the demineralized enamel regions, oral tissue images, caries, periodontal diseases, and oral cancers [25,26]. In addition, infrared light with long wavelengths were used in OCT for clinical applications owing to the high depth penetration [27].

In this paper, we performed an initial *ex vivo* study using a 1.3 μm wavelength laser utilized spectral domain OCT (SD-OCT) system to introduce a quantitative method to calculate the thickness and volume of remaining enamel region (enamel residual). Furthermore, we developed an algorithm to analyze the total intensity fluctuation in depth direction of OCT images, which can be useful to identify the progression of initial caries. As a result, the proposed quantification can be implemented to identify the reduction of enamel region along with the progression of the demineralization. Moreover, the capability of our SD-OCT system to perform the proposed method was validated by obtaining images of *ex vivo* caries with a high resolution and a high depth penetration.

2. Materials and Methods

2.1. Optical Frequency Domain Imaging (OFDI) Technique

The implemented optical frequency domain imaging technique was a customized 1.3 μm SD-OCT system. The speed of the SD-OCT system was 120 frames/s when the image size was 1024 × 500 pixels, and the average output power of the system was 16 mW. In Figure 1, the broadband light source that was used for light emission is a superluminescent diode (SLED) (Denselight Semiconductors, Singapore) with 1.3 μm central wavelength and 135 nm bandwidth. The axial resolution of the system was 6 μm (in air) and 3.61 μm (in tissue). The transverse resolution of the system was 25 μm. The detector was a 14-bit complementary metal-oxide semiconductor (CMOS) line scan camera (SU-1024LDM Compact; Goodrich, Charlotte, NC, USA) with 1024 pixels. A 50:50 optical fiber coupler was used to split the broadband light beam into the sample and reference arms. A galvanoscanner (GVS002, Thorlabs, Newton, NJ, USA) connected to the sample arm was used to scan the tooth samples. All the samples were scanned with a sufficient cross-sectional scanning range of 1 mm × 1 mm × 1 mm dimensions. A compact spectrometer was designed and contained a collimator, a diffraction grating, an achromatic doublet lens, and a line scan camera. The spectrometer was calibrated to compensate the distortion of the point spread function (PSF), and to improve the signal-to-noise ratio (SNR) up to 110 dB using previous literature reports [28,29]. Further details about the system configuration can be found in Table 1.

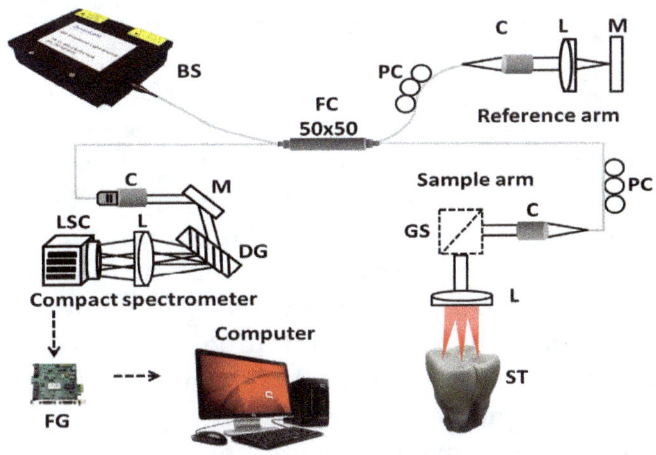

Figure 1. Schematic diagram of the spectral-domain optical coherence tomography (SD-OCT) system. Note the use of the following acronyms in the figure: BS: broadband source, C: collimator, DG: diffraction grating, FC: fiber coupler, FG: frame grabber, GS: galvanoscanner, L: lens, LSC: line scan camera, M: mirror, PC: polarization controller, and ST: sample tooth.

Table 1. The details of the optical frequency domain imaging system.

System Parameters	Specification
Central Wavelength	1310 nm
Spectral bandwidth	135 nm
Axial resolution air/tissue	6 μm/3.61 μm
Transverse resolution	25 μm
Maximum imaging width	8 mm
Maximum imaging depth	>6 mm
Optical power variation	±5%

2.2. *Specimen Preparation*

For the proposed preliminary study, four types of *ex vivo* tooth samples, including partially demineralized canine tooth sample, partially demineralized pre-molar tooth sample, partially demineralized molar tooth sample, completely demineralized (carious) molar tooth sample, and *in vivo* healthy molar tooth sample were involved in the experiment. All tooth specimens were examined in patients before extraction. The experimented *ex vivo* tooth specimens were extracted after performing early childhood caries (ECC) surgeries for four orthodontic patients at different age groups (10–12 years) of the dental clinic of the Faculty of Dentistry, Kyungpook National University, Daegu, Korea. The details of the experimented volunteers and tooth specimens are illustrated in Table 2. Prior to the OCT inspection, all *ex vivo* tooth specimens were preserved in sterile filtered de-ionized water solution for 24 h at 30 °C to eliminate any possible superficial enamel cracks and maintain a standard smooth surface after the extraction. The experiments were performed in accordance with the guidelines of the Institutional Animal Care and Use Committee of Kyungpook National University (Daegu, Korea) and approvals from the human ethics committees of the Institute for Bio-diagnostics, Kyungpook National University (Daegu, Korea) were obtained prior to sample collection.

Table 2. The details of the experimented tooth specimens.

Experimented Volunteer	Tooth Classification	Inspection Category
11-year-old male	Molar tooth	Healthy
11-year-old female	Molar tooth	Partially demineralized
10-year-old male	Molar tooth	Carious
11-year-old male	Canine tooth	Partially demineralized
12-year-old female	Pre-molar tooth	Partially demineralized

2.3. *Intensity Fluctuation Analysis*

To evaluate the proposed method precisely, the obtained cross-sectional images were involved in an amplitude scan (A-scan) depth profile analysis to verify the microstructural comparison between healthy, partially demineralized, and carious molar tooth samples. For the A-scan profile analysis, a software-based program was coded using Matlab (Mathworks, Natick, MA, USA) to search the intensity peaks in the depth direction. The acquired 2D OCT image was loaded and a peak search algorithm-based cropped window with 15 intensity signals (A-scan lines) was applied. The developed algorithm detects the maximum intensity in each individual A-scan line to search the peak position, and all the peak positions in all 15 A-scan lines were rearranged while matching the peak intensity index in the A-scans to flatten the region of interest. Owing to the non-flattened region of interest, the maximum intensity index positions vary, and therefore, the index positions with higher intensity values should be rearranged and matched linearly to obtain a flattened image. Finally, all the rearranged and flattened A-scan lines were summed up, averaged, and normalized to obtain a single A-scan depth profile of the region of interest. The applied refractive index of a tooth structure, which affects the depth scale of 2D OCT images was 1.63 [30,31]. Moreover, we performed an additional quantification method to analyze the total intensity fluctuation in deep microstructures according to imaging depth. Thus, an additional automated program was coded using Matlab to analyze the total pixel intensity of each depth range of demodulated 2D OCT images. The analysis was performed for the entire visible depth range of 1 mm, and the total pixel intensity was evaluated for each 250 μm depth range of the cross-sectional image to identify the depth dependent total intensity fluctuation of each tooth specimen category. Then, the entire total pixel intensity of each depth range was summed and averaged for each 2D OCT image. This study was a preliminary observational study, and the data analysis was primarily descriptive. A continuous variation of the optical laser source power was observed, which was compensated afterward. Due to the instability of the laser optical power, the entire intensity of 2D OCT images was compensated by multiplying $\pm 5\%$.

2.4. *Volumetric Analysis*

The volumetric measurements of enamel residual was obtained using 2D OCT image based 3D OCT volumetric images by implementing a pixel intensity based automated calculation method, which was performed through a software program coded in Matlab. Figure 2a shows the volumetric calculation algorithm of enamel residual of a single 2D OCT image along with the obtained 3D OCT volumetric image containing 500 2D OCT images (Figure 2c). In the developed algorithm based program, demodulated raw data was loaded and the intensity of the entire cross-sectional region was analyzed. An image window was applied to select the enamel residual region. For the precise selection (filter the region of interest) of the enamel residual region, we approximated the pixel intensity difference between the enamel residual region and other cross-sectional regions, and provided a pre-determined intensity threshold range for a separate evaluation of the enamel residual region.

The entire cross-sectional intensity varies from 0 to 255, and the pre-determined enamel threshold ($TH_{(en)}$) range can be expressed as, $45 \leq TH_{(en)} \leq 255$. The selected threshold range contains the intensity range of the enamel region and excludes the dark black region of the selected image window. The area of a single pixel, which belongs to the selected image window in Figure 2b can be expressed as

$$l_x \times l_y = A_{pix}, \tag{1}$$

where l_x *is* the pixel size in the *x*-direction, l_y *is* the pixel size in the *y*-direction, and A_{pix} is the area of a single pixel. The pixel sizes in the *x*-, *y*-, and *z*-directions can be expressed as

$$l_x = l_y = 12\ \mu\text{m, and } l_z = 7\ \mu\text{m.}$$

The total number of *z*-direction pixels (B-mode images) is 500 owing to the composition of the 3D OCT image. Therefore, the enamel residual volume (volume of the remaining enamel) of 500 2D OCT images (3D volumetric image) can be calculated as

$$(N_1 \times l_x \times l_y) \times l_z + (N_2 \times l_x \times l_y) \times l_z + (N_3 \times l_x \times l_y) \times l_z + \ldots (N_{500} \times l_x \times l_y) \times l_z = V_{tot}, \tag{2}$$

where N_i (i = 1, 2, 3, ... , 500) is the number of image window pixels in each respective window, which satisfies the pre-determined threshold value range, and V_{tot} is the evaluated volume of the enamel residual. $N_1, N_2, \ldots, N_{500}$ represent the sequential number of respective image window pixels. The accuracy of the developed algorithm can be enhanced by providing a precise pre-determined threshold value range to detect the gradual changes of enamel structure as a result of demineralization.

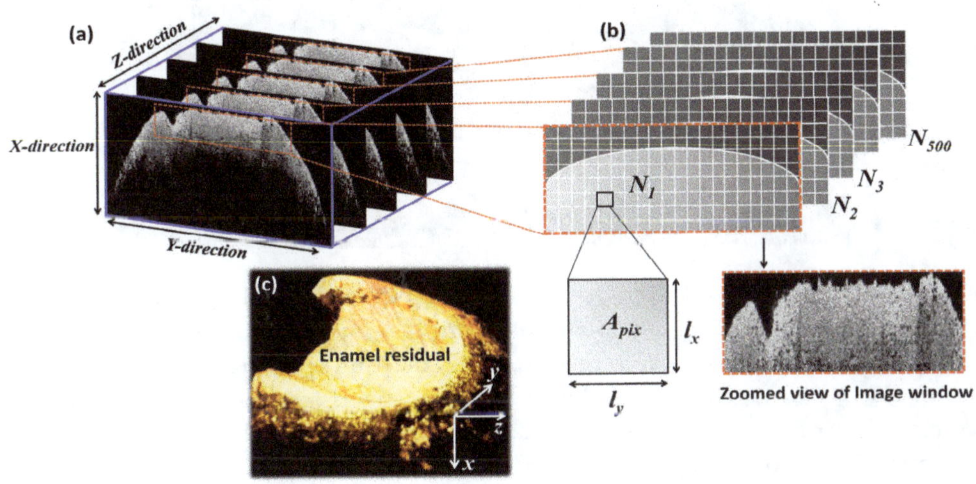

Figure 2. Volumetric evaluation algorithm for enamel residual. (**a**) Sequential 2D OCT images along with the applied image window; (**b**) Detected pixels, which satisfy the applied pre-determined threshold range; (**c**) Acquired 3D OCT volumetric image.

3. Results and Discussion

3.1. *Morphological Analysis of Dental Caries along with Quantitative Evaluations*

Figure 3a–c show the cross-sectional comparison between healthy, partially demineralized, and completely demineralized (carious) molar tooth samples. Figure 3d,e present the three-dimensional volumetric images of partially demineralized and carious molar tooth samples for a better view. In Figure 3a, the structural layers such as, enamel, dentino-enamel junction, and dentin can be visualized along with the depth ranges of 250 μm, 600 μm, and 800 μm, respectively. The progression of the demineralization can be identified in Figure 3b due to the demineralized enamel region and the formation of pits region in the depth range of 500 μm below the enamel range, and the remaining dentino-junction and dentin layer thickness was about 300 μm. Moreover, a clearly distinguishable demineralized enamel and dentino-junction (in the depth range of 800 μm), which leads to a formation of a carious region including pits and fissures were identified in Figure 3c. In addition, the remaining dentin thickness was about 100 μm. The three-dimensional images (Figure 3d,e) emphasize the top view of the partially demineralized and carious molar teeth samples. The infected microstructures, formation of pits and fissures, as well as the enamel loss, can be clearly visualized through the obtained volumetric images, owing to the high depth penetration. The desired morphological changes owing to demineralization mostly occurred in the enamel and dentin regions, which belong to a depth range that can be sufficiently achieved from the developed OFDI technique, and therefore, the necessity of histological images could be minimized by using the two-dimensional cross-sectional images acquired from the developed non-invasive OCT system [32–35]. Although the customized SD-OCT system implemented in this preliminary study improves the anatomical evaluation of the enamel and dentin, due to the low image acquisition speed and low sensitivity, the image quality has a limitation in SD-OCT compared to optical frequency domain imaging based high-speed swept source OCT (SS-OCT) [36]. Though the implementation of high-speed 1.3 μm SS-OCT can be beneficial, the customized cost effective OFDI system of this preliminary study was capable of obtaining a sufficient depth visibility to confirm the desired morphological results.

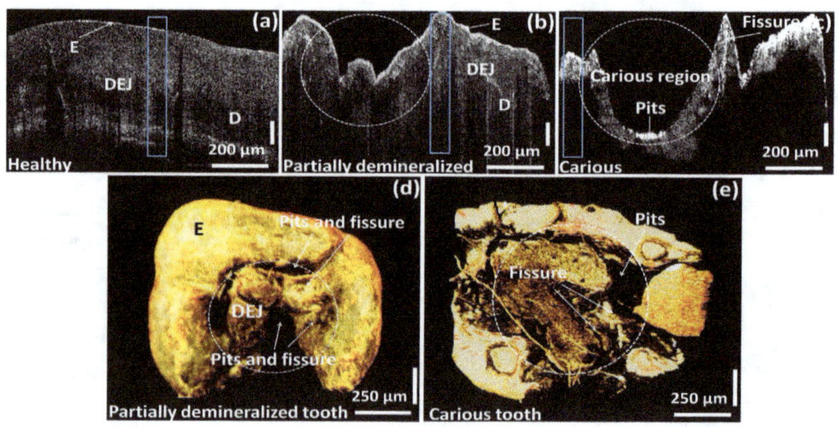

Figure 3. Two-dimensional OCT image comparison between healthy, partially demineralized, and completely demineralized (carious) molar tooth samples along with three-dimensional OCT images. (**a**) 2D OCT image of a healthy molar tooth region; (**b**) 2D OCT image of a partially demineralized molar tooth region; (**c**) 2D OCT image of a completely demineralized (carious) molar tooth region; (**d**) 3D OCT volumetric image of a partially demineralized molar tooth sample; and (**e**) 3D OCT volumetric image of a carious molar tooth sample.

The blue color box regions of Figure 3a–c depict the averaged A-scan depth profile regions. In Figure 4a, the blue solid line, red dotted line, and black dashed line represent the A-scan depth profiles of healthy, partially demineralized, and carious samples, respectively. Owing to the high scattering coefficient of the healthy structure region, a high backscattered signal intensity can be identified compared to partially demineralized and carious samples. In addition, it is difficult to detect dentin enamel junction and dentin regions of the partially demineralized and carious samples (within depth range of 500 μm to 1000 μm) due to low signal intensity from the structure. The demineralization mainly affects the hard calcium based structural surface of the tooth enamel region by decreasing the calcium constitution and simultaneously increase the progression of caries, which contain soft tissues and blood vessels. Owing to the aforementioned increase of the soft tissue region containing blood vessels, light scattering coefficient decreases. Therefore, the degree of demineralization affects the OCT signal in depth direction. As a consequence, low signal intensity could be detected from partially demineralized samples compared to healthy samples.

The aforementioned depth dependent intensity fluctuation according to each sample within each depth range is shown in the Figure 4b graph. The total intensity fluctuation of the healthy sample, partially demineralized sample, and carious sample are illustrated in blue, red, and gray color plots, respectively. Owing to the high optical scattering coefficient, the healthy sample performs the highest total intensity in all depth ranges, and the least intensity values could be identified in the carious sample. Furthermore, the partially demineralized sample performed less total intensity than the healthy sample and a higher intensity than the carious sample, which confirms the progression of dental caries. All the obtained intensity values are shown along with the corresponding graph bars. Furthermore, the enamel thickness was evaluated, and the next bar graph shown in Figure 4c represents the depth direction enamel thickness values of the aforementioned three samples using two-dimensional cross-sectional image based A-scan depth profile analysis. The thickness of the healthy enamel region was measured as 255.45 ± 15.03 μm, a partially demineralized molar specimen was measured as 150.30 ± 10.02 μm (with a reduction of 41.1% compared to the healthy sample), and the enamel residual of the carious region was measured as 100.20 ± 6.68 μm (with a reduction of 60.8% compared to the healthy sample), respectively.

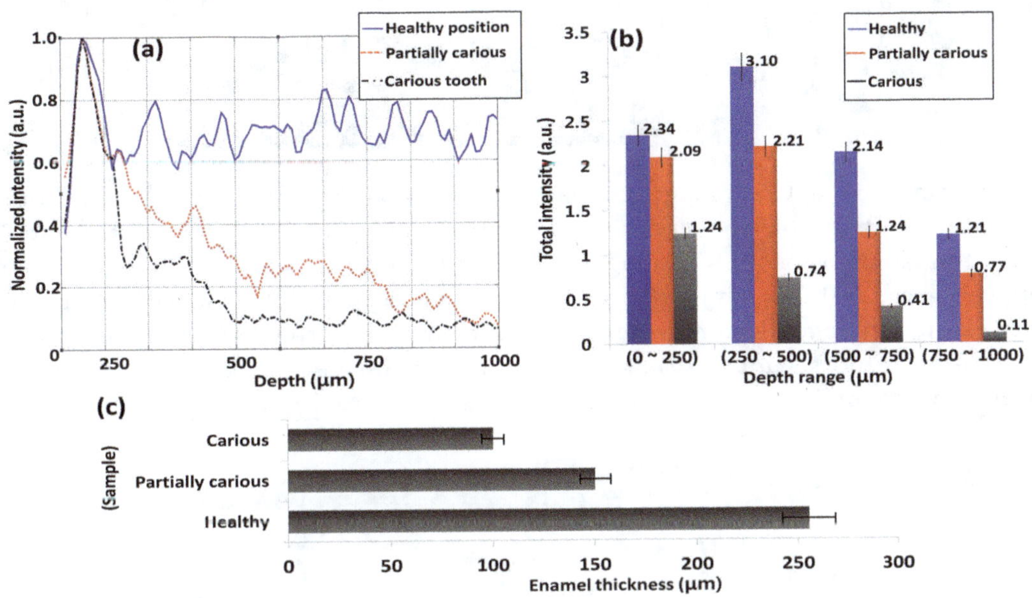

Figure 4. The quantitative evaluation method for healthy, partially demineralized, and completely demineralized (carious) molar tooth samples. (**a**) A-scan depth profiles of healthy, partially demineralized, and carious samples; (**b**) The total intensity fluctuation of healthy, partially demineralized molar, and completely demineralized (carious) molar tooth samples for the entire visible depth range of 1 mm with a gap of 250 μm depth range; (**c**) The depth direction enamel thickness values of the healthy, partially carious, and carious samples.

To gain a better understanding about the enamel demineralization, we repeated the aforementioned similar experimental method using partially demineralized canine and pre-molar tooth samples, which have a healthy appearance externally. Figure 5a,c emphasize the 2D OCT images along with the acquired 3D OCT volumetric images (Figure 5b,d) and sample photographs. The scanned positions of the samples are shown by red dashed lines. Although the samples have a healthy appearance, the formation of the demineralized enamel and root cavity region were identified in cross-sectional images and 3D OCT images of both canine and pre-molar tooth samples. Moreover, the enamel of the pre-molar tooth sample was demineralized towards a 750 μm depth to form the cavity region, which can be quantitatively evaluated using A-scan depth profile analysis. To acquire the most accurate quantification of enamel residual and the demineralized enamel region, we repeated the previous quantitative methods under the same experimental conditions.

The obtained A-scans of partially demineralized canine tooth sample and partially demineralized pre-molar tooth sample were compared with a healthy sample and shown in Figure 6a. In the A-scan profile, the blue solid line, black dashed line, and green dotted line represent the A-scan depth profiles of healthy sample, canine sample, and pre-molar sample, respectively. Similar signal intensity behavior was confirmed as before, owing to the low scattering coefficient of partially demineralized samples, which confirms the changes of the sample composition compared to the healthy sample. Then, we analyzed and compared the total intensity fluctuation of both partially demineralized samples according to each imaging depth range (Figure 6b).

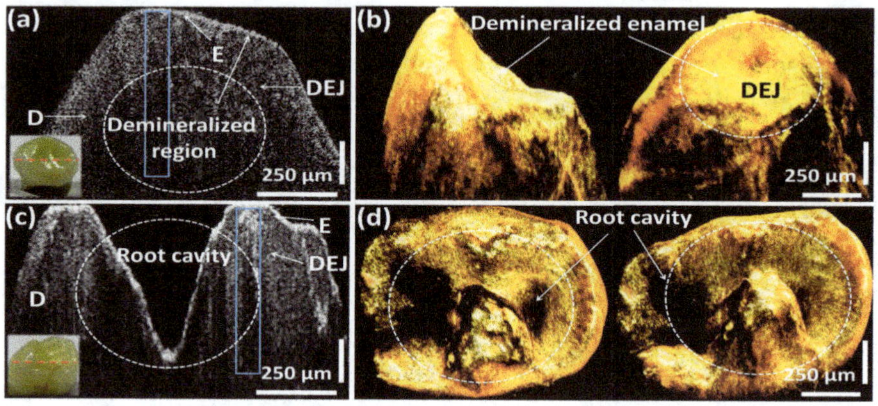

Figure 5. Two-dimensional OCT image comparison between a partially demineralized but healthy appearing canine tooth sample and a partially demineralized but healthy appearing pre-molar tooth sample with three-dimensional OCT images. (**a**) 2D OCT image of a partially demineralized but healthy appearing canine tooth sample; (**b**) 3D OCT volumetric image of a partially demineralized but healthy appearing canine tooth sample; (**c**) 2D OCT image of a partially demineralized but healthy appearing pre-molar tooth sample; (**d**) 3D OCT volumetric image of a partially demineralized but healthy appearing pre-molar tooth sample.

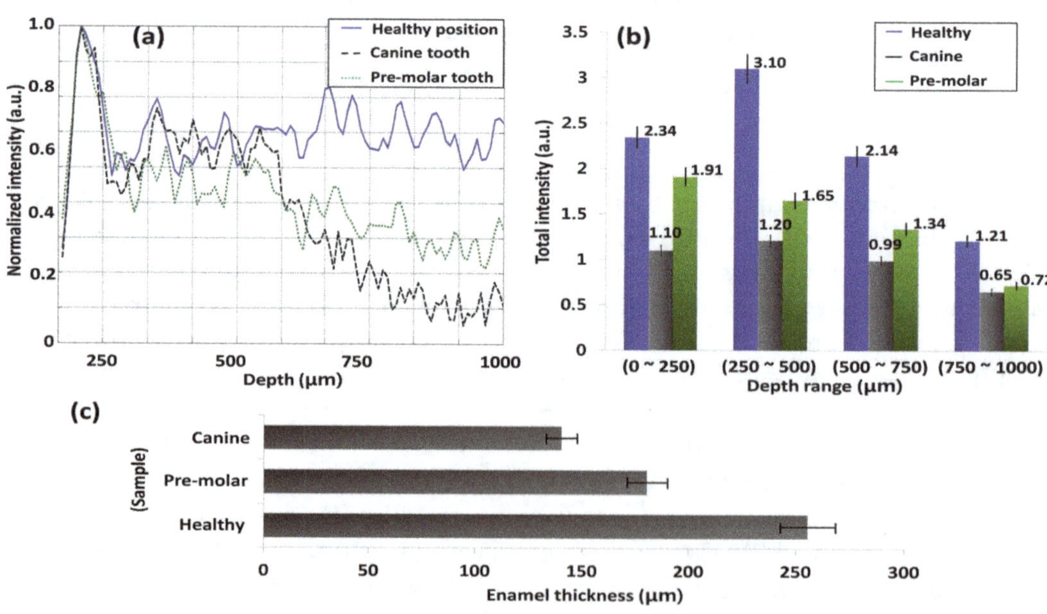

Figure 6. The quantitative evaluation for a healthy sample and partially demineralized but healthy appearing canine and pre-molar tooth samples. (**a**) A-scan depth profiles of healthy and partially demineralized but healthy appearing canine and pre-molar tooth samples; (**b**) the total intensity fluctuation of healthy, canine, and pre-molar tooth samples for the entire visible depth range of 1 mm with a gap of 250 µm depth range; (**c**) the depth direction enamel thickness values of the healthy, partially demineralized but healthy appearing canine and pre-molar tooth samples.

All the obtained intensity values are shown along with the corresponding graph bars. Although a reduction of the total intensity was noticed in partially demineralized samples (compared to the healthy sample), all the intensity levels were comparatively higher than the intensity levels of the carious sample. Therefore, the results confirm that the experimentally tested samples were neither healthy nor carious and verify the progression of demineralization. Next, we analyzed and compared enamel thickness of all three samples, and the bar graph shown in Figure 6c represents the obtained depth direction enamel thickness. The thickness of the healthy enamel region was measured as 255.45 ± 15.03 μm, partially demineralized pre-molar tooth sample was measured as 180.36 ± 12.02 μm (reduction of 29.4% compared to the healthy sample), and partially demineralized canine tooth sample was measured as 140.28 ± 9.35 μm (reduction of 45.1% compared to the healthy sample), respectively. Therefore, the obtained quantitative evaluations confirm the progression of early caries, and, moreover, the obtained quantitative evaluations can be utilized as threshold parameters to detect the progression of early caries. To gain a better understanding about the quantified thickness values and total intensity fluctuations of the experimented tooth specimens, the summarized quantifications are illustrated in Table 3.

Table 3. The quantified enamel thickness and depth direction total intensity fluctuations.

Specimen Category	Enamel Thickness (μm)	Total Intensity Fluctuation in Each Depth Range (a.u.)			
		0–250 μm	250–500 μm	500–750 μm	750–1000 μm
Healthy molar	255.45 ± 15.03	2.34 ± 0.2	3.10 ± 0.2	2.14 ± 0.2	1.21 ± 0.2
Dem. molar	150.30 ± 10.02	2.09 ± 0.2	2.21 ± 0.2	1.24 ± 0.2	0.77 ± 0.1
Carious molar	100.20 ± 6.68	1.24 ± 0.1	0.74 ± 0.05	0.41 ± 0.02	0.11 ± 0.01
Dem. canine	140.28 ± 9.35	1.10 ± 0.1	1.21 ± 0.1	0.99 ± 0.1	0.65 ± 0.1
Dem. premolar	180.36 ± 12.02	1.91 ± 0.1	1.65 ± 0.1	1.34 ± 0.1	0.72 ± 0.05

3.2. *Volumetric Evaluation Technique to Identify Initial Caries*

We quantified the volume of the enamel residual by applying the described volumetric algorithm in Section 2.4. Thus, we calculated the enamel residual of a selected particular position determined by the expert orthodontist for the healthy tooth specimen, three partially demineralized but healthy appearing tooth specimens, and the carious tooth specimen. All the performed calculations were based on the refractive index of 1.63, and the calculated enamel residual volume evaluations are illustrated along with the parameters in Table 4.

Table 4. The volumetric evaluation results of the enamel residual.

Tooth Specimen	Total Number of 2D OCT Images	Total Number of Enamel Residual Pixels	Enamel Residual Volume (mm^3)
Healthy molar tooth	500	2.13×10^7	28.72
Part.dem. molar	500	1.31×10^7	17.70
Carious molar	500	0.91×10^7	12.26
Part.dem. canine	500	1.28×10^7	17.20
Part.dem. pre-molar	500	1.42×10^7	19.15

Hence, the obtained results confirmed that the proposed volumetric evaluation method will be more useful to detect the progression of caries, since the gradual reduction of the enamel volume owing to the gradual growth of caries can be detected quantitatively in advance. Therefore, medical treatments can be initiated immediately in order to obstruct the progression of caries, once the volume reduction of teeth is identified.

3.3. Structural Comparison between OCT and Conventional Methods

Figure 7 shows the structural analysis of a carious molar tooth sample and a comparison between imaging results obtained from various inspection methods. Figure 7a shows the *in vivo* radiographic image of the carious tooth, which was captured before early childhood caries (ECC) surgery performed on a 10-year-old male volunteer. The images were acquired to inspect the dental caries and cavity filling portions using a system that is currently applied in standard clinical practice: ultra speed (D-speed) film (Kodak, Rochester, NY, USA), 150 kVp, 15 mA, and 20 impulses. In this radiographic method, resolving a sub-millimeter tissue structure proves to be difficult, and only the surface structures of the cavity fillings, carious region, partially demineralized regions, pulps, and root canals along with healthy tooth were visualized. Thus, the obtained results were neither quantitative nor sensitive, and the cavity depths could not be imaged as well. Hence, precise radiographic detection of demineralization is a challenging task, since minimally demineralized regions are unable to reach the threshold of resolution. Figure 7b shows the photograph of the carious tooth, which was obtained after early childhood caries (ECC) surgery. Figure 7c,d represent the *ex vivo* 3D OCT images of the same sample and show the top and the side views of the sample. A precise enhancement could be identified, compared to radiographic images. Both 3D OCT figures give a clear view of the distinguishable anatomical structures e.g., dentin tubules, pulp, root canals, and cement owing to the high axial and lateral resolutions. Therefore, the applicability and the reliability of our system were verified because the dental caries, demineralization, and the inner microstructures of dentin were confirmed simultaneously through the obtained results.

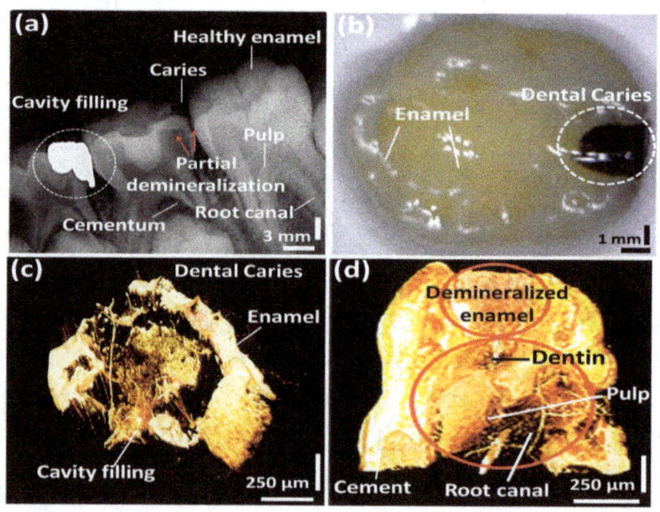

Figure 7. Structural analysis of the carious tooth sample using various inspection methods. (**a**) Radiographic image of the carious tooth sample before the surgery; (**b**) Photograph of the carious tooth sample after the surgery; (**c**,**d**) top and side views of 3D OCT images of the carious tooth sample.

4. Conclusions

We have demonstrated an optical frequency-domain imaging technique based quantitative evaluation method as an initial *ex vivo* study to detect the progression of dental caries by comparing partially and completely demineralized tooth samples with healthy tooth specimens. The quantification techniques were carried out by evaluating precise volume and thickness of enamel residual. Next, the total intensity fluctuation in each imaging depth range of all the specimens was quantified to confirm the changes that occurred in the internal composition of partially and completely demineralized tooth samples compared to a healthy sample. The performed study was a preliminary descriptive observational study, which was performed to confirm the feasibility of the three developed quantification techniques. The representative *ex vivo* tooth specimens as well as the experimental procedure was conducted according to the guidelines provided by an expert orthodontist. The results obtained using our high-resolution OFDI system revealed anatomic and quantitative information in a relatively nondestructive manner. The threshold parameters to detect the progression of early caries were determined on the basis of the quantitative results obtained from partially demineralized samples. Therefore, the physicians were able to diagnose the tooth volumetric and thickness changes at an initial stage by considering the obtained results as promising threshold parameters, which will be useful to barricade the progression of caries. To enhance the accuracy of the threshold parameters, quantitative (thickness and volumetric) information of multiple *in vivo* specimens will be evaluated, averaged, and normalized along with clinical trials in future studies.

Acknowledgments: This research was supported by the Industrial Strategic Technology Development Program, Grant No. 10047943; the "Development of Micro-Surgical Apparatus Based on 3D Tomographic Operating Microscope" program, funded by the Ministry of Trade, Industry and Energy (MI, Korea, No. 10047943). This study was also supported by the BK21 Plus project funded by the Ministry of Education, Korea (21A20131600011).

Author Contributions: R.E.W. and N.H.C. conducted the experiment, and analyzed and drafted the manuscript. K.P. designed the experimental setup with software and hardware components. M.J. and J.K. designed the study and critically revised and finalized the intellectual contents of manuscript.

References

1. Selwitz, R.H.; Ismail, A.I.; Pitts, N.B. Dental caries. *Lancet* **2007**, *369*, 51–59. [CrossRef]
2. Fejerskov, O. Changing paradigms in concepts on dental caries: Consequences for oral health care. *Caries Res.* **2004**, *38*, 182–191. [CrossRef] [PubMed]
3. Dove, S.B.; McDavid, W. A comparison of conventional intra-oral radiography and computer imaging techniques for the detection of proximal surface dental caries. *Dentomaxillofac. Radiol.* **1992**, *21*, 127–134. [CrossRef] [PubMed]
4. Fercher, A.F. Optical coherence tomography. *J. Biomed. Opt.* **1996**, *1*, 157–173. [CrossRef] [PubMed]
5. Ding, Z.; Ren, H.; Zhao, Y.; Nelson, J.S.; Chen, Z. High-resolution optical coherence tomography over a large depth range with an axicon lens. *Opt. Lett.* **2002**, *27*, 243–245. [CrossRef] [PubMed]
6. Boppart, S.A.; Herrmann, J.; Pitris, C.; Stamper, D.L.; Brezinski, M.E.; Fujimoto, J.G. High-resolution optical coherence tomography-guided laser ablation of surgical tissue. *J. Surg. Res.* **1999**, *82*, 275–284. [CrossRef] [PubMed]
7. Nassif, N.; Cense, B.; Park, B.; Pierce, M.; Yun, S.; Bouma, B.; Tearney, G.; Chen, T.; de Boer, J. In vivo high-resolution video-rate spectral-domain optical coherence tomography of the human retina and optic nerve. *Opt. Express* **2004**, *12*, 367–376. [CrossRef] [PubMed]
8. Wijesinghe, R.E.; Park, K.; Kim, P.; Oh, J.; Kim, S.-W.; Kim, K.; Kim, B.-M.; Jeon, M.; Kim, J. Optically deviated focusing method based high-speed sd-oct for in vivo retinal clinical applications. *Opt. Rev.* **2016**, *23*, 307–315. [CrossRef]
9. Welzel, J. Optical coherence tomography in dermatology: A review. *Skin Res. Technol.* **2001**, *7*, 1–9. [CrossRef] [PubMed]
10. Cho, N.H.; Lee, J.W.; Cho, J.-H.; Kim, J.; Jang, J.H.; Jung, W. Evaluation of the usefulness of three-dimensional optical coherence tomography in a guinea pig model of endolymphatic hydrops induced by surgical obliteration of the endolymphatic duct. *J. Biomed. Opt.* **2015**, *20*, 036009. [CrossRef] [PubMed]
11. Lee, J.; Kim, K.; Wijesinghe, R.E.; Jeon, D.; Lee, S.H.; Jeon, M.; Jang, J.H. Decalcification using ethylenediaminetetraacetic acid for clear microstructure imaging of cochlea through optical coherence tomography. *J. Biomed. Opt.* **2016**, *21*, 081204. [CrossRef] [PubMed]
12. Akkaya, N.; Kansu, Ö.; Kansu, H.; Çağirankaya, L.; Arslan, U. Comparing the accuracy of panoramic and intraoral radiography in the diagnosis of proximal caries. *Dentomaxillofac. Radiol.* 2014. [CrossRef] [PubMed]
13. Seneadza, V.; Koob, A.; Kaltschmitt, J.; Staehle, H.; Duwenhoegger, J.; Eickholz, P. Digital enhancement of radiographs for assessment of interproximal dental caries. *Dentomaxillofac. Radiol.* 2014. [CrossRef] [PubMed]
14. Featherstone, J.; Ten Cate, J.; Shariati, M.; Arends, J. Comparison of artificial caries-like lesions by quantitative microradiography and microhardness profiles. *Caries Res.* **1983**, *17*, 385–391. [CrossRef] [PubMed]
15. Bühler, C.M.; Ngaotheppitak, P.; Fried, D. Imaging of occlusal dental caries (decay) with near-ir light at 1310-nm. *Opt. Express* **2005**, *13*, 573–582. [CrossRef] [PubMed]

16. Cochrane, N.J.; Iijima, Y.; Shen, P.; Yuan, Y.; Walker, G.D.; Reynolds, C.; MacRae, C.M.; Wilson, N.C.; Adams, G.G.; Reynolds, E.C. Comparative study of the measurement of enamel demineralization and remineralization using transverse microradiography and electron probe microanalysis. *Microsc. Microanal.* **2014**, *20*, 937–945. [CrossRef] [PubMed]

17. Fried, D.; Xie, J.; Shafi, S.; Featherstone, J.D.; Breunig, T.M.; Le, C. Imaging caries lesions and lesion progression with polarization sensitive optical coherence tomography. *J. Biomed. Opt.* **2002**, *7*, 618–627. [CrossRef] [PubMed]

18. Ishibashi, K.; Ozawa, N.; Tagami, J.; Sumi, Y. Swept-source optical coherence tomography as a new tool to evaluate defects of resin-based composite restorations. *J. Dent.* **2011**, *39*, 543–548. [CrossRef] [PubMed]

19. Baumgartner, A.; Dichtl, S.; Hitzenberger, C.; Sattmann, H.; Robl, B.; Moritz, A.; Fercher, A.; Sperr, W. Polarization–sensitive optical coherence tomography of dental structures. *Caries Res.* **1999**, *34*, 59–69. [CrossRef]

20. Huynh, G.D.; Darling, C.L.; Fried, D. Changes in the optical properties of dental enamel at 1310 nm after demineralization. In Proceedings of the Biomedical Optics 2004, San Jose, CA, USA, 28 May 2004; pp. 118–124.

21. Cahill, L.; Lee, A.M.; Pahlevaninezhad, H.; Ng, S.; MacAulay, C.E.; Poh, C.; Lane, P. Passive endoscopic polarization sensitive optical coherence tomography with completely fiber based optical components. In Proceedings of the SPIE BiOS, San Francisco, CA, USA, 2 March 2015; p. 930413.

22. Jones, R.S.; Staninec, M.; Fried, D. Imaging artificial caries under composite sealants and restorations. *J. Biomed. Opt.* **2004**, *9*, 1297–1304. [CrossRef] [PubMed]

23. Popescu, D.P.; Sowa, M.G.; Hewko, M.D. Assessment of early demineralization in teeth using the signal attenuation in optical coherence tomography images. *J. Biomed. Opt.* **2008**, *13*, 054053. [CrossRef] [PubMed]

24. Shimada, Y.; Sadr, A.; Burrow, M.F.; Tagami, J.; Ozawa, N.; Sumi, Y. Validation of swept-source optical coherence tomography (ss-oct) for the diagnosis of occlusal caries. *J. Dent.* **2010**, *38*, 655–665. [CrossRef] [PubMed]

25. Cara, A.C.; Zezell, D.M.; Ana, P.A.; Maldonado, E.P.; Freitas, A.Z. Evaluation of two quantitative analysis methods of optical coherence tomography for detection of enamel demineralization and comparison with microhardness. *Lasers Surg. Med.* **2014**, *46*, 666–671. [CrossRef] [PubMed]

26. Hsieh, Y.-S.; Ho, Y.-C.; Lee, S.-Y.; Chuang, C.-C.; Tsai, J.-C.; Lin, K.-F.; Sun, C.-W. Dental optical coherence tomography. *Sensors* **2013**, *13*, 8928–8949. [CrossRef] [PubMed]

27. Keane, P.A.; Ruiz-Garcia, H.; Sadda, S.R. Clinical applications of long-wavelength (1000-nm) optical coherence tomography. *Ophthalmic Surg. Lasers Imaging Retin.* **2011**, *42*, S67–S74. [CrossRef] [PubMed]

28. Jeon, M.; Kim, J.; Jung, U.; Lee, C.; Jung, W.; Boppart, S.A. Full-range k-domain linearization in spectral-domain optical coherence tomography. *Appl. Opt.* **2011**, *50*, 1158–1163. [CrossRef] [PubMed]

29. Jung, U.-S.; Cho, N.-H.; Kim, S.-H.; Jeong, H.-S.; Kim, J.-H.; Ahn, Y.-C. Simple spectral calibration method and its application using an index array for swept source optical coherence tomography. *J. Opt. Soc. Korea* **2011**, *15*, 386–393. [CrossRef]

30. Lee, C.; Lee, S.-Y.; Kim, J.-Y.; Jung, H.-Y.; Kim, J. Optical sensing method for screening disease in melon seeds by using optical coherence tomography. *Sensors* **2011**, *11*, 9467–9477. [CrossRef] [PubMed]

31. Wijesinghe, R.E.; Lee, S.-Y.; Kim, P.; Jung, H.-Y.; Jeon, M.; Kim, J. Optical inspection and morphological analysis of diospyros kaki plant leaves for the detection of circular leaf spot disease. *Sensors* **2016**, *16*, 1282. [CrossRef] [PubMed]

32. Shellis, R. Relationship between human enamel structure and the formation of caries-like lesions in vitro. *Arch. Oral Biol.* **1984**, *29*, 975–981. [CrossRef]

33. Silverstone, L.; Poole, D. The effect of saliva and calcifying solutions upon the histological appearance of enamel caries. *Caries Res.* **1968**, *2*, 87–96. [CrossRef] [PubMed]

34. Ekstrand, K.; Kuzmina, I.; Bjørndal, L.; Thylstrup, A. Relationship between external and histologic features of progressive stages of caries in the occlusal fossa. *Caries Res.* **1995**, *29*, 243–250. [CrossRef] [PubMed]

35. Go, E.-J.; Jung, H.-S.; Kim, E.-S.; Jung, I.-Y.; Lee, S.-J. Histology of dental pulp healing after tooth replantation in rats. *J. Korean Acad. Conserv. Dent.* **2010**, *35*, 273–284. [CrossRef]

36. Yun, S.; Tearney, G.; de Boer, J.; Iftimia, N.; Bouma, B. High-speed optical frequency-domain imaging. *Opt. Express* **2003**, *11*, 2953–2963. [CrossRef] [PubMed]

Permissions

All chapters in this book were first published by MDPI; hereby published with permission under the Creative Commons Attribution License or equivalent. Every chapter published in this book has been scrutinized by our experts. Their significance has been extensively debated. The topics covered herein carry significant findings which will fuel the growth of the discipline. They may even be implemented as practical applications or may be referred to as a beginning point for another development.

The contributors of this book come from diverse backgrounds, making this book a truly international effort. This book will bring forth new frontiers with its revolutionizing research information and detailed analysis of the nascent developments around the world.

We would like to thank all the contributing authors for lending their expertise to make the book truly unique. They have played a crucial role in the development of this book. Without their invaluable contributions this book wouldn't have been possible. They have made vital efforts to compile up to date information on the varied aspects of this subject to make this book a valuable addition to the collection of many professionals and students.

This book was conceptualized with the vision of imparting up-to-date information and advanced data in this field. To ensure the same, a matchless editorial board was set up. Every individual on the board went through rigorous rounds of assessment to prove their worth. After which they invested a large part of their time researching and compiling the most relevant data for our readers.

The editorial board has been involved in producing this book since its inception. They have spent rigorous hours researching and exploring the diverse topics which have resulted in the successful publishing of this book. They have passed on their knowledge of decades through this book. To expedite this challenging task, the publisher supported the team at every step. A small team of assistant editors was also appointed to further simplify the editing procedure and attain best results for the readers.

Apart from the editorial board, the designing team has also invested a significant amount of their time in understanding the subject and creating the most relevant covers. They scrutinized every image to scout for the most suitable representation of the subject and create an appropriate cover for the book.

The publishing team has been an ardent support to the editorial, designing and production team. Their endless efforts to recruit the best for this project, has resulted in the accomplishment of this book. They are a veteran in the field of academics and their pool of knowledge is as vast as their experience in printing. Their expertise and guidance has proved useful at every step. Their uncompromising quality standards have made this book an exceptional effort. Their encouragement from time to time has been an inspiration for everyone.

The publisher and the editorial board hope that this book will prove to be a valuable piece of knowledge for researchers, students, practitioners and scholars across the globe.

List of Contributors

Mallika Asar and Mette Soendergaard
Department of Chemistry, Western Illinois University, 214 Currens Hall, Macomb, IL 61455, USA

Jessica Newton-Northup
Department of Biochemistry, University of Missouri, 117 Schweitzer Hall, Columbia, MO 65211, USA

Susan Deutscher
Department of Biochemistry, University of Missouri, 117 Schweitzer Hall, Columbia, MO 65211, USA
Harry S. Truman Memorial Veterans Hospital, 1 Hospital Drive, Columbia, MO 65201, USA

Arturo Armone Caruso
ENT Department, AIAS Structure of Afragola, Contrada Leutrec snc, 80021 Naples, Italy

Veronica Viola and Daniele Naviglio
Department of Chemical Sciences, University of Naples Federico II, via Cintia, 21, 80126 Naples, Italy

Salvatore Del Prete and Daniela Marasco
Service Biotech s.r.l., 80132 Napoli, Italy

Sabato Leo
ENT Outpatient Clinic at Scafati Hospital ASL SA, 84018 Salerno, Italy

Andrea Fulgione
Department of Agricultural Science, University of Naples Federico II, Via Università 100, 80045 Portici (NA), Italy

Monica Gallo
Department of Molecular Medicine and Medical Biotechnology, University of Naples Federico II, via Pansini, 5, 80131 Naples, Italy

Dario Di Stasio, Antonio Romano, Enrica Gentile and Alberta Lucchese
Multidisciplinary Department of Medical-Surgical and Dental Specialties, University of Campania—Luigi Vanvitelli, 80138 Naples, Italy

Dorina Lauritano
Department of Medicine and Surgery, Centre of Neuroscience of Milan, University of Milano-Bicocca, 20126 Milan, Italy

Hasan Iquebal
ECU School of Dental Medicine, 1851 MacGregor Downs Road, Greenville, NC 27834, USA

Marzena Hirsch, Daria Majchrowicz, Paweł Wierzba and Małgorzata Jędrzejewska-Szczerska
Department of Metrology and Optoelectronics, Faculty of Electronics, Telecommunications and Informatics, Gdańsk University of Technology, Narutowicza Street 11/12, 80-233 Gdańsk, Poland

Matthieu Weber and Mikhael Bechelany
Institut Européen des Membranes, UMR-5635, Université de Montpellier, École Nationale Supérieure de Chimie de Montpellier, Centre national de la recherche scientifique, Place Eugène Bataillon, Montpellier 34095, France

Ksenia Kandurova, Elena Potapova and Andrey Dunaev
Research and Development Center of Biomedical Photonics, Orel State University, 302026 Orel, Russia

Evgeny Zherebtsov
Research and Development Center of Biomedical Photonics, Orel State University, 302026 Orel, Russia
Faculty of Information Technology and Electrical Engineering, University of Oulu, Optoelectronics and Measurement Techniques Unit, 90570 Oulu, Finland

Marina Zajnulina, Sergei Sokolovski and Edik U. Rafailov
Aston Institute of Photonic Technologies, Aston University, Birmingham B4 7ET, UK

Viktor Dremin
Research and Development Center of Biomedical Photonics, Orel State University, 302026 Orel, Russia
Aston Institute of Photonic Technologies, Aston University, Birmingham B4 7ET, UK

Andrian Mamoshin
Research and Development Center of Biomedical Photonics, Orel State University, 302026 Orel, Russia
Department of X-ray Surgical Methods of Diagnosis and Treatment, Orel Regional Clinical Hospital, 302028 Orel, Russia

Jong Yoon Shin, Kilwha Pi and Dong-il "Dan" Cho
ISRC/ASRI, Department of Electrical and Computer Engineering, Seoul National University, 1 Gwanak-ro, Gwanak-gu, Seoul 08826, Korea

Zhyldyz Musakulova
Computer Information Systems, International University of Kyrgyzstan, Bishkek 720007, Kyrgyzstan

Suk Won Jung
ISRC/ASRI, Department of Electrical and Computer Engineering, Seoul National University, 1 Gwanak-ro, Gwanak-gu, Seoul 08826, Korea
Human Care System Research Center, Convergence System R&D Division, Korea Electronics Technology Institute, 25 Saenari-ro, Bundang-gu, Seongnam-si, Gyeonggi-do 13509, Korea

Yong Sook Goo
Department of Physiology, College of Medicine, Chungbuk National University, 1 Chungdae-ro, Seowon-gu, Cheongju, Chungbuk 28644, Korea

Brigitte Pajic-Eggspuehler
Eye Clinic Orasis, Swiss Eye Research Foundation, 5734 Reinach AG, Switzerland

Zeljka Cvejic
Department of Physics, Faculty of Sciences, University of Novi Sad, Trg Dositeja Obradovica 4, 21000 Novi Sad, Serbia

Bojan Pajic
Eye Clinic Orasis, Swiss Eye Research Foundation, 5734 Reinach AG, Switzerland
Department of Physics, Faculty of Sciences, University of Novi Sad, Trg Dositeja Obradovica 4, 21000 Novi Sad, Serbia
Division of Ophthalmology, Department of Clinical Neurosciences, Geneva University Hospitals, Rue Gabrielle-Perret-Gentil 4, 1205 Genève, Switzerland
Faculty of Medicine of the Military Medical academy, University of Defense, 11000 Belgrade, Serbia

Janis Spigulis
Biophotonics Laboratory, Institute of Atomic Physics and Spectroscopy, University of Latvia, Riga, LV-1586, Latvia

Ekaterina Savchenko, Ilya Kolokolnikov and Elena Velichko
Institute of Physics, Nanotechnology and Telecommunications, Peter the Great St. Petersburg Polytechnic University, 195251 St. Petersburg, Russia

Victor Osovskikh and Lyubov Kiseleva
Department of Anesthesiology and Resuscitation Russian Research Center for Radiology and Surgical Technologies, 197758 St. Petersburg, Russia

Joerg Mueller
Swiss Eye Research Foundation, Eye Clinic ORASIS, 5734 Reinach AG, Switzerland

Zeljka Cvejic and Zoran Mijatovic
Faculty of Sciences, Department of Physics, University of Novi Sad, Trg Dositeja Obradovica 4, Novi Sad 21000, Serbia

Dragan Indjin
School of Electronic and Electrical Engineering, University of Leeds, Leeds LS2 9JT, UK

Mohesh Moothanchery and Manojit Pramanik
School of Chemical and Biomedical Engineering, Nanyang Technological University, 62 Nanyang Drive, Singapore 637459, Singapore

Alexander S. Machikhin and Demid D. Khokhlov
Laboratory of Acousto-optical Spectroscopy, Scientific and Technological Center of Unique Instrumentation, Russian Academy of Sciences, 117342 Moscow, Russia

Mikhail V. Volkov and Andrey V. Potemkin
Department of Applied Optics, University ITMO, 190000 Saint Petersburg, Russia

Alexander B. Burlakov
Department of Ichthyology, Faculty of Biology, Lomonosov Moscow State University, 119991 Moscow, Russia

Chia-Nan Wang, Ming-Hsun Lin, Yao-Lang Chang and Chia-Ming Kuo
Industrial Engineering and Management, National Kaohsiung University of Applied Sciences, Kaohsiung 80778, Taiwans

Jing-Wein Wang
Institute of Photonics and Communications, National Kaohsiung University of Applied Sciences, Kaohsiung 80778, Taiwan

Christian Pfitzner
Department of Electrical Engineering, Precision Engineering, Information Technology at the Techniche Hochschule Nürnberg Georg Simon Ohm; Keßlerplatz 12, 90489 Nuremberg, Germany
Department of Informatics VII: Robotics and Telematics at the Julius-Maximilians University Würzburg, Am Hubland, 97074 Wuerzburg, Germany

Stefan May
Department of Electrical Engineering, Precision Engineering, Information Technology at the Techniche Hochschule Nürnberg Georg Simon Ohm; Keßlerplatz 12, 90489 Nuremberg, Germany

Andreas Nüchter
Department of Informatics VII: Robotics and Telematics at the Julius-Maximilians University Würzburg, Am Hubland, 97074 Wuerzburg, Germany

Sidra Batool and Fabrizio Frezza
Department of Information Engineering, Electronics and Telecommunications, Sapienza University of Rome, Via Eudossiana 18, 00184 Rome, Italy

Mehwish Nisar
Department of Information Engineering, Electronics and Telecommunications, Sapienza University of Rome, Via Eudossiana 18, 00184 Rome, Italy
Department of Fundamental and Applied Sciences for Engineering, Sapienza University of Rome, Via A. Scarpa 16, 00161 Rome, Italy

Eugenio Fazio
Department of Fundamental and Applied Sciences for Engineering, Sapienza University of Rome, Via A. Scarpa 16, 00161 Rome, Italy

Fabio Mangini
Department of Information Engineering, University of Brescia, Via Branze 59, 25123 Brescia, Italy

Laura Rey-Barroso, Francisco J. Burgos-Fernández, Xana Delpueyo, Miguel Ares, Santiago Royo and Meritxell Vilaseca
Centre for Sensors, Instruments and Systems Development, Technical University of Catalonia, Terrassa 08222, Spain

Josep Malvehy and Susana Puig
Dermatology Department of the Hospital Clinic of Barcelona, IDIBAPS; Barcelona 08036, Spain

Konstantin S. Yashin
University Clinic, Privolzhsky Research Medical University, 603950 Nizhny Novgorod, Russia

Ekaterina V. Gubarkova, Elena B. Kiseleva, Marina A. Sirotkina, Ksenia A. Achkasova, Anton A. Plekhanov and Natalia D. Gladkova
Institute of Experimental Oncology and Biomedical Technologies, Privolzhsky Research Medical University, 603950 Nizhny Novgorod, Russia

Dmitry A. Vorontsov and Alexey Y. Vorontsov
Department of Oncology, Nizhny Novgorod Regional Oncologic Hospital, 603126 Nizhny Novgorod, Russia

Sergey S. Kuznetsov
Department of Pathology, Privolzhsky Research Medical University, 603950 Nizhny Novgorod, Russia

Aleksander L. Matveyev
Laboratory of Multidimensional Signal Processing, Institute of Applied Physics of the Russian Academy of Sciences, 603950 Nizhny Novgorod, Russia

Aleksander A. Sovetsky, Lev A. Matveev and Vladimir Y. Zaitsev
Laboratory of Wave Methods for Studying Structurally Inhomogeneous Media, Institute of Applied Physics of the Russian Academy of Sciences, 603950 Nizhny Novgorod, Russia

Ruchire Eranga Wijesinghe, Kibeom Park, Mansik Jeon and Jeehyun Kim
School of Electronics Engineering, College of IT Engineering, Kyungpook National University, 80, Daehak-ro, Buk-gu, Daegu 41566, Korea

Nam Hyun Cho
Eaton-Peabody Laboratories, Massachusetts Eye and Ear Infirmary(MEEI), 243, Charles Street, Boston, MA 02114, USA
Department of Otology and Laryngology, Harvard Medical School, 243, Charles Street, Boston, MA 02114, USA

Index

R

S

T

Z

www.ingramcontent.com/pod-product-compliance
Lightning Source LLC
LaVergne TN
LVHW081029210926
848485LV00004B/985